First FRCR Anatomy

Practice Cases

SECOND EDITION

First FRCR Anatomy

Practice Cases

SECOND EDITION

Edited by

Eunjong Yoo MBBS MMedSc BASc EngSci FRCR
Radiology Registrar
Leeds & West Yorkshire Radiology Academy, UK

Claire Exley MBBS FRCR
Consultant Radiologist
Mid Yorkshire Hospitals NHS Trust, UK

David Minks MBBS BSc FRCR
Consultant Neurointerventionist and Neuroradiologist
North Bristol NHS Trust, UK

Constantinos Tingerides MBBS BSc MRCS FRCR
Consultant Vascular and Interventional Radiologist
Leeds Teaching Hospitals NHS Trust, UK

Ashley Uttley MBBS BSc FRCR
Consultant Radiologist
Harrogate and District NHS Foundation Trust, UK

JP medical publishers

London • New Delhi

Published by JP Medical Ltd
83 Victoria Street, London, SW1H 0HW, UK
Tel: +44 (0)20 3170 8910 Email: info@jpmedpub.com
Web: www.jpmedpub.com

EU GPSR Authorised Representative
Logos Europe, 9 rue Nicolas Poussin
17000, La Rochelle, France
Phone: +33 (0) 6 67 93 73 78
E-mail: Contact@logoseurope.eu

ISBN: 978-1-78779-179-4

British Library Cataloguing in Publication Data
A catalogue record for this book is available from the British Library

Library of Congress Cataloging in Publication Data
A catalog record for this book is available from the Library of Congress

Development Editor: Dr Meenakshi Tripathi

Editorial Assistant: Keshav Kumar

Cover Design: Seema Dogra

Preface to the second edition

Welcome to the Second Edition of *'First FRCR Anatomy: Practice Cases'*. Since the release of the first edition over a decade ago, the landscape of radiology has undergone significant transformations. However, the key to success in radiology remains the same – a strong foundation in radiological anatomy knowledge.

In this edition, we have meticulously updated the content to provide radiology trainees with a reliable resource for mastering radiological anatomy essential to the First FRCR examination and day-to-day practice.

As with any educational endeavour, this edition has been a collaborative effort. I extend my heartfelt gratitude to all those who have contributed to shaping this edition and helping it reach fruition. It is my hope that this revised edition serves as a valuable companion in your journey towards excellence in radiology.

Eunjong Yoo
Claire Exley
David Minks
Constantinos Tingerides
Ashley Uttley

Preface to the first edition

In 2010, the Royal College of Radiologists introduced the radiological anatomy module into the First FRCR examination. The module is designed to test a candidate's knowledge of radiological anatomy, as demonstrated in various different modalities and planes. This book is specifically designed as a tool to help candidates revising for it. The book is a compilation of over 200 images, which provide an excellent demonstration of human anatomy, using a wide range of different radiological investigations. Each case is followed by descriptive text discussing the salient points that can be taken from the case, as well as hints and tips to improve examination success. Where appropriate, artworks are included to help to explain the anatomy that is being demonstrated.

The images are presented in a similar format to those in the examination, allowing readers to become familiar with the examination structure. Each chapter focusses on a single anatomical area matched to the syllabus, allowing readers to consolidate knowledge as they progress through the book. Once the main chapters have been worked through, there are two practice papers at the end for self-assessment. Each of these papers comprises 20 cases to be answered within 75 minutes, with further explanatory answers and references to the main chapters. These practice papers allow readers to test knowledge and practise timings before the real examination.

This book is an excellent revision tool to help trainees to develop confidence and improve technique for the First FRCR Anatomy module. It provides a wide variety of images and a thorough grounding for candidates preparing to sit the examination.

Constantinos Tingerides
Ashley Uttley
David Minks
Claire Exley

Preface to the first edition

Contents

Contributors

Edem Barnor-Ahiaku MBChB BSc FRCR
Consultant Vascular and Interventional Radiologist
York and Scarborough Teaching Hospitals NHS Foundation Trust, UK

Emily Holt MBChB BSc FRCR
Consultant Radiologist
Bradford Teaching Hospitals NHS Foundation Trust, UK

Acknowledgement

We wish to thank the authors of the first edition for their guidance and reviewing the contents of the second edition.

Exam revision hints and tips

The examination

The First FRCR Anatomy module comprises 100 images and associated questions. A single structure on each image will be indicated by one or more arrows with a single question on that structure. The examination lasts for 90 minutes. The cases are viewed on an individual computer workstation, with a mouse and keyboard to navigate between the images and record their answers. Details of the viewing software and sample questions can be found on the Royal College of Radiologists website (http://www.rcr.ac.uk).

What can you do to prepare?

One of the most important methods to prepare for the anatomy module is to gain a breadth of experience of normal images. An understanding of normal anatomy as seen in different modalities and in different planes is essential. Testing yourself during normal day-to-day practice is a good way to develop knowledge and understanding.

There are various 'classic' images that can be found in anatomy atlases and are important when studying for the examination. It is worthwhile learning the details of these anatomical sections, since they demonstrate the relationship between structures and are likely to appear in the examination.

An understanding of anatomical relationships is the first step in learning radiological anatomy. However, knowledge of the imaging acquisition process will help to build on this and will greatly enhance the understanding of how anatomy is demonstrated radiologically. It is important not only to understand the relationship between anatomical structures and their surroundings, but also how they appear on different modalities and how they enhance. This background knowledge can be invaluable in the examination. For example, recognising whether an image has been acquired in the arterial or venous phase, or whether an image is T1 or T2 weighted can be very helpful when defining anatomy. When comparing the appearance of structures on different modalities, it is also worthwhile learning how the density, signal and echogenicity compare between neighbouring structures, e.g. that the liver typically appears slightly more dense than the spleen, or that it is usually more echogenic than the neighbouring renal cortex.

To prepare for the examination, it can also be helpful to attend a revision course specifically designed for this examination. Courses can consolidate learning and offer a simulated examination environment to practise timings and technique. It is important to practise mock examinations before the real one, since they provide an idea of how long is needed to complete the examination and will help you to manage time appropriately. If you perform well in a simulated examination environment, it will improve your confidence when sitting the real examination.

In the examination

Make sure you read the questions accurately and identify the arrow properly. There may be extra information on the image, e.g. side markers–pay attention to these, since they can provide extra detail.

Put as much detail into the answer as you can, while maintaining accuracy. It is important to add 'left' and 'right' to answers when appropriate, since this can contribute significantly to the mark. When labelling a structure, ask yourself whether there could be any more detail in the answer. For example, if labelling the aorta, add more detail by describing which part of the aorta is indicated, i.e. ascending, descending thoracic or abdominal.

Good luck! We hope that you find this book a useful tool in your preparation for the anatomy examination!

Chapter 1

Head and neck

Brain

Case 1.1

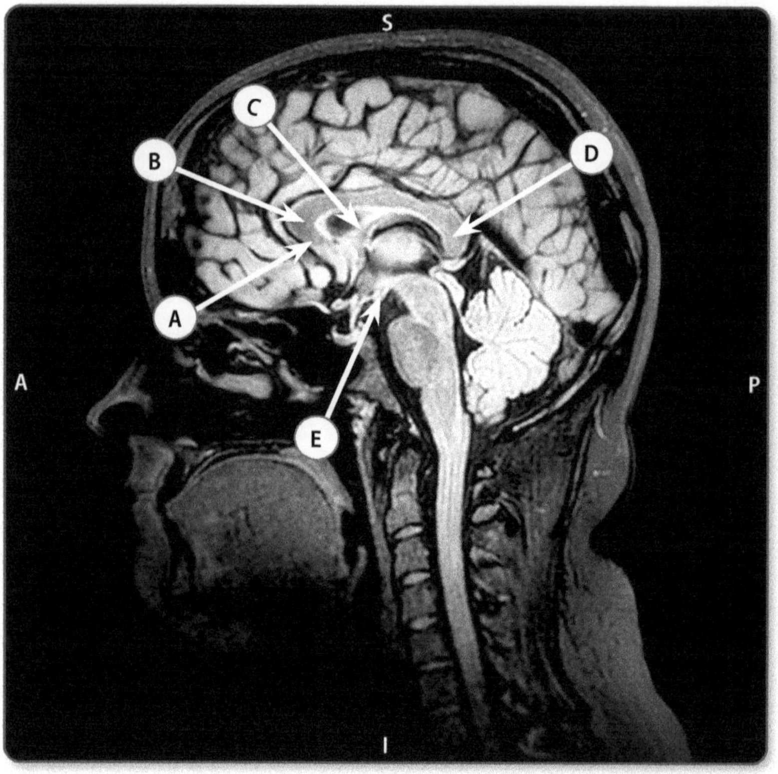

Case 1.1

QUESTION		WRITE YOUR ANSWER HERE
A	Name the structure labelled A.	
B	Name the structure labelled B.	
C	Name the structure labelled C.	
D	Name the structure labelled D.	
E	Name the structure labelled E.	

Case 1.2

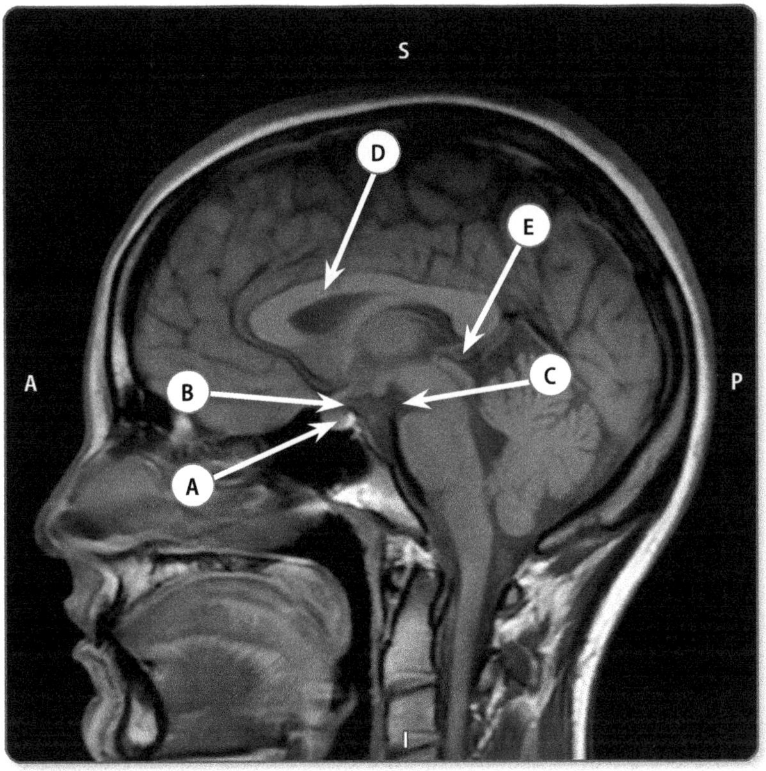

Case 1.2		
QUESTION		WRITE YOUR ANSWER HERE
A	Name the structure labelled A.	
B	Name the structure labelled B.	
C	Name the structure labelled C.	
D	Name the structure labelled D.	
E	Name the structure labelled E.	

Case 1.3

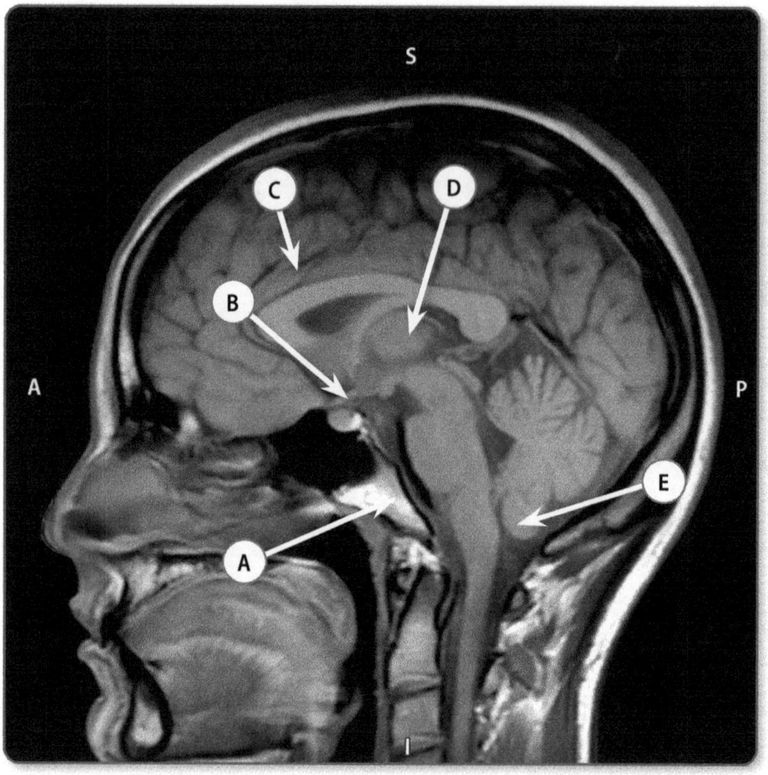

Case 1.3

QUESTION		WRITE YOUR ANSWER HERE
A	Name the structure labelled A.	
B	Name the structure labelled B.	
C	Name the structure labelled C.	
D	Name the structure labelled D.	
E	Name the structure labelled E.	

Case 1.4

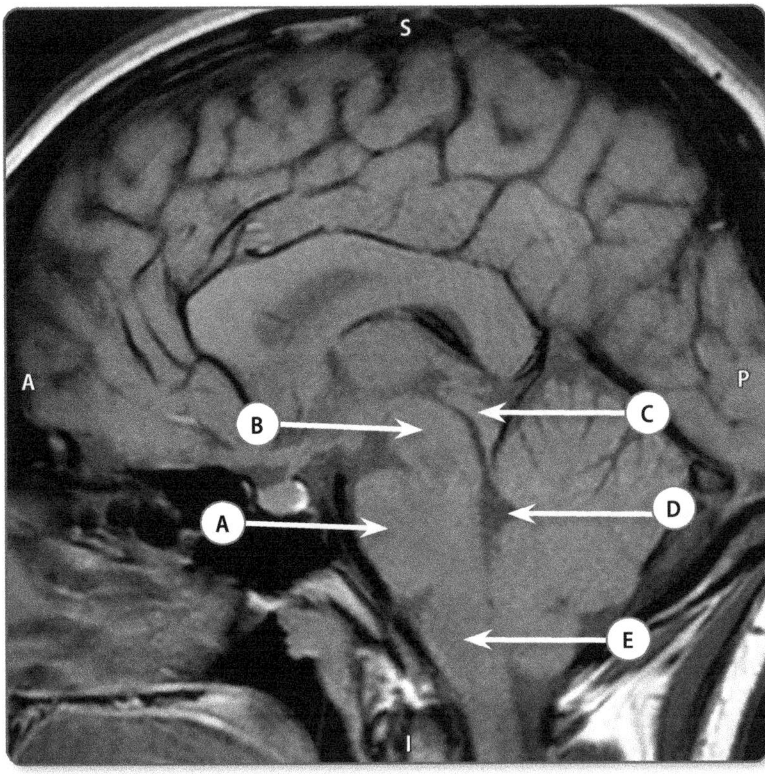

Case 1.4		
QUESTION		WRITE YOUR ANSWER HERE
A	Name the structure labelled A.	
B	Name the structure labelled B.	
C	Name the structure labelled C.	
D	Name the structure labelled D.	
E	Name the structure labelled E.	

Case 1.5

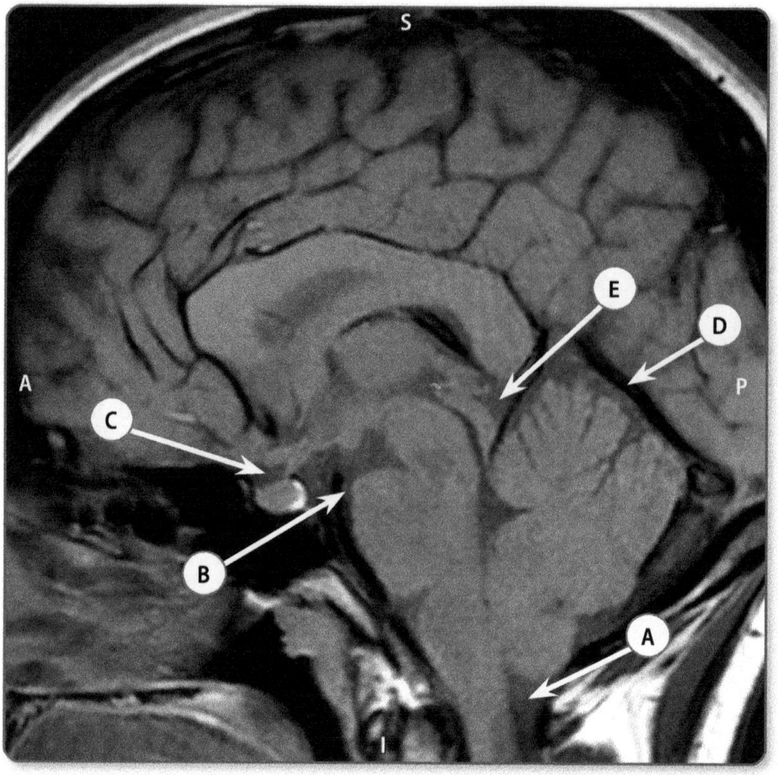

Case 1.5

QUESTION		WRITE YOUR ANSWER HERE
A	Name the structure labelled A.	
B	Name the structure labelled B.	
C	Name the structure labelled C.	
D	Name the structure labelled D.	
E	Name the structure labelled E.	

Case 1.6

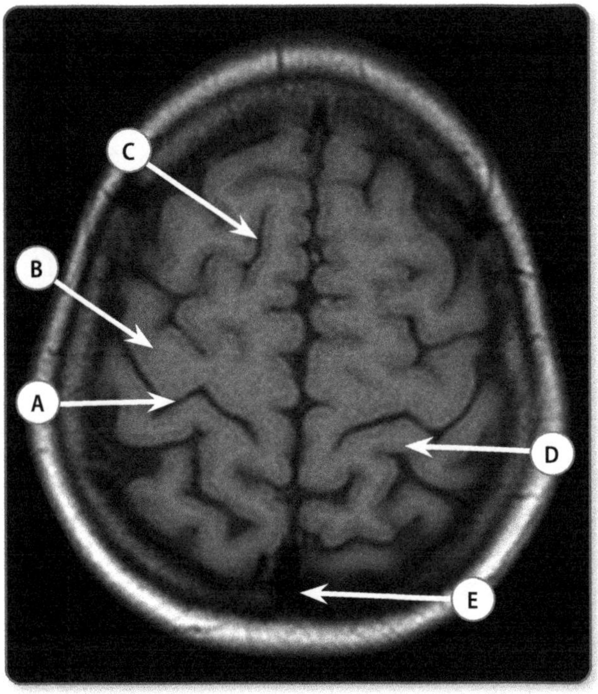

Case 1.6

QUESTION		WRITE YOUR ANSWER HERE
A	Name the structure labelled A.	
B	Name the structure labelled B.	
C	Name the structure labelled C.	
D	Name the structure labelled D.	
E	Name the structure labelled E.	

Case 1.7

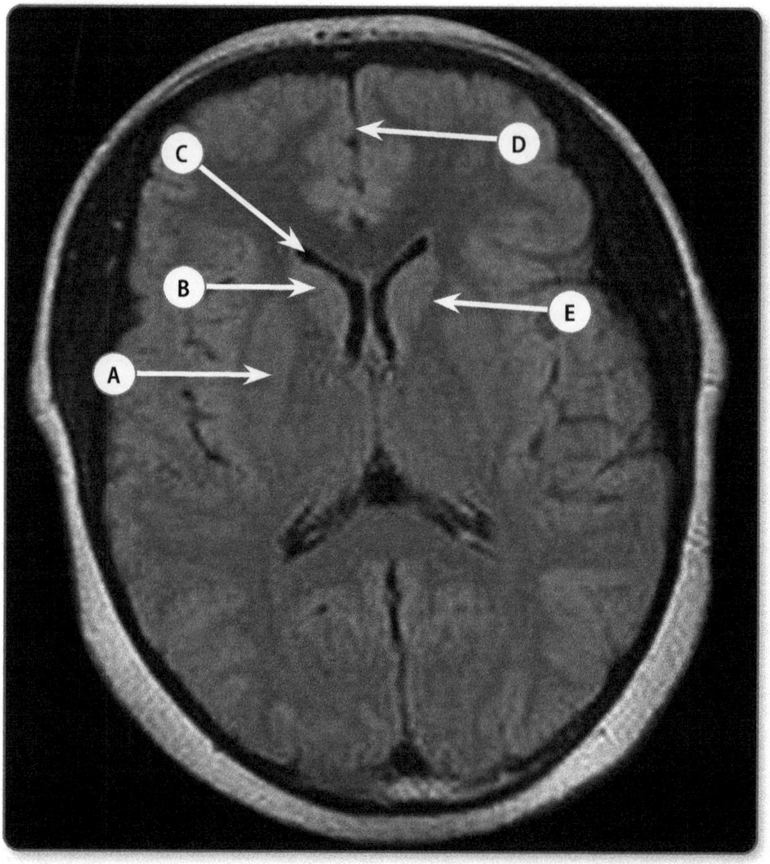

Case 1.7

QUESTION		WRITE YOUR ANSWER HERE
A	Name the structure labelled A.	
B	Name the structure labelled B.	
C	Name the structure labelled C.	
D	Name the structure labelled D.	
E	Name the structure labelled E.	

Case 1.8

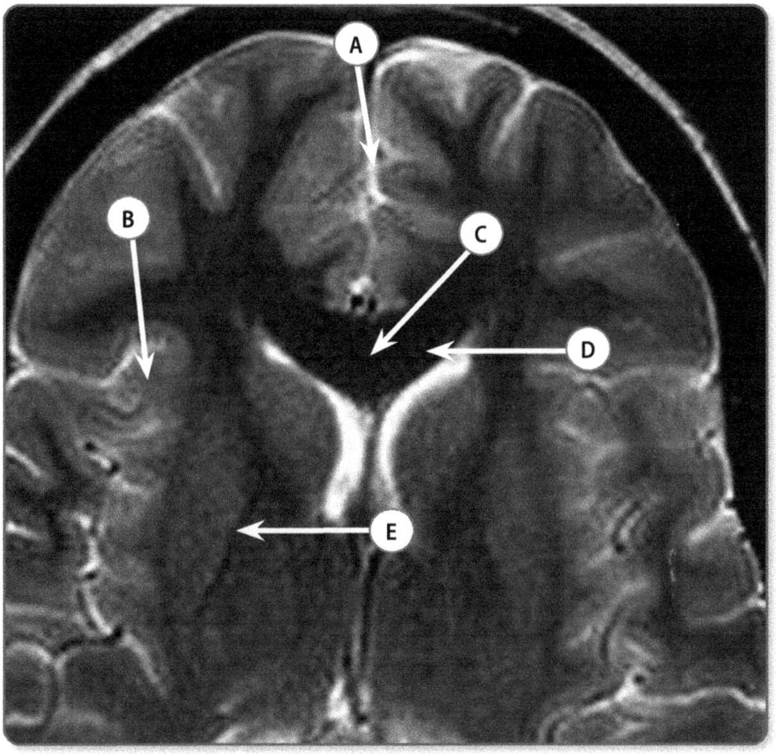

Case 1.8

QUESTION		WRITE YOUR ANSWER HERE
A	Name the structure labelled A.	
B	Name the structure labelled B.	
C	Name the structure labelled C.	
D	Name the structure labelled D.	
E	Name the structure labelled E.	

Case 1.9

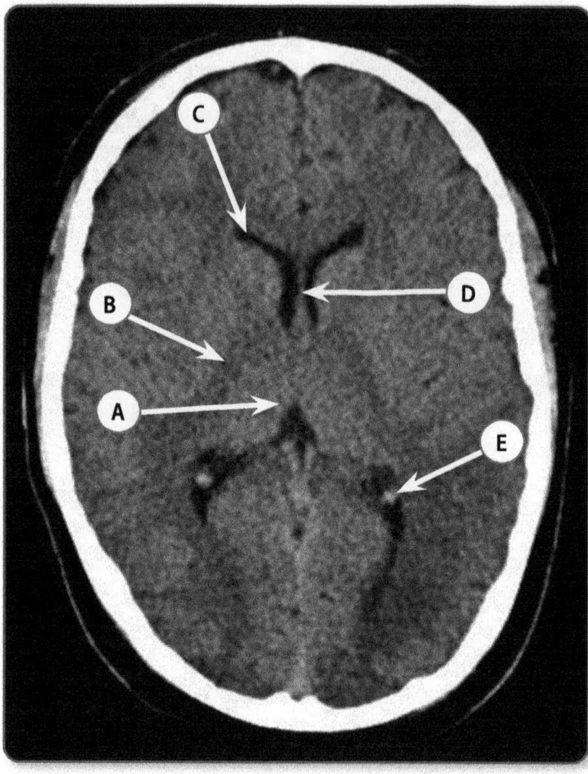

Case 1.9

QUESTION		WRITE YOUR ANSWER HERE
A	Name the structure labelled A.	
B	Name the structure labelled B.	
C	Name the structure labelled C.	
D	Name the structure labelled D.	
E	Name the structure labelled E.	

Case 1.10

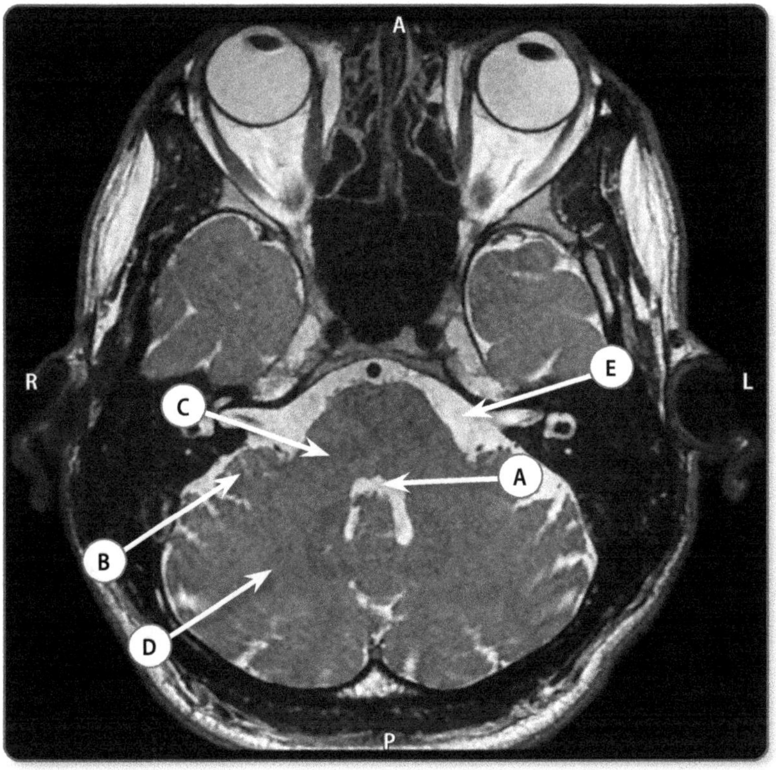

Case 1.10

	QUESTION	WRITE YOUR ANSWER HERE
A	Name the structure labelled A.	
B	Name the structure labelled B.	
C	Name the structure labelled C.	
D	Name the structure labelled D.	
E	Name the structure labelled E.	

Case 1.11

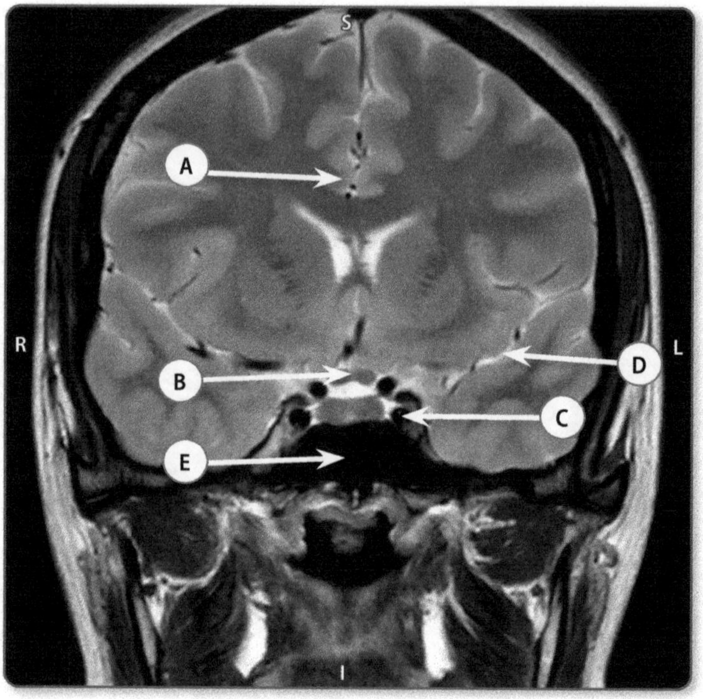

Case 1.11

QUESTION		WRITE YOUR ANSWER HERE
A	Name the structure labelled A.	
B	Name the structure labelled B.	
C	Name the structure labelled C.	
D	Name the structure labelled D.	
E	Name the structure labelled E.	

Case 1.12

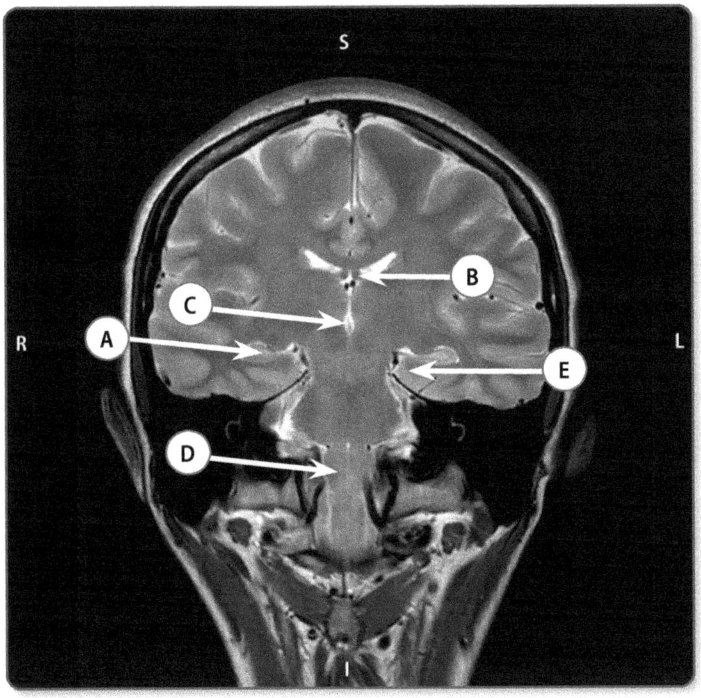

Case 1.12

QUESTION		WRITE YOUR ANSWER HERE
A	Name the structure labelled A.	
B	Name the structure labelled B.	
C	Name the structure labelled C.	
D	Name the structure labelled D.	
E	Name the structure labelled E.	

Case 1.13

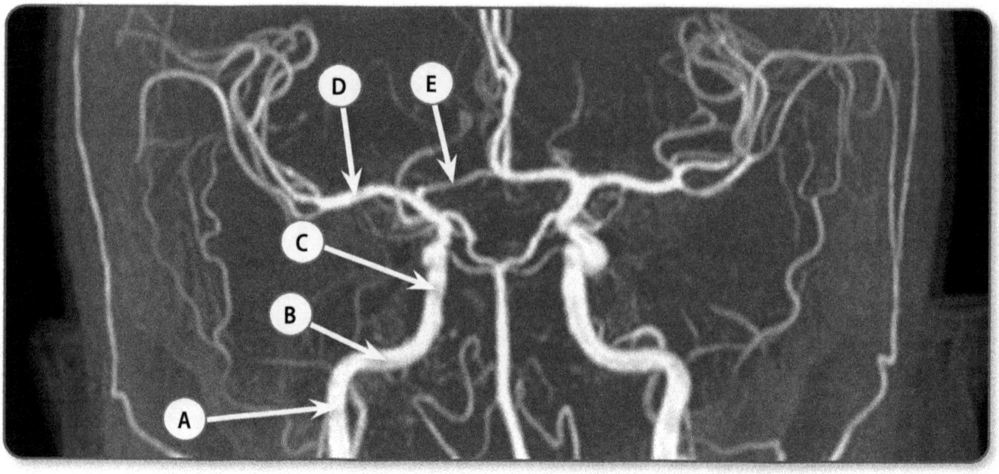

Case 1.13

QUESTION		WRITE YOUR ANSWER HERE
A	Name the structure labelled A.	
B	Name the structure labelled B.	
C	Name the structure labelled C.	
D	Name the structure labelled D.	
E	Name the structure labelled E.	

Case 1.14

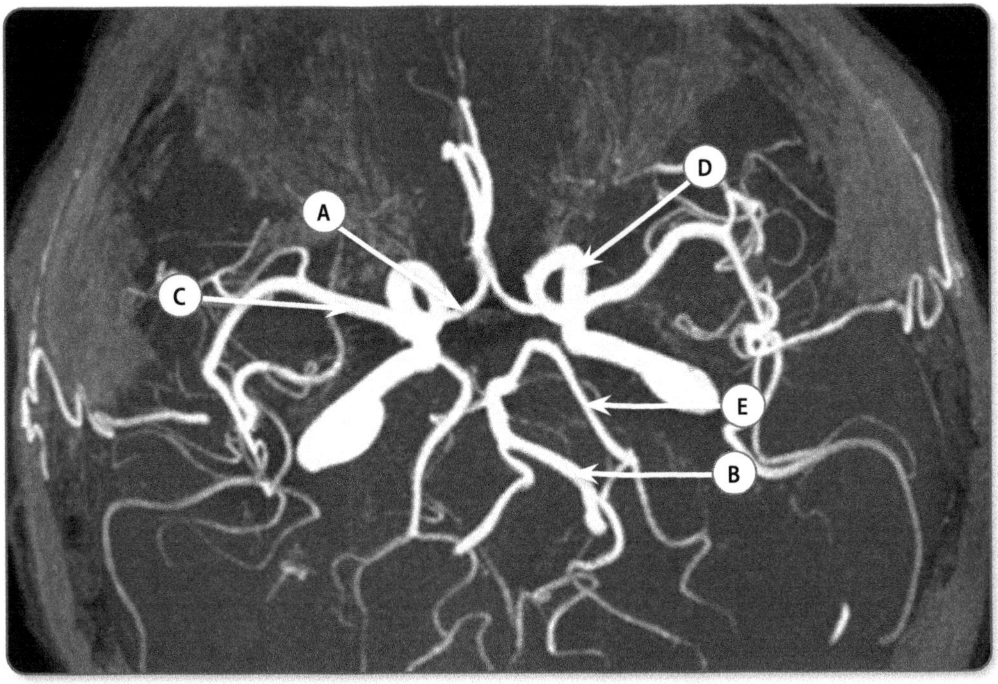

Case 1.14

QUESTION		WRITE YOUR ANSWER HERE
A	Name the structure labelled A.	
B	Name the structure labelled B.	
C	Name the structure labelled C.	
D	Name the structure labelled D.	
E	Name the structure labelled E.	

Case 1.15

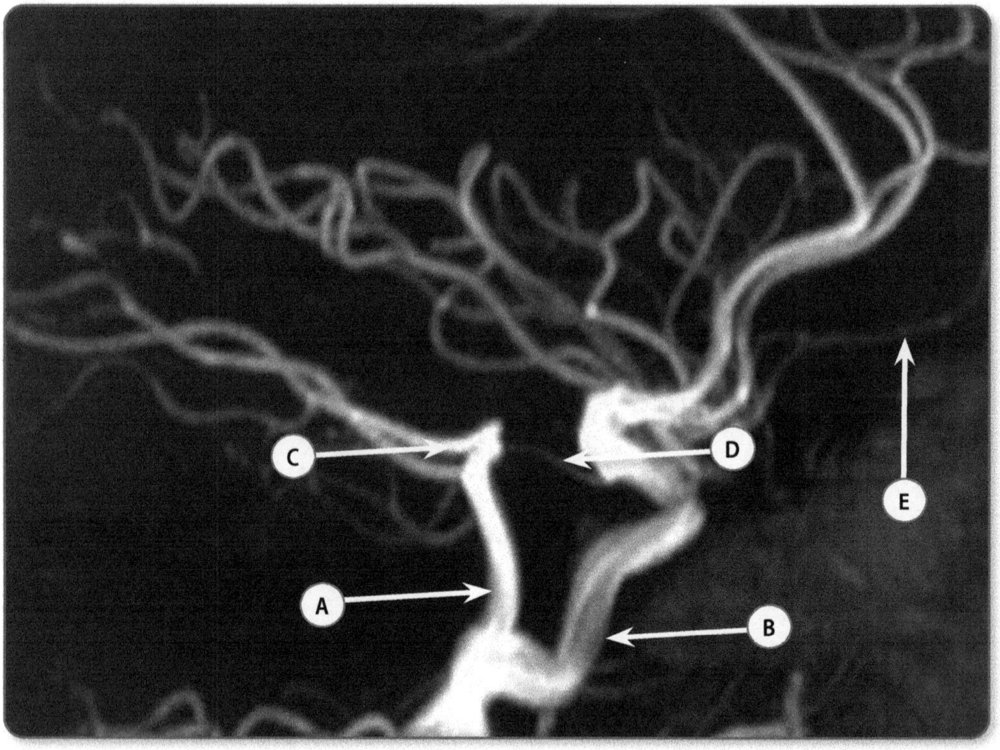

Case 1.15

QUESTION		WRITE YOUR ANSWER HERE
A	Name the structure labelled A.	
B	Name the structure labelled B.	
C	Name the structure labelled C.	
D	Name the structure labelled D.	
E	Name the structure labelled E.	

Case 1.16

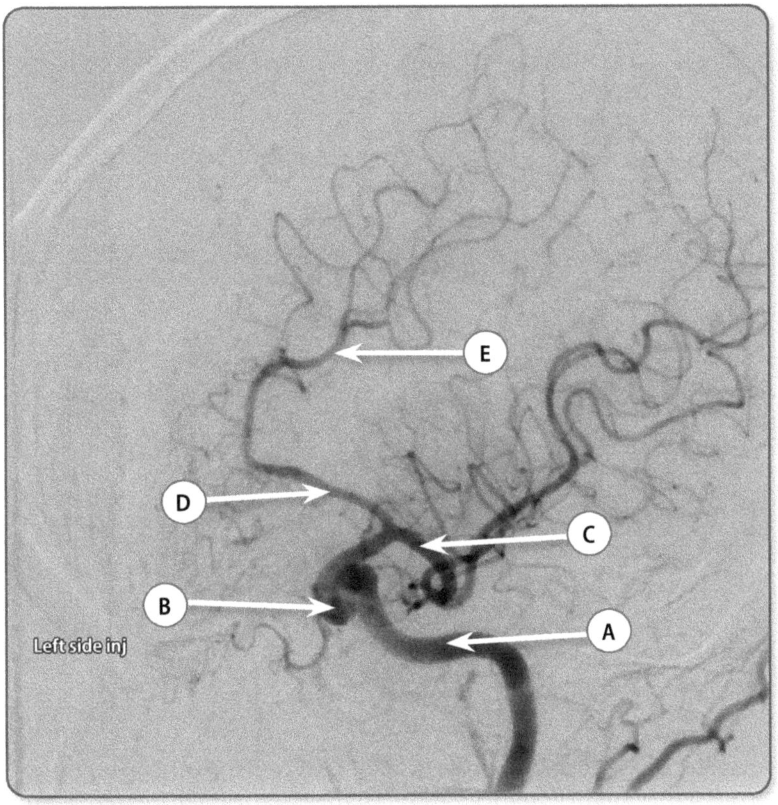

Case 1.16

QUESTION		WRITE YOUR ANSWER HERE
A	Name the structure labelled A.	
B	Name the structure labelled B.	
C	Name the structure labelled C.	
D	Name the structure labelled D.	
E	Name the structure labelled E.	

Case 1.17

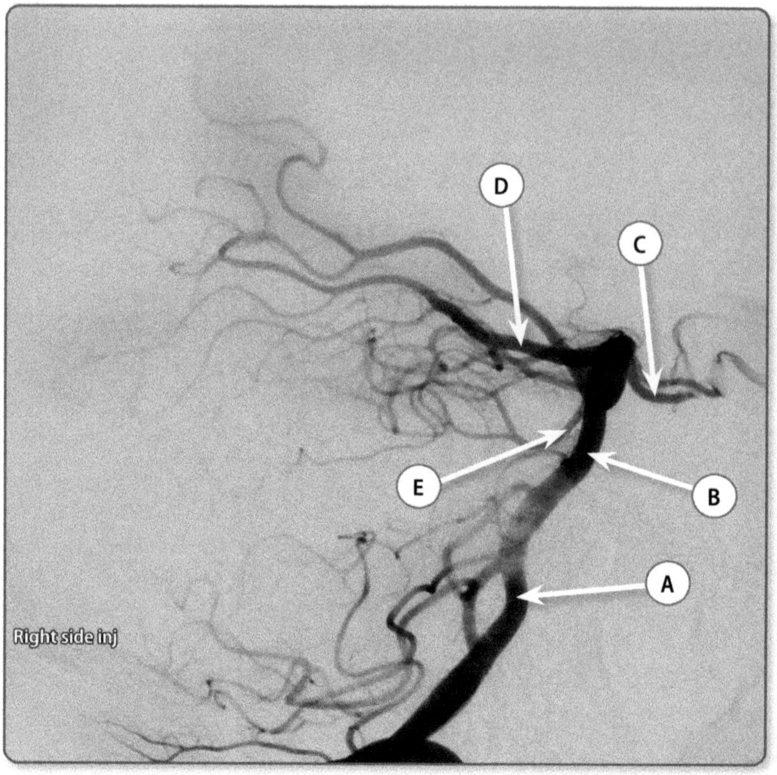

Case 1.17

QUESTION		WRITE YOUR ANSWER HERE
A	Name the structure labelled A.	
B	Name the structure labelled B.	
C	Name the structure labelled C.	
D	Name the structure labelled D.	
E	Name the structure labelled E.	

Case 1.18

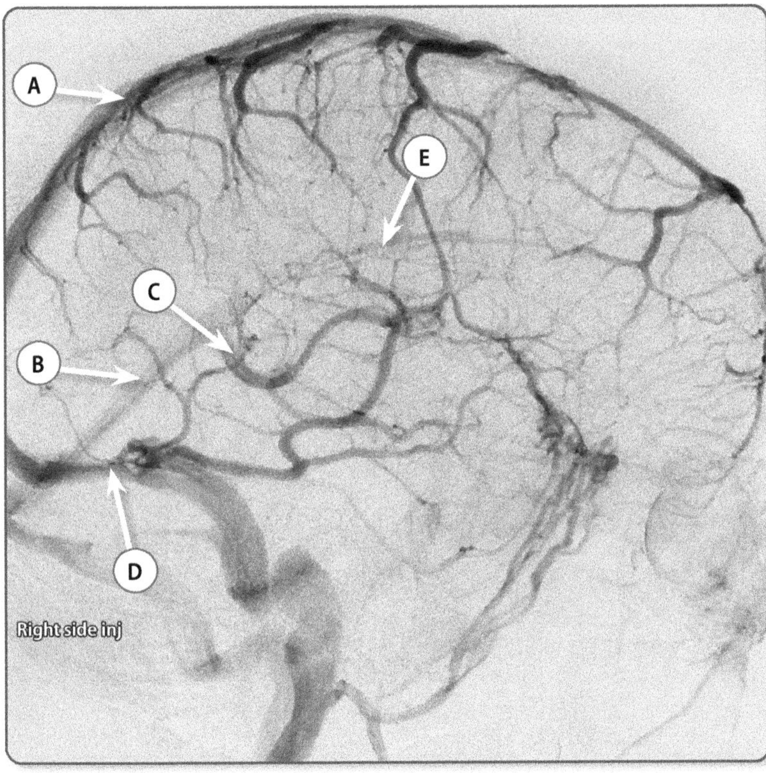

Case 1.18

QUESTION		WRITE YOUR ANSWER HERE
A	Name the structure labelled A.	
B	Name the structure labelled B.	
C	Name the structure labelled C.	
D	Name the structure labelled D.	
E	Name the structure labelled E.	

Case 1.19

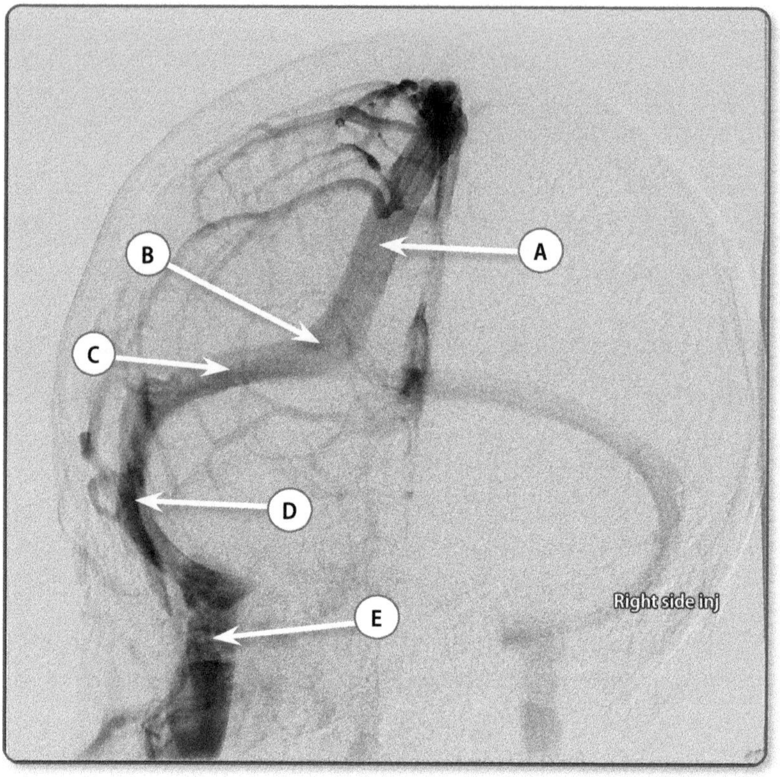

Case 1.19

	QUESTION	WRITE YOUR ANSWER HERE
A	Name the structure labelled A.	
B	Name the structure labelled B.	
C	Name the structure labelled C.	
D	Name the structure labelled D.	
E	Name the structure labelled E.	

Face and neck

Case 1.20

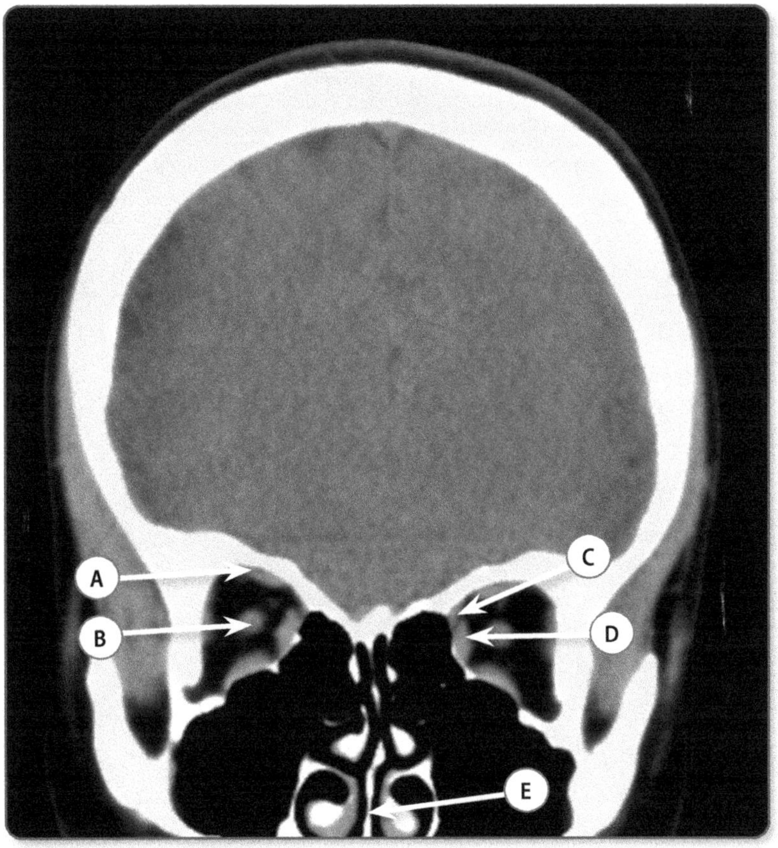

Case 1.20

QUESTION		WRITE YOUR ANSWER HERE
A	Name the structure labelled A.	
B	Name the structure labelled B.	
C	Name the structure labelled C.	
D	Name the structure labelled D.	
E	Name the structure labelled E.	

Case 1.21

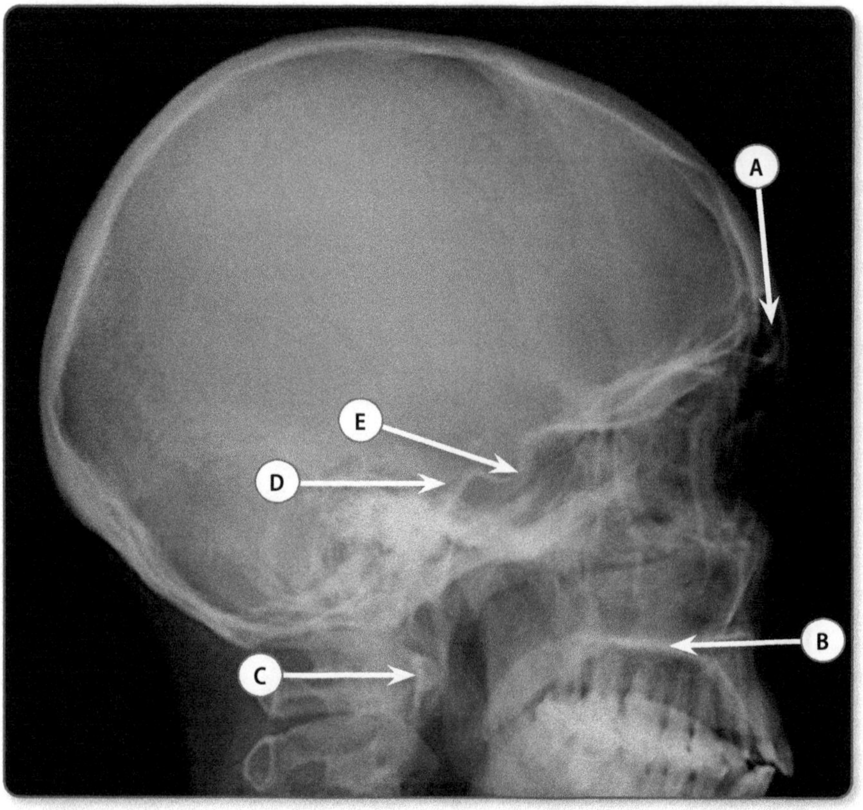

Case 1.21

QUESTION		WRITE YOUR ANSWER HERE
A	Name the structure labelled A.	
B	Name the structure labelled B.	
C	Name the structure labelled C.	
D	Name the structure labelled D.	
E	Name the structure labelled E.	

Case 1.22

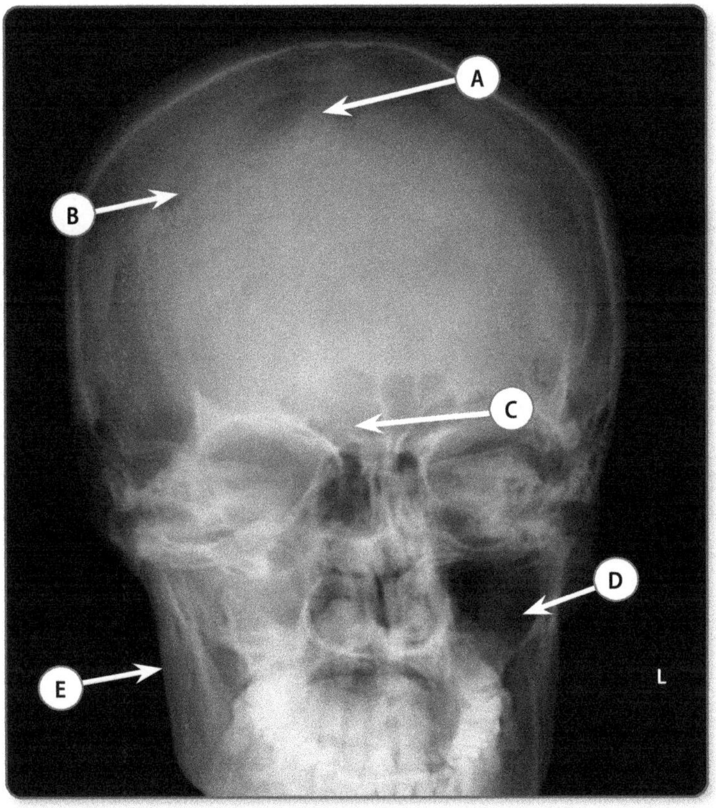

Case 1.22

QUESTION		WRITE YOUR ANSWER HERE
A	Name the structure labelled A.	
B	Name the structure labelled B.	
C	Name the structure labelled C.	
D	Name the structure labelled D.	
E	Name the structure labelled E.	

Case 1.23

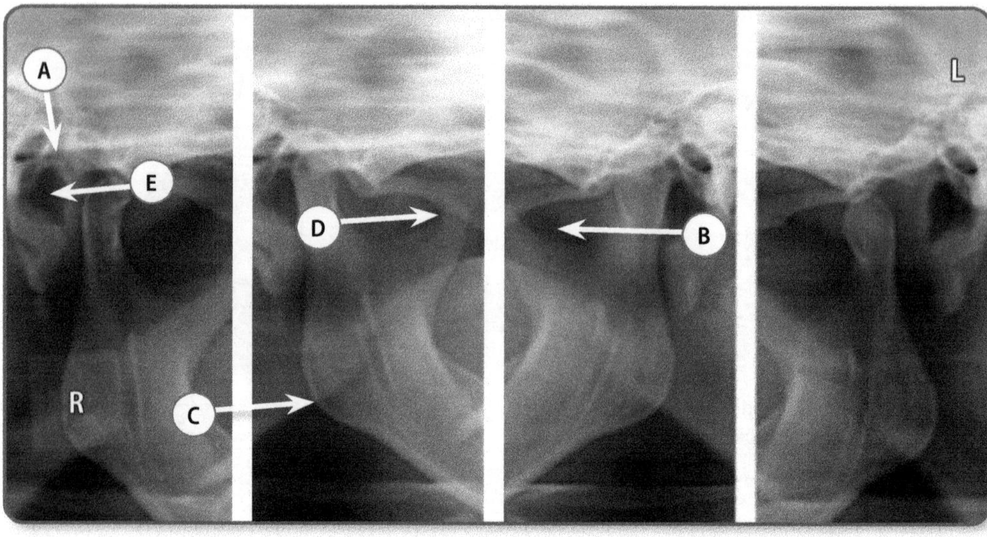

Case 1.23

QUESTION		WRITE YOUR ANSWER HERE
A	Name the structure labelled A.	
B	Name the structure labelled B.	
C	Name the structure labelled C.	
D	Name the structure labelled D.	
E	Name the structure labelled E.	

Case 1.24

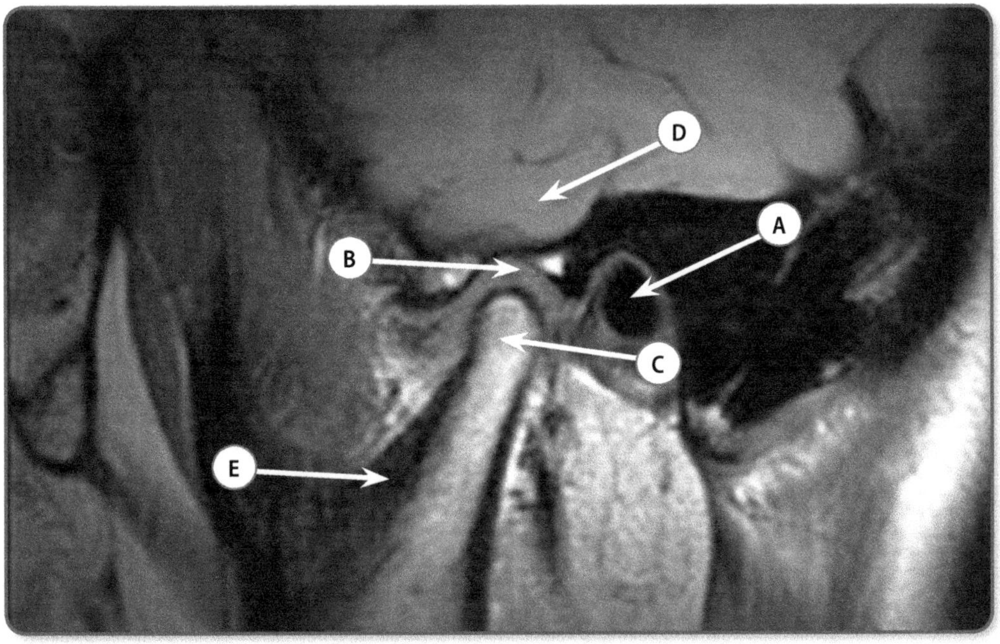

Case 1.24

QUESTION		WRITE YOUR ANSWER HERE
A	Name the structure labelled A.	
B	Name the structure labelled B.	
C	Name the structure labelled C.	
D	Name the structure labelled D.	
E	Name the structure labelled E.	

Case 1.25

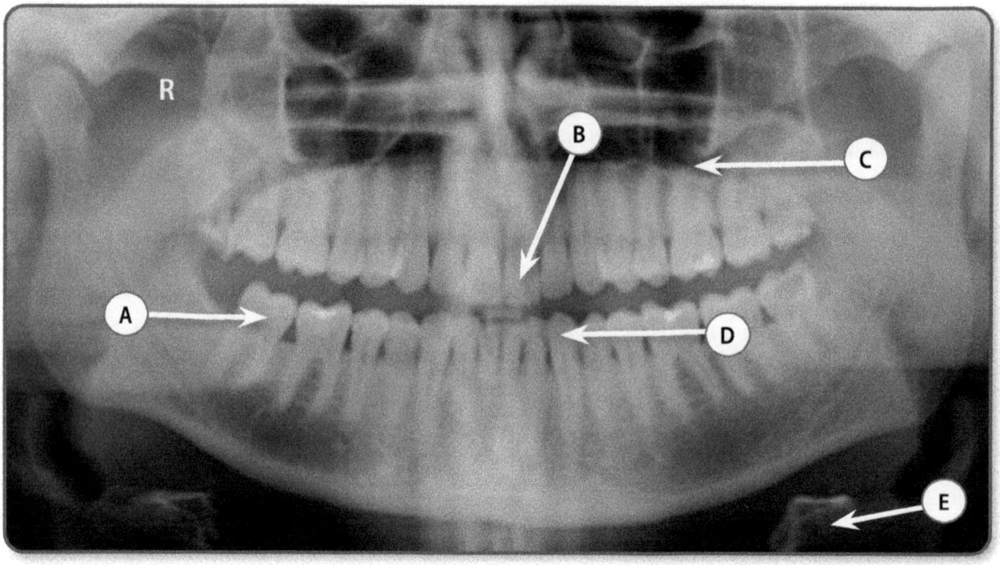

Case 1.25

QUESTION		WRITE YOUR ANSWER HERE
A	Name the structure labelled A.	
B	Name the structure labelled B.	
C	Name the structure labelled C.	
D	Name the structure labelled D.	
E	Name the structure labelled E.	

Case 1.26

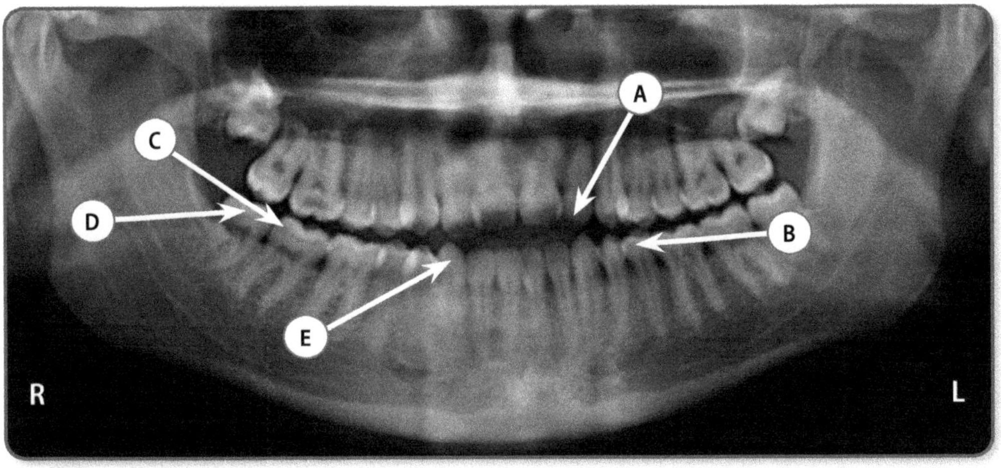

Case 1.26

QUESTION		WRITE YOUR ANSWER HERE
A	Name the structure labelled A.	
B	Name the structure labelled B.	
C	Name the structure labelled C.	
D	Name the structure labelled D.	
E	Name the structure labelled E.	

Case 1.27

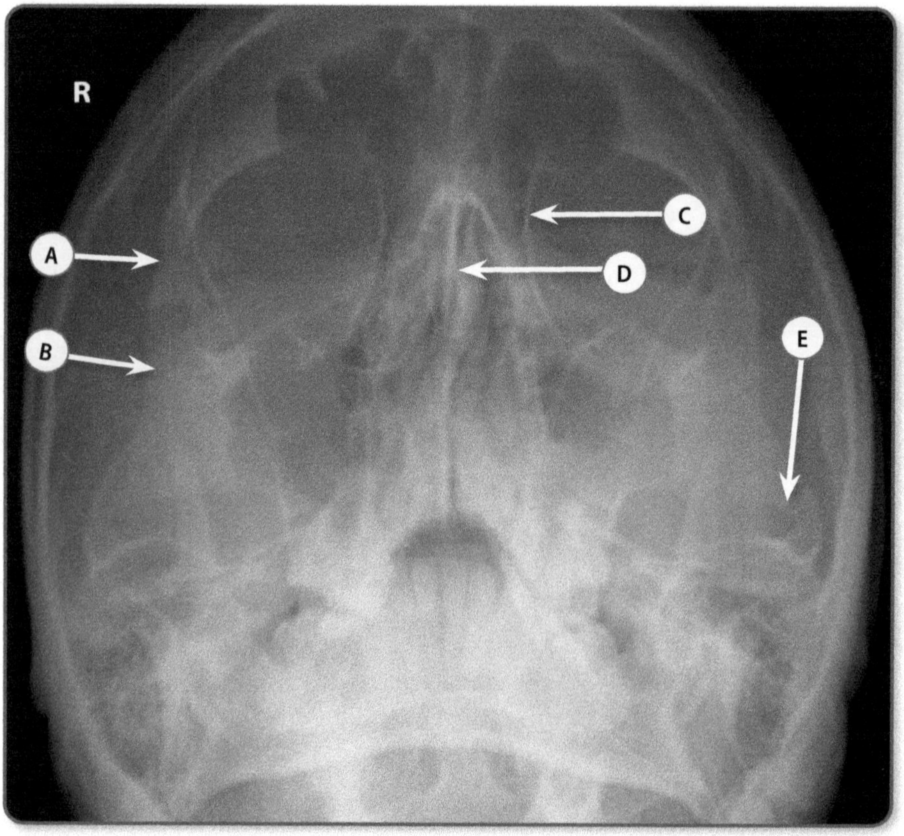

Case 1.27

QUESTION		WRITE YOUR ANSWER HERE
A	Name the structure labelled A.	
B	Name the structure labelled B.	
C	Name the structure labelled C.	
D	Name the structure labelled D.	
E	Name the structure labelled E.	

Case 1.28

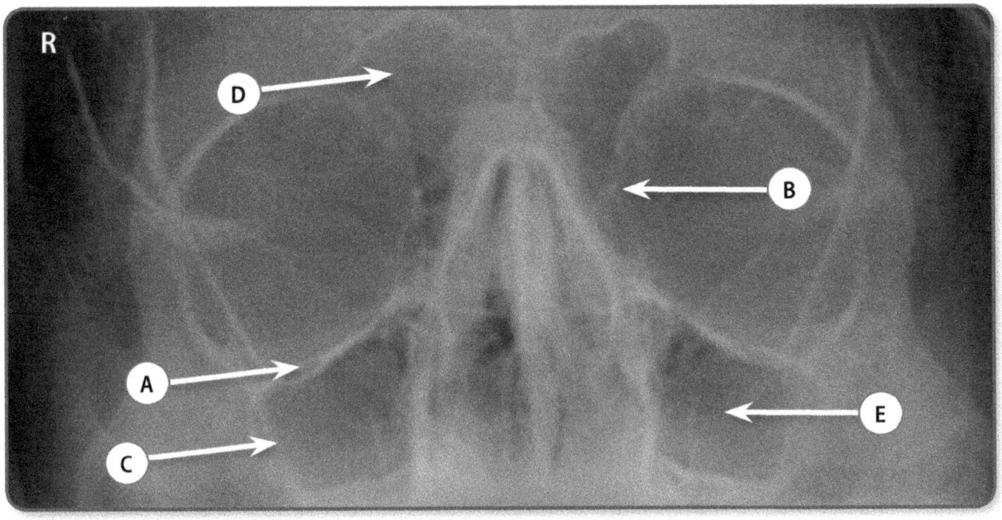

Case 1.28

QUESTION		WRITE YOUR ANSWER HERE
A	Name the structure labelled A.	
B	Name the structure labelled B.	
C	Name the structure labelled C.	
D	Name the structure labelled D.	
E	Name the structure labelled E.	

Case 1.29

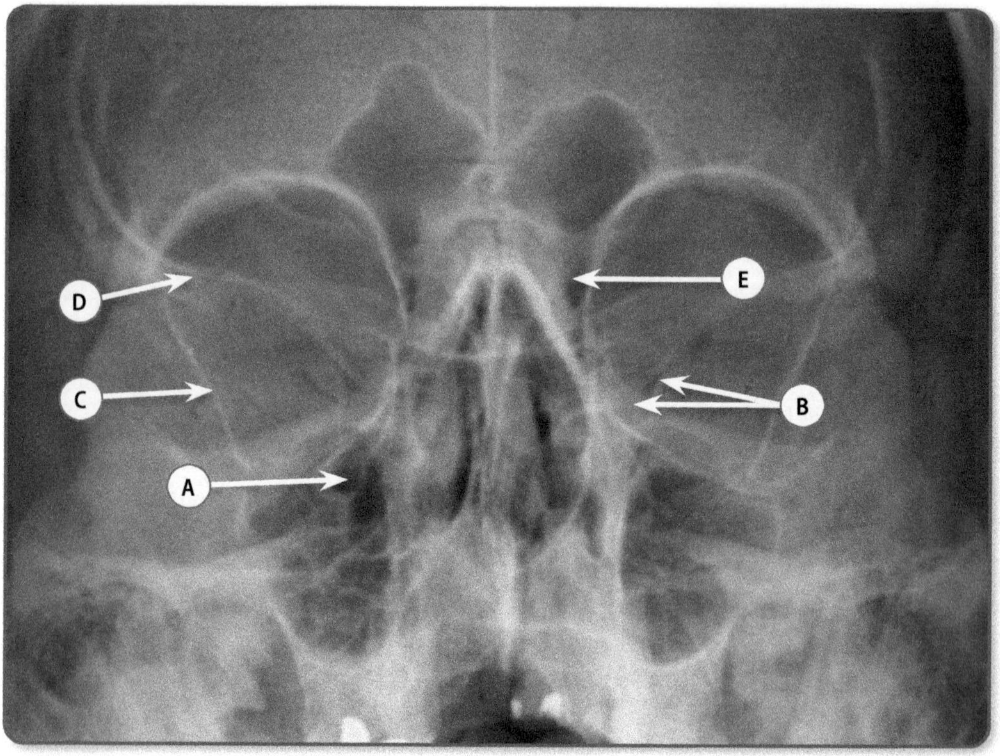

Case 1.29

QUESTION		WRITE YOUR ANSWER HERE
A	Name the structure labelled A.	
B	Name the structure labelled B.	
C	Name the structure labelled C.	
D	Name the structure labelled D.	
E	Name the structure labelled E.	

Case 1.30

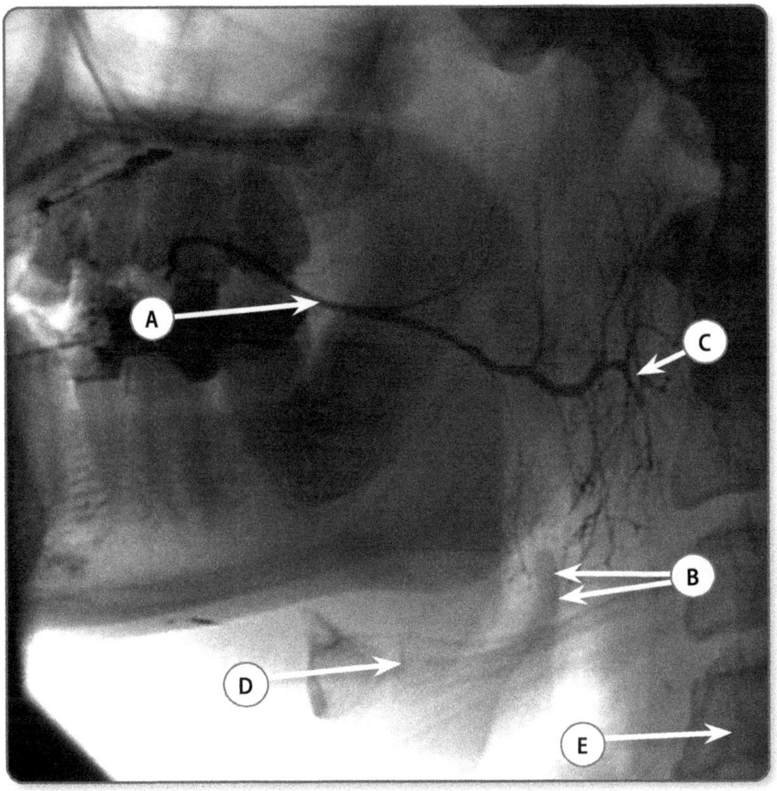

Case 1.30

QUESTION		WRITE YOUR ANSWER HERE
A	Name the structure labelled A.	
B	Name the structure labelled B.	
C	Name the structure labelled C.	
D	Name the structure labelled D.	
E	Name the structure labelled E.	

Case 1.31

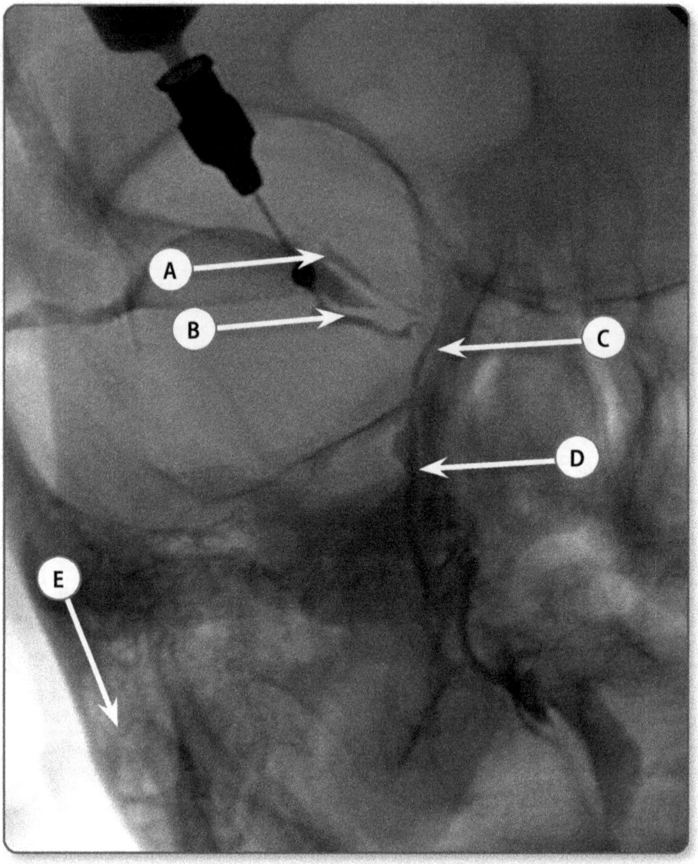

Case 1.31

QUESTION		WRITE YOUR ANSWER HERE
A	Name the structure labelled A.	
B	Name the structure labelled B.	
C	Name the structure labelled C.	
D	Name the structure labelled D.	
E	Name the structure labelled E.	

Case 1.32

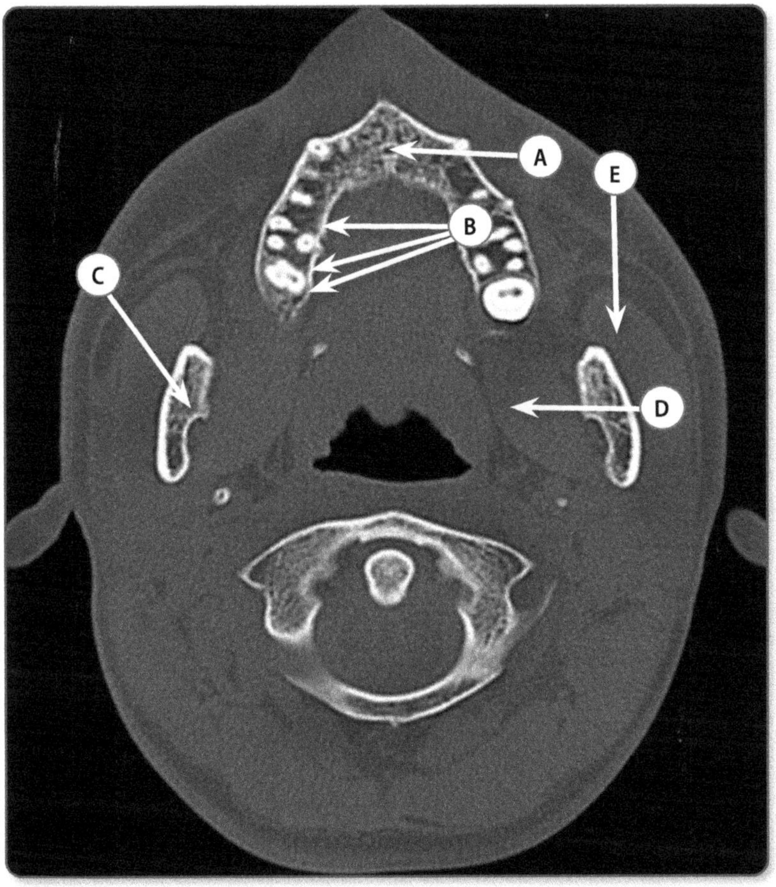

Case 1.32

QUESTION		WRITE YOUR ANSWER HERE
A	Name the structure labelled A.	
B	Name the structure labelled B.	
C	Name the structure labelled C.	
D	Name the structure labelled D.	
E	Name the structure labelled E.	

Case 1.33

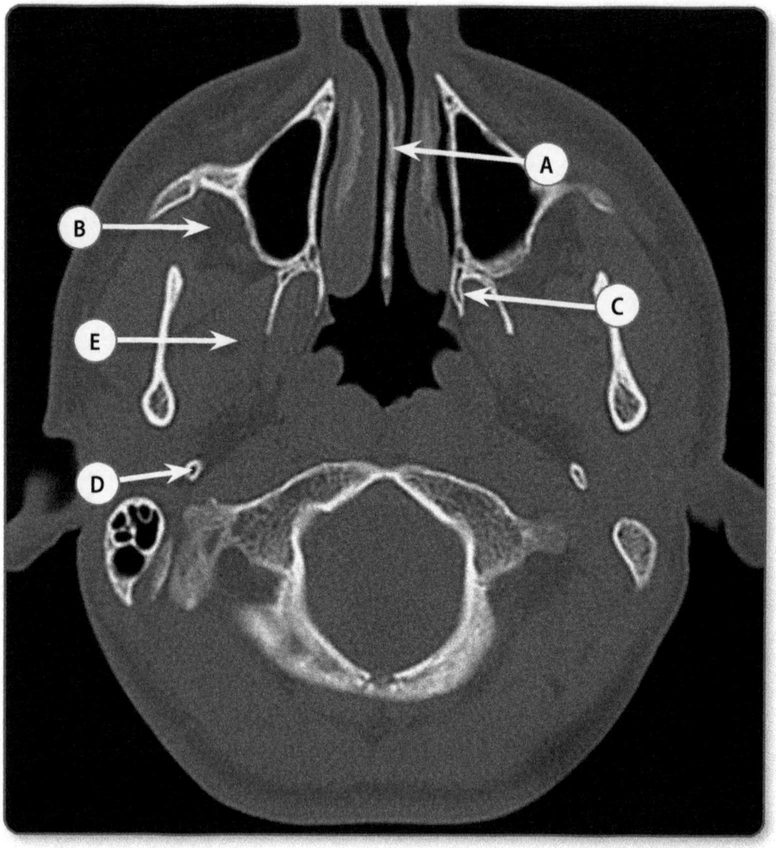

Case 1.33

QUESTION		WRITE YOUR ANSWER HERE
A	Name the structure labelled A.	
B	Name the structure labelled B.	
C	Name the structure labelled C.	
D	Name the structure labelled D.	
E	Name the structure labelled E.	

Case 1.34

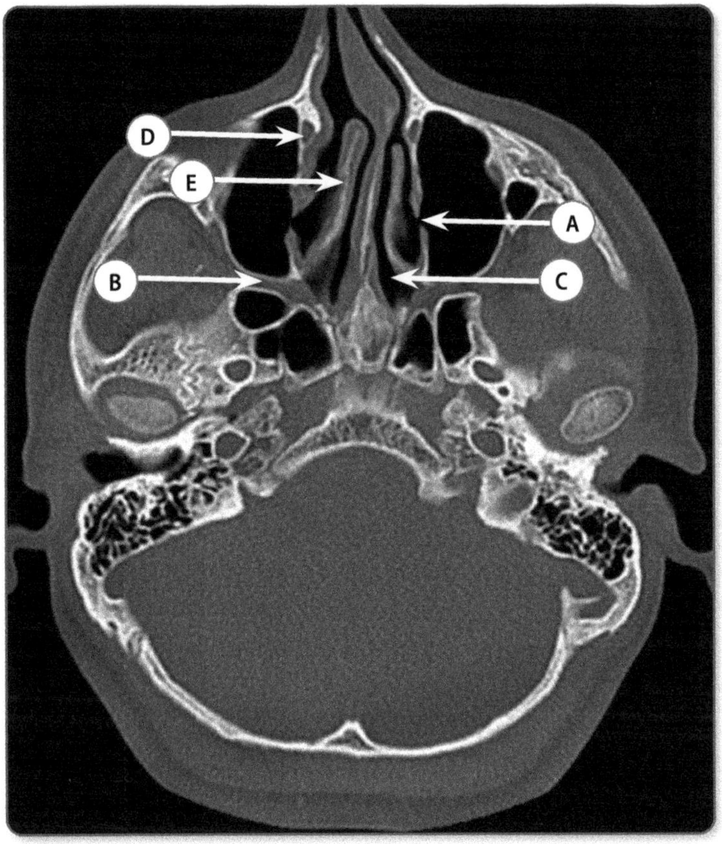

Case 1.34

QUESTION		WRITE YOUR ANSWER HERE
A	Name the structure labelled A.	
B	Name the structure labelled B.	
C	Name the structure labelled C.	
D	Name the structure labelled D.	
E	Name the structure labelled E.	

Case 1.35

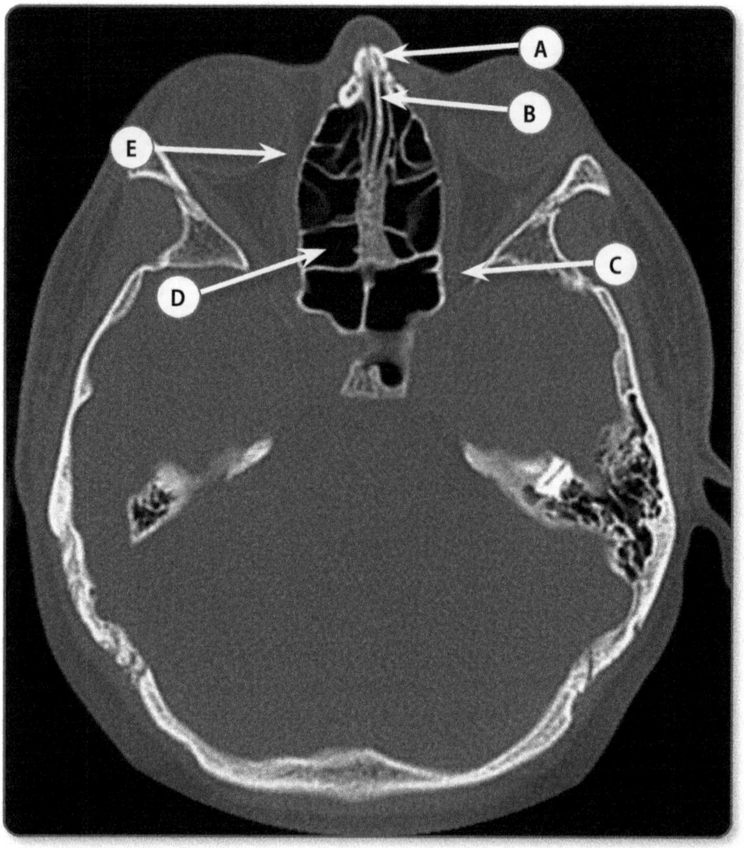

Case 1.35

QUESTION		WRITE YOUR ANSWER HERE
A	Name the structure labelled A.	
B	Name the structure labelled B.	
C	Name the structure labelled C.	
D	Name the structure labelled D.	
E	Name the structure labelled E.	

Case 1.36

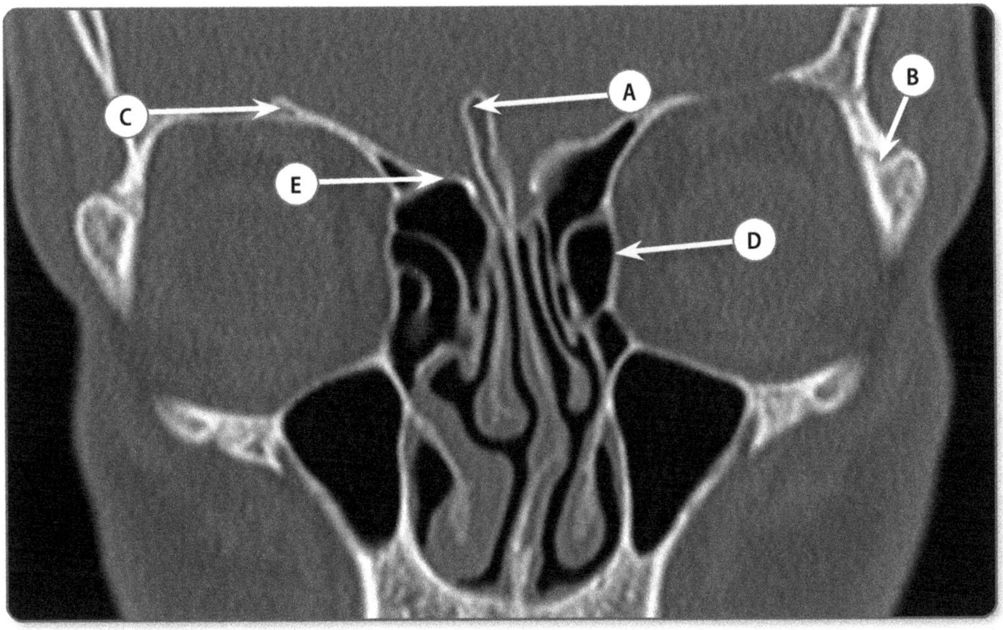

Case 1.36

QUESTION		WRITE YOUR ANSWER HERE
A	Name the structure labelled A.	
B	Name the structure labelled B.	
C	Name the structure labelled C.	
D	Name the structure labelled D.	
E	Name the structure labelled E.	

Case 1.37

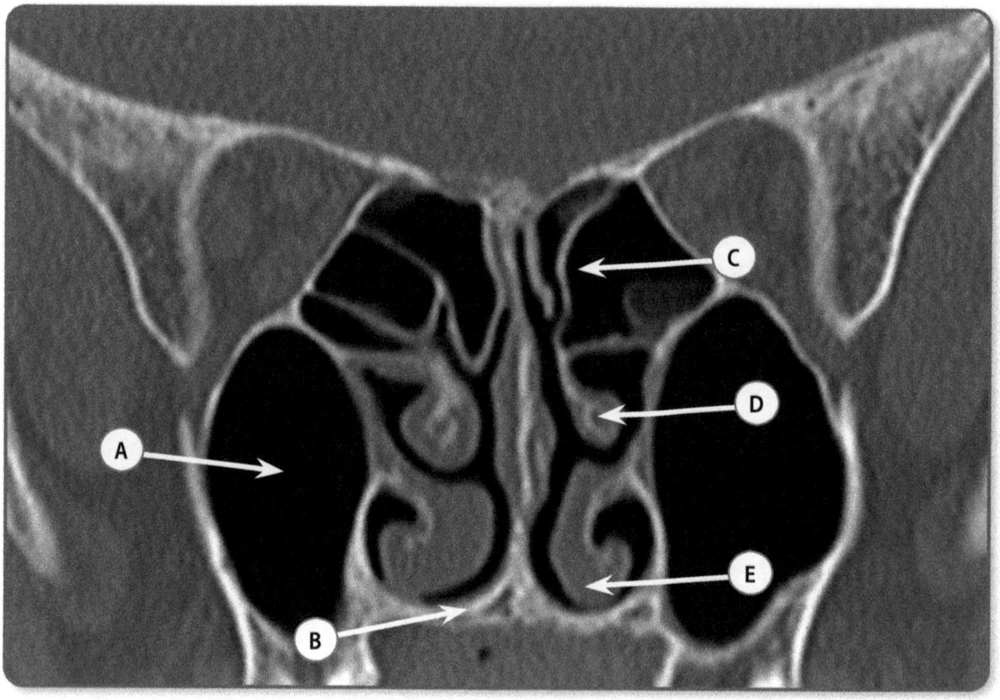

Case 1.37

QUESTION		WRITE YOUR ANSWER HERE
A	Name the structure labelled A.	
B	Name the structure labelled B.	
C	Name the structure labelled C.	
D	Name the structure labelled D.	
E	Name the structure labelled E.	

Case 1.38

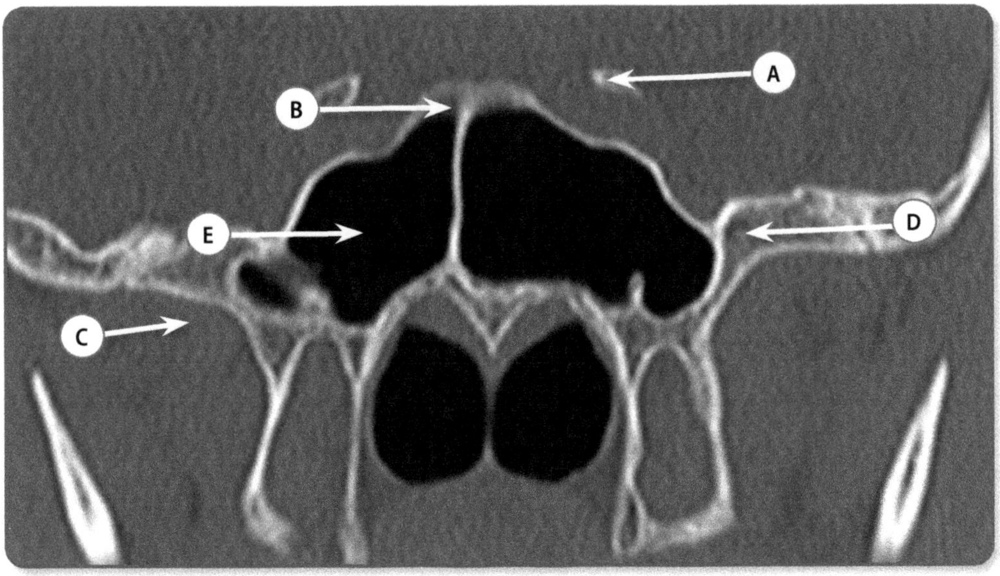

Case 1.38

QUESTION		WRITE YOUR ANSWER HERE
A	Name the structure labelled A.	
B	Name the structure labelled B.	
C	Name the structure labelled C.	
D	Name the structure labelled D.	
E	Name the structure labelled E.	

Case 1.39

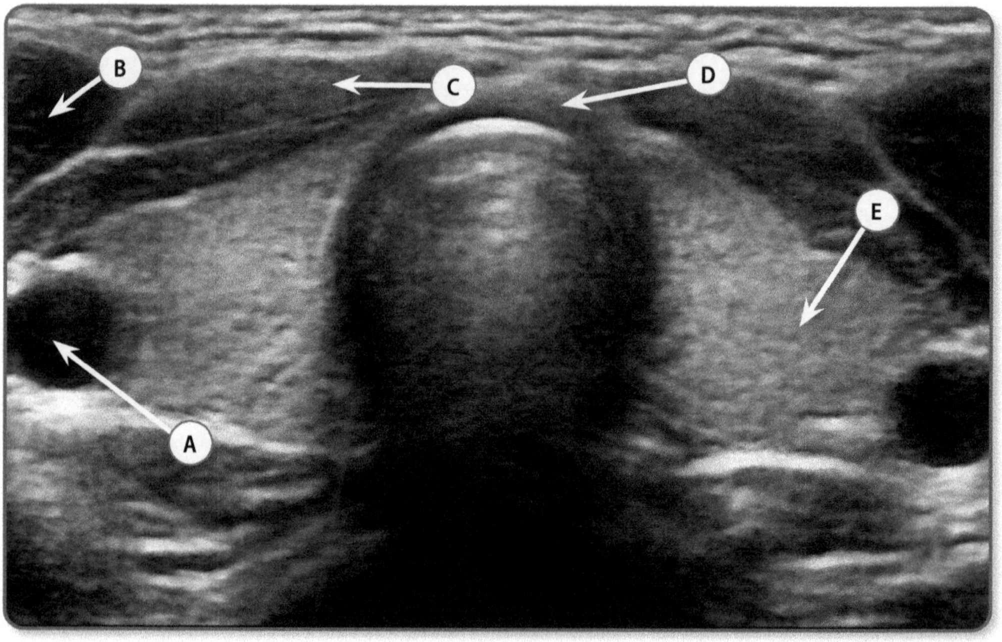

Case 1.39

QUESTION		WRITE YOUR ANSWER HERE
A	Name the structure labelled A.	
B	Name the structure labelled B.	
C	Name the structure labelled C.	
D	Name the structure labelled D.	
E	Name the structure labelled E.	

Case 1.40

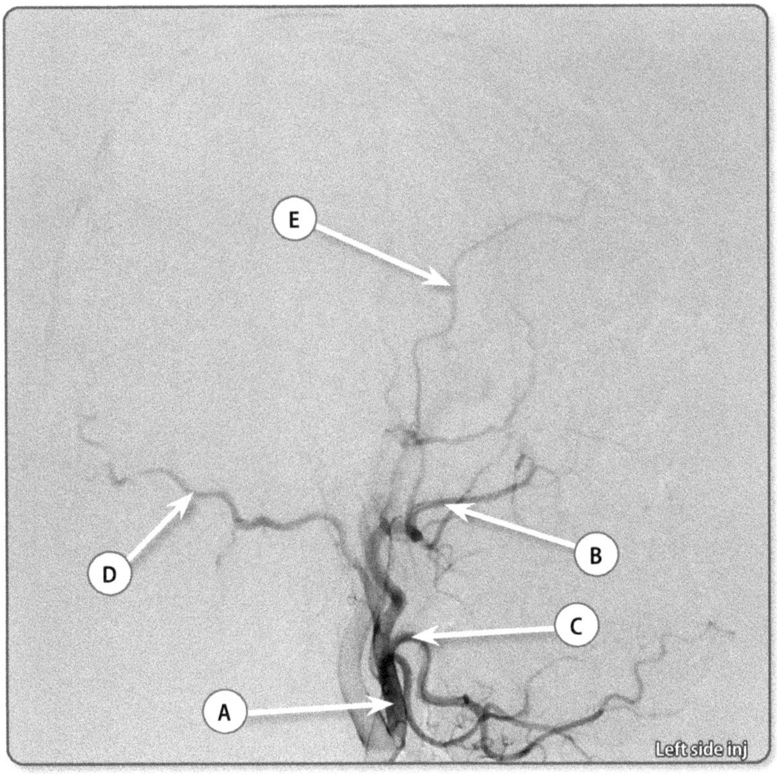

Case 1.40

QUESTION		WRITE YOUR ANSWER HERE
A	Name the structure labelled A.	
B	Name the structure labelled B.	
C	Name the structure labelled C.	
D	Name the structure labelled D.	
E	Name the structure labelled E.	

Case 1.41

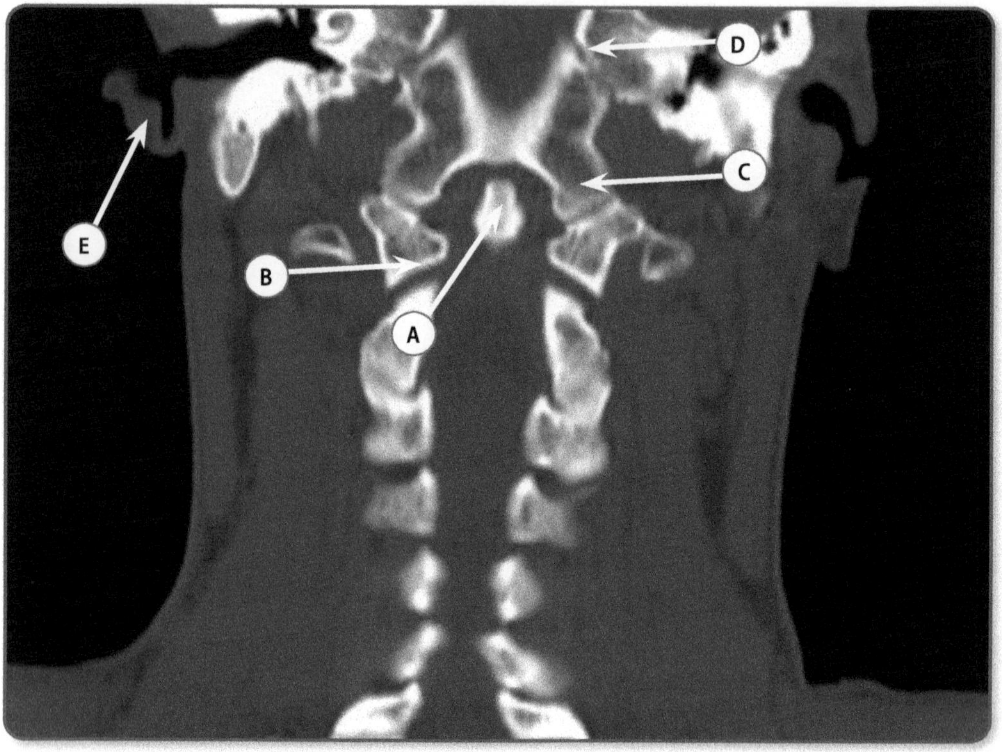

Case 1.41

QUESTION		WRITE YOUR ANSWER HERE
A	Name the structure labelled A.	
B	Name the structure labelled B.	
C	Name the structure labelled C.	
D	Name the structure labelled D.	
E	Name the structure labelled E.	

Case 1.42

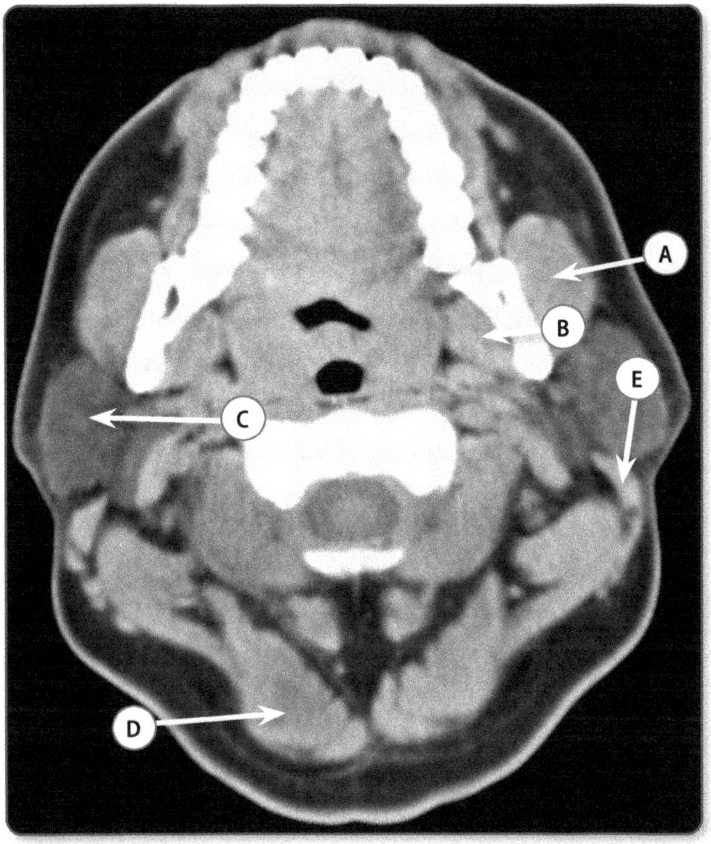

Case 1.42

QUESTION		WRITE YOUR ANSWER HERE
A	Name the structure labelled A.	
B	Name the structure labelled B.	
C	Name the structure labelled C.	
D	Name the structure labelled D.	
E	Name the structure labelled E.	

Case 1.43

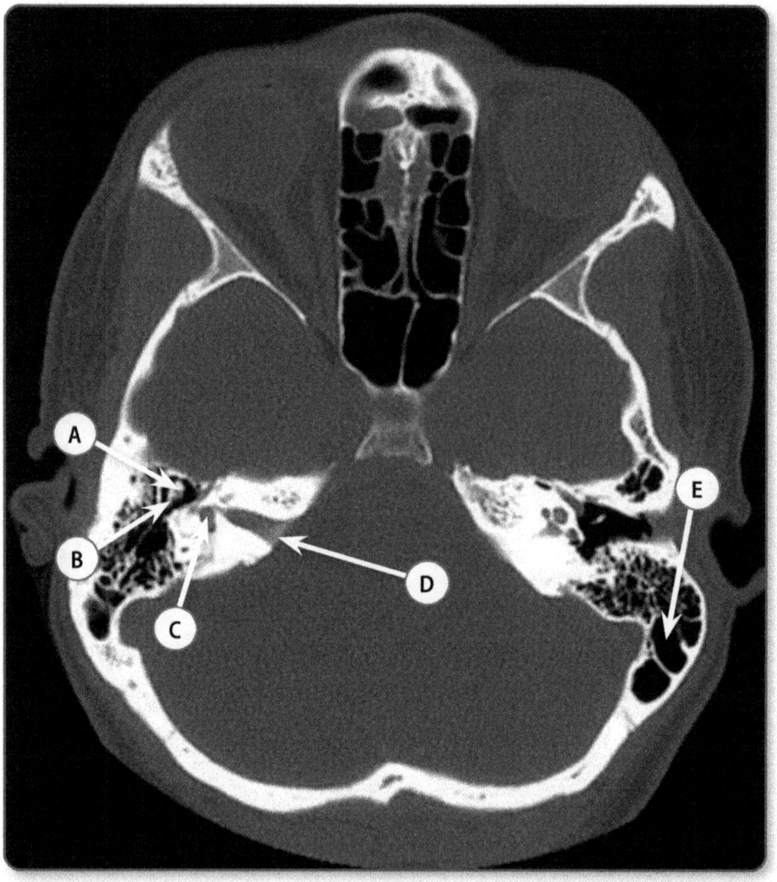

Case 1.43

QUESTION		WRITE YOUR ANSWER HERE
A	Name the structure labelled A.	
B	Name the structure labelled B.	
C	Name the structure labelled C.	
D	Name the structure labelled D.	
E	Name the structure labelled E.	

Case 1.44

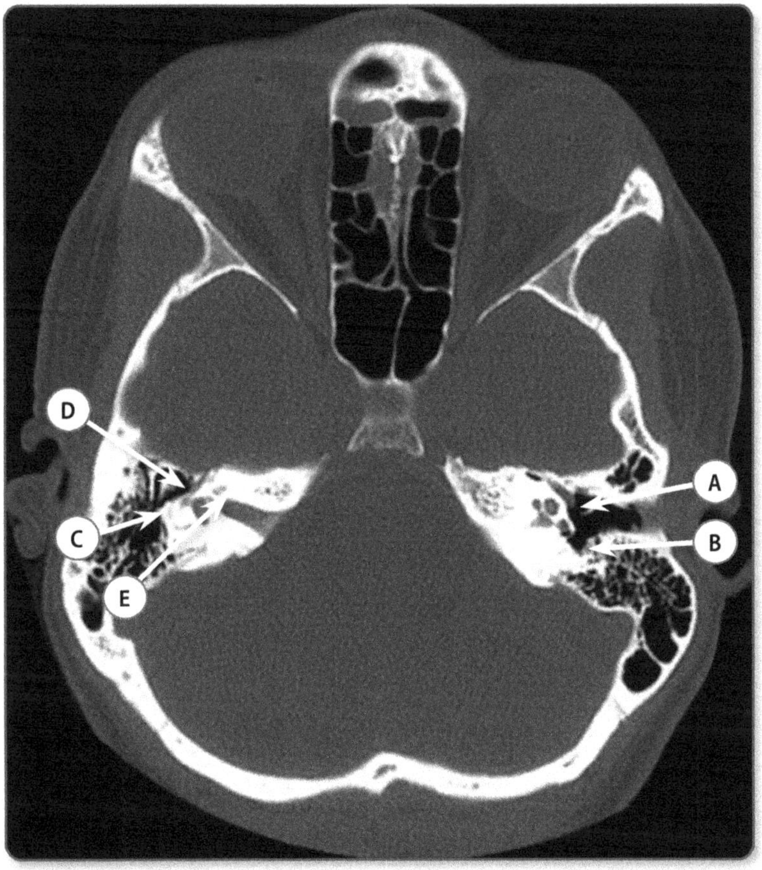

Case 1.44

QUESTION		WRITE YOUR ANSWER HERE
A	Name the structure labelled A.	
B	Name the structure labelled B.	
C	Name the structure labelled C.	
D	Name the structure labelled D.	
E	Name the structure labelled E.	

Case 1.45

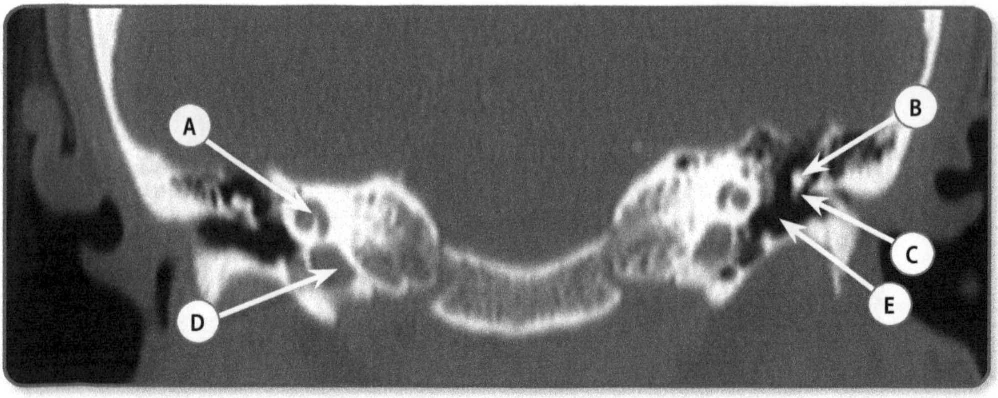

Case 1.45

QUESTION		WRITE YOUR ANSWER HERE
A	Name the structure labelled A.	
B	Name the structure labelled B.	
C	Name the structure labelled C.	
D	Name the structure labelled D.	
E	Name the structure labelled E.	

Case 1.46

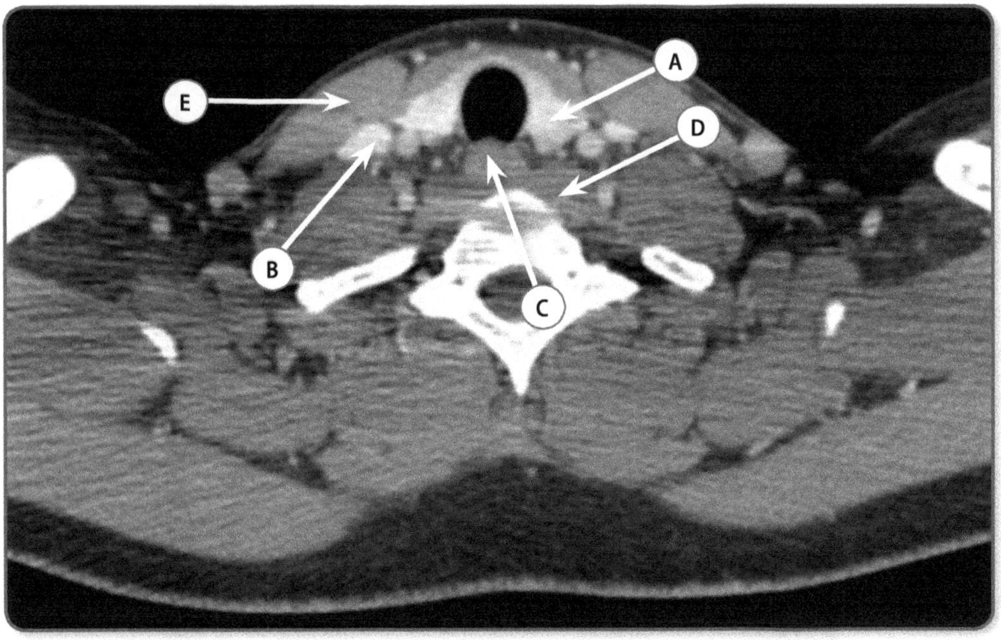

Case 1.46

QUESTION		WRITE YOUR ANSWER HERE
A	Name the structure labelled A.	
B	Name the structure labelled B.	
C	Name the structure labelled C.	
D	Name the structure labelled D.	
E	Name the structure labelled E.	

Case 1.47

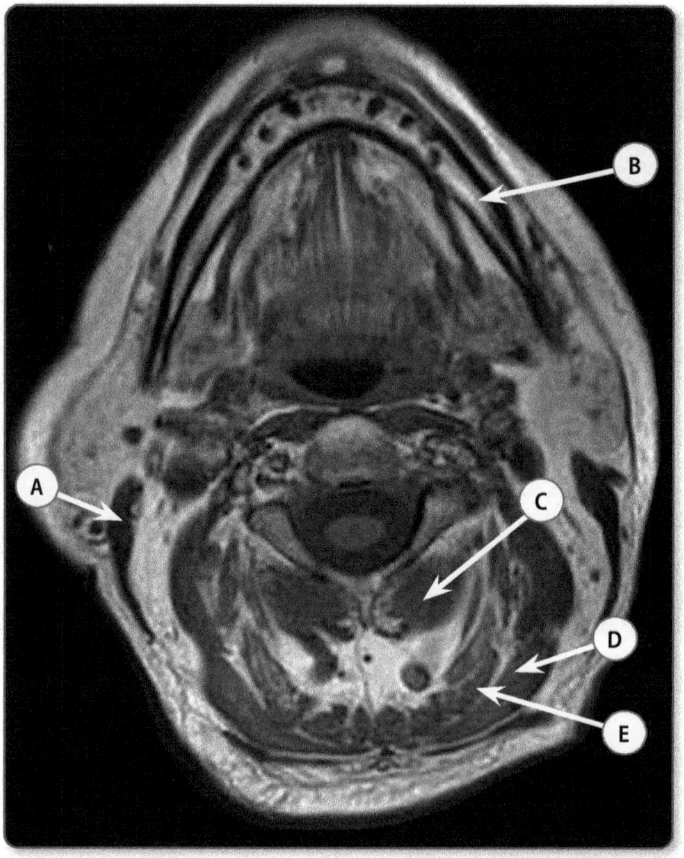

Case 1.47

QUESTION		WRITE YOUR ANSWER HERE
A	Name the structure labelled A.	
B	Name the structure labelled B.	
C	Name the structure labelled C.	
D	Name the structure labelled D.	
E	Name the structure labelled E.	

Case 1.48

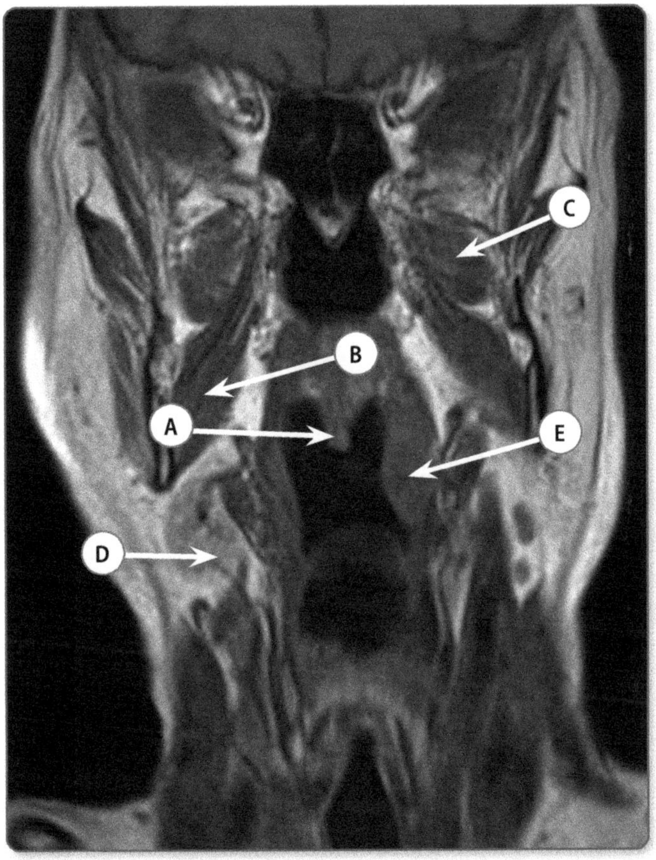

Case 1.48

QUESTION		WRITE YOUR ANSWER HERE
A	Name the structure labelled A.	
B	Name the structure labelled B.	
C	Name the structure labelled C.	
D	Name the structure labelled D.	
E	Name the structure labelled E.	

Case 1.49

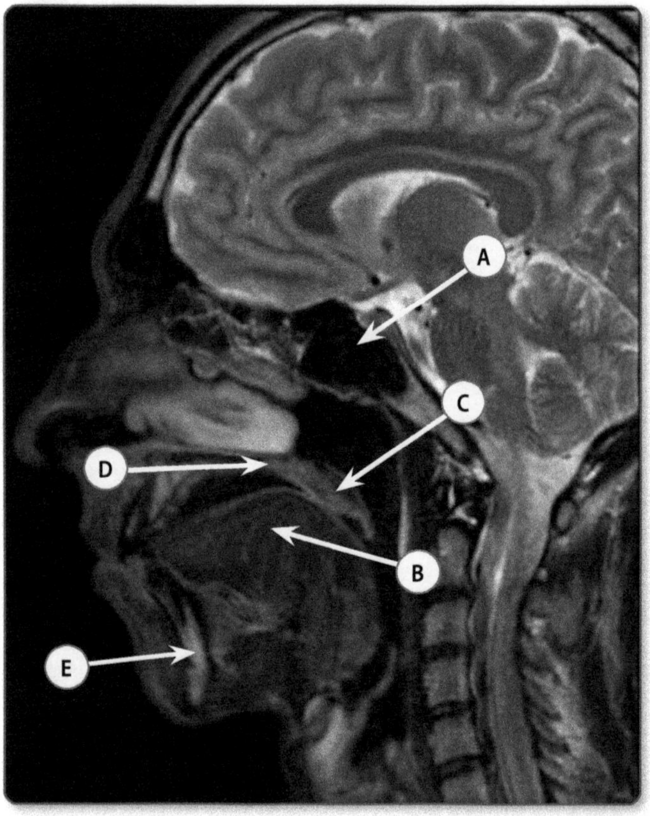

Case 1.49

QUESTION		WRITE YOUR ANSWER HERE
A	Name the structure labelled A.	
B	Name the structure labelled B.	
C	Name the structure labelled C.	
D	Name the structure labelled D.	
E	Name the structure labelled E.	

Case 1.50

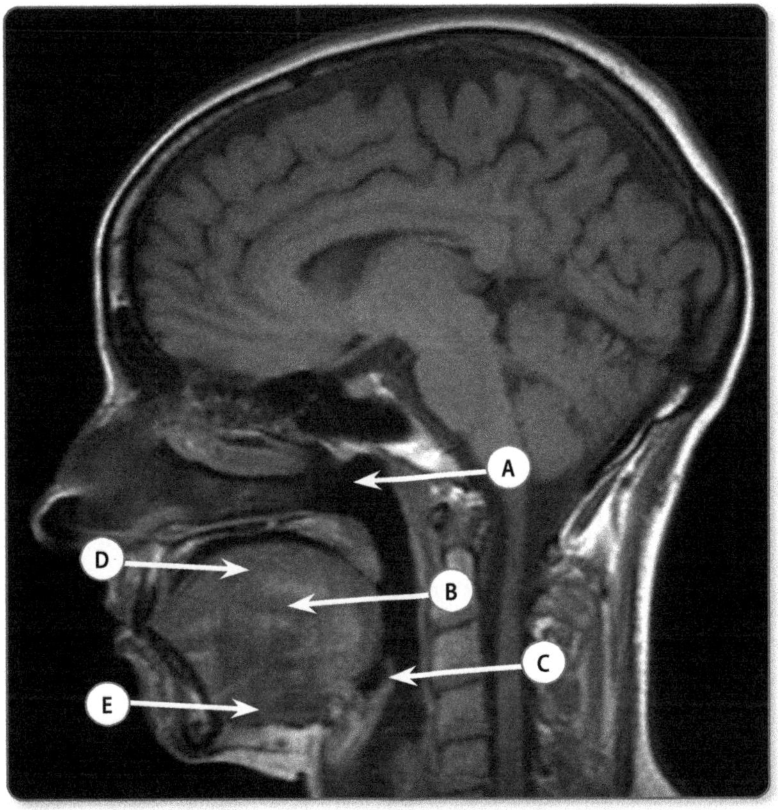

Case 1.50

QUESTION		WRITE YOUR ANSWER HERE
A	Name the structure labelled A.	
B	Name the structure labelled B.	
C	Name the structure labelled C.	
D	Name the structure labelled D.	
E	Name the structure labelled E.	

Case 1.51

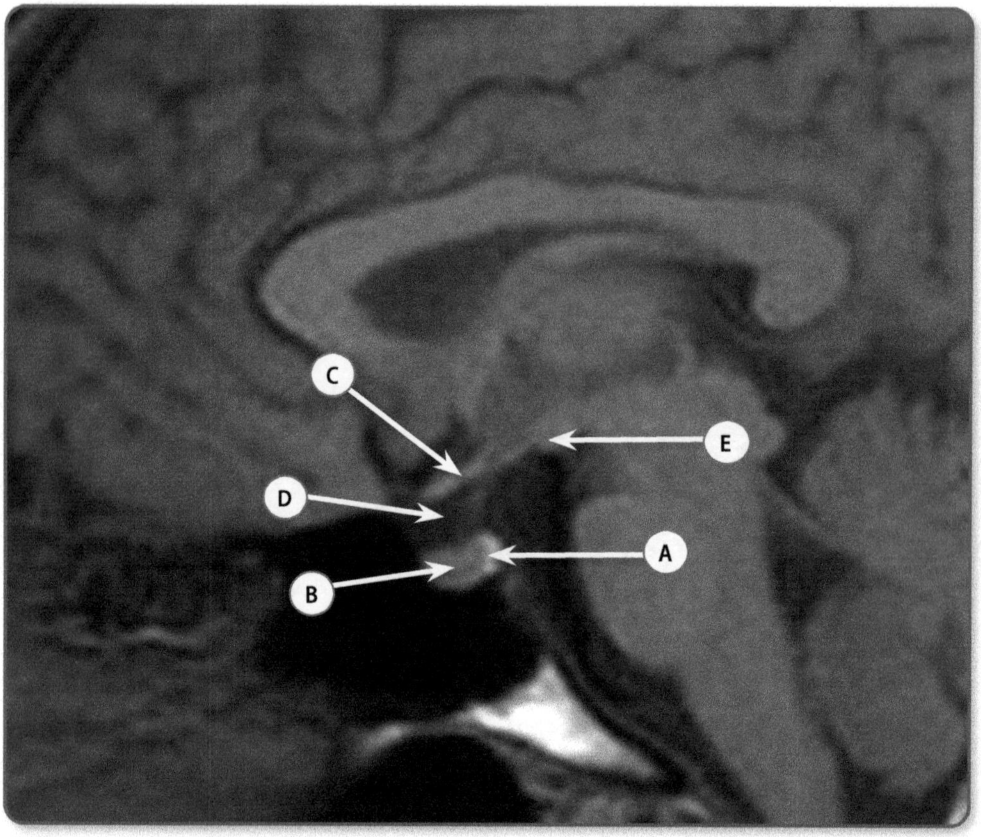

Case 1.51

QUESTION		WRITE YOUR ANSWER HERE
A	Name the structure labelled A.	
B	Name the structure labelled B.	
C	Name the structure labelled C.	
D	Name the structure labelled D.	
E	Name the structure labelled E.	

Case 1.52

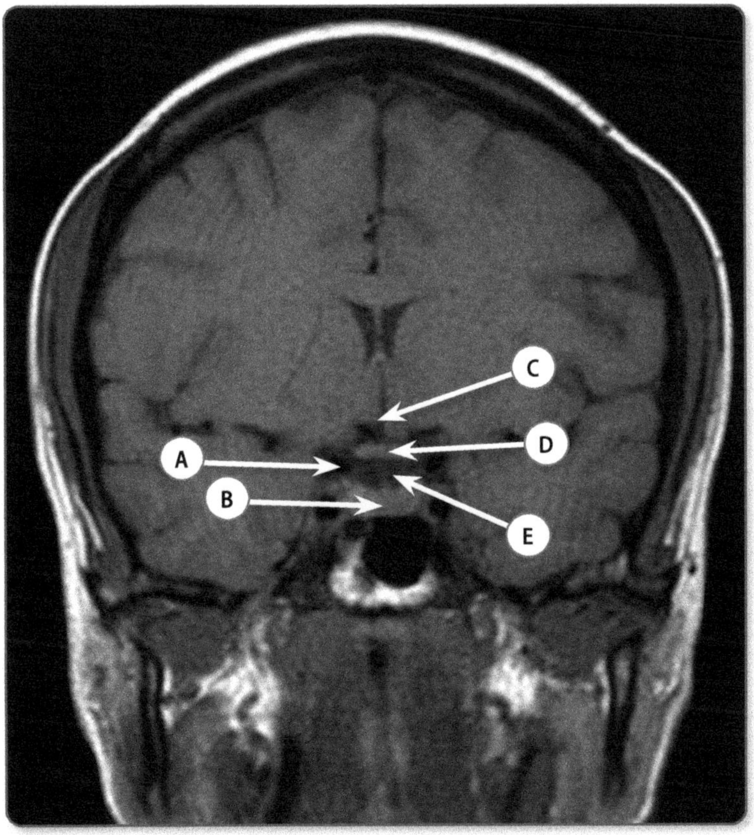

Case 1.52

QUESTION		WRITE YOUR ANSWER HERE
A	Name the structure labelled A.	
B	Name the structure labelled B.	
C	Name the structure labelled C.	
D	Name the structure labelled D.	
E	Name the structure labelled E.	

Case 1.53

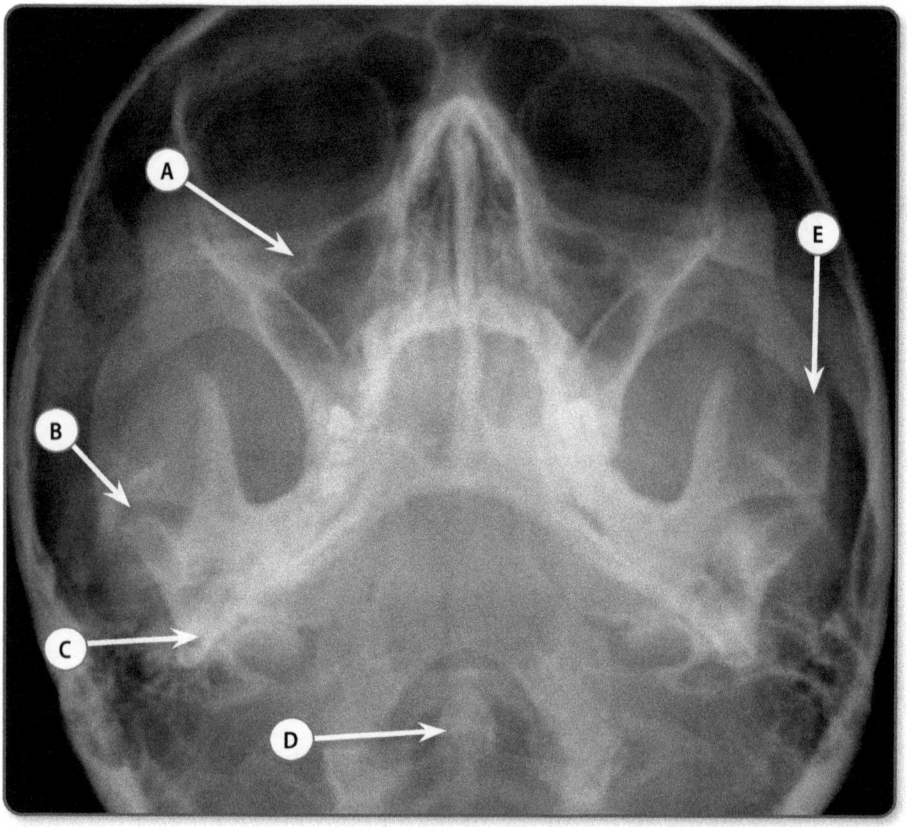

Case 1.53

QUESTION		WRITE YOUR ANSWER HERE
A	Name the structure labelled A.	
B	Name the structure labelled B.	
C	Name the structure labelled C.	
D	Name the structure labelled D.	
E	Name the structure labelled E.	

Case 1.54

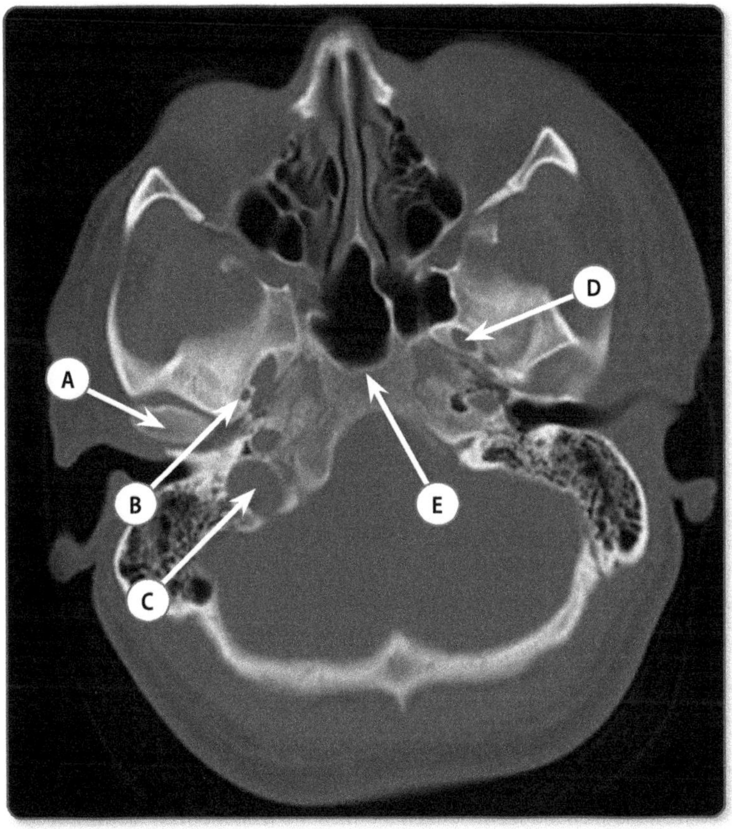

Case 1.54

QUESTION		WRITE YOUR ANSWER HERE
A	Name the structure labelled A.	
B	Name the structure labelled B.	
C	Name the structure labelled C.	
D	Name the structure labelled D.	
E	Name the structure labelled E.	

Case 1.55

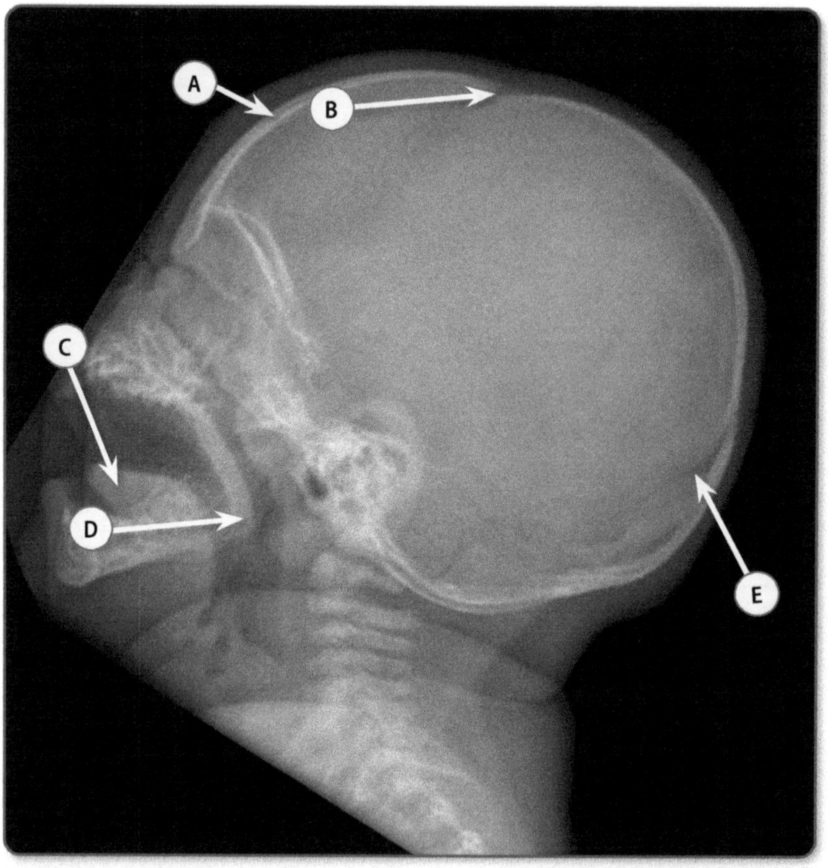

Case 1.55

QUESTION		WRITE YOUR ANSWER HERE
A	Name the structure labelled A.	
B	Name the structure labelled B.	
C	Name the structure labelled C.	
D	Name the structure labelled D.	
E	Name the structure labelled E.	

Case 1.56

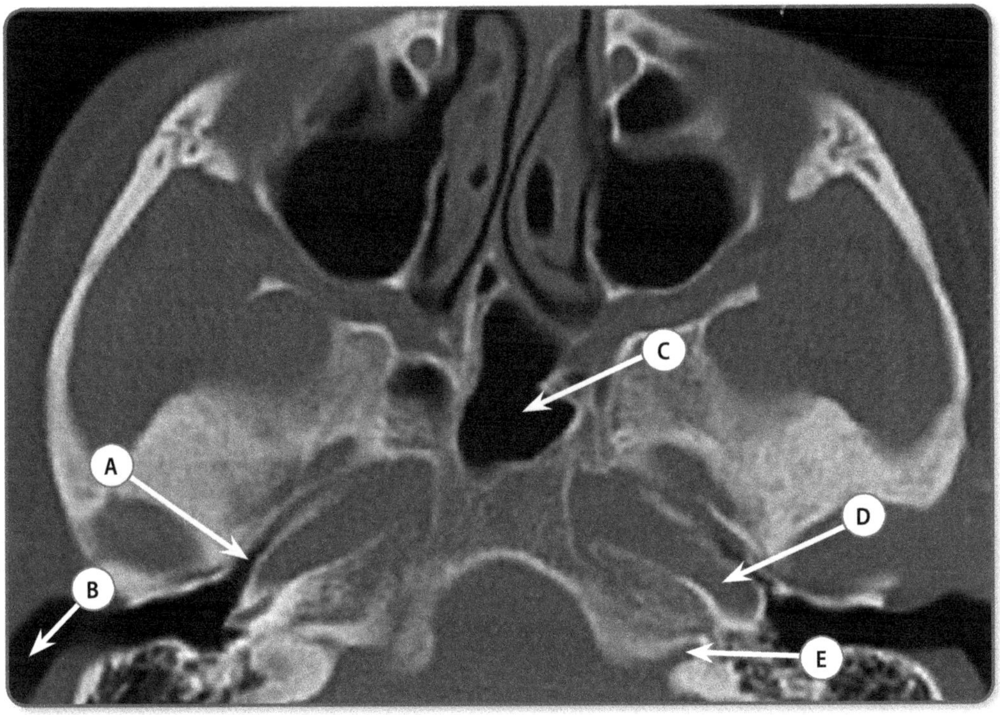

Case 1.56

QUESTION		WRITE YOUR ANSWER HERE
A	Name the structure labelled A.	
B	Name the structure labelled B.	
C	Name the structure labelled C.	
D	Name the structure labelled D.	
E	Name the structure labelled E.	

Case 1.57

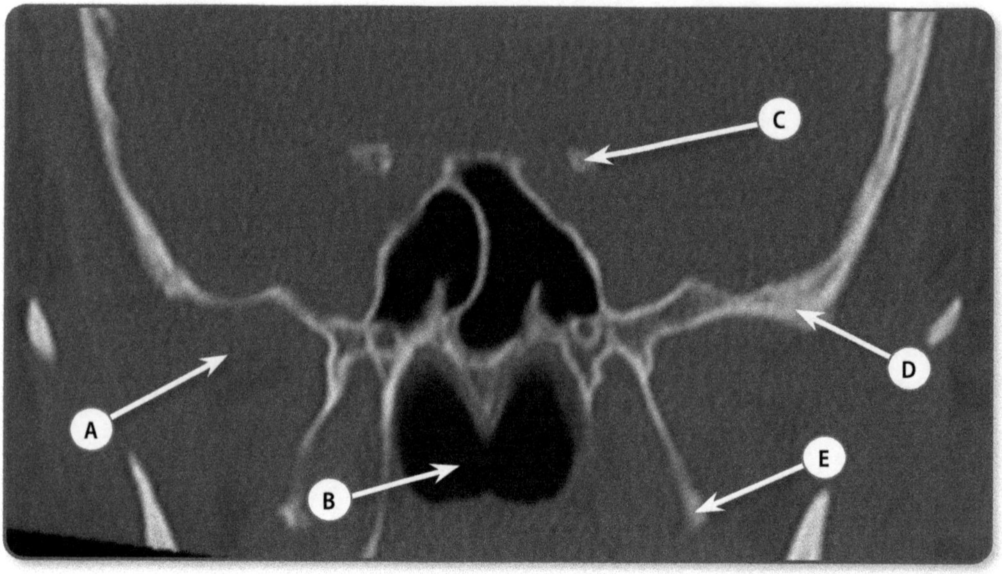

Case 1.57

QUESTION		WRITE YOUR ANSWER HERE
A	Name the structure labelled A.	
B	Name the structure labelled B.	
C	Name the structure labelled C.	
D	Name the structure labelled D.	
E	Name the structure labelled E.	

Case 1.58

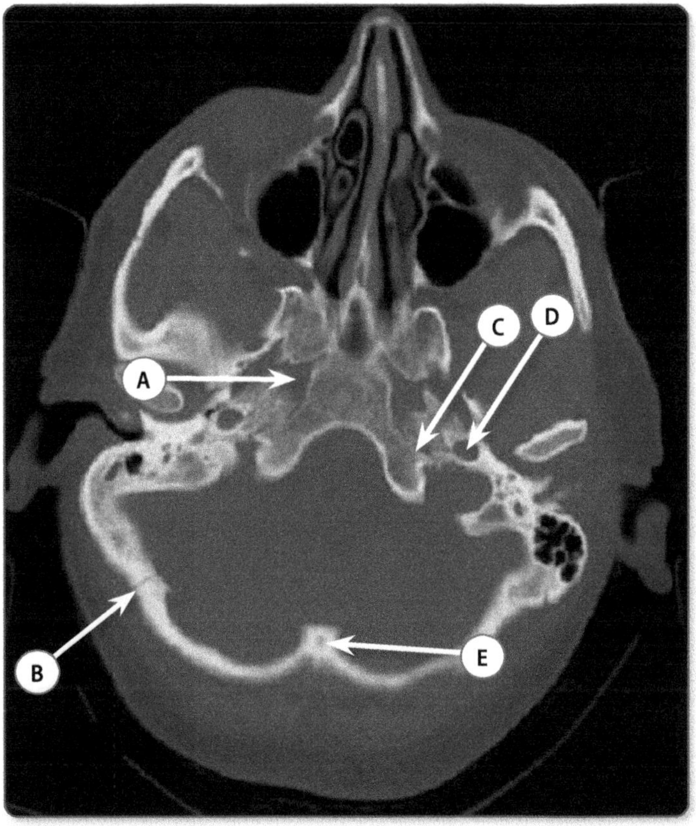

Case 1.58

QUESTION		WRITE YOUR ANSWER HERE
A	Name the structure labelled A.	
B	Name the structure labelled B.	
C	Name the structure labelled C.	
D	Name the structure labelled D.	
E	Name the structure labelled E.	

Case 1.59

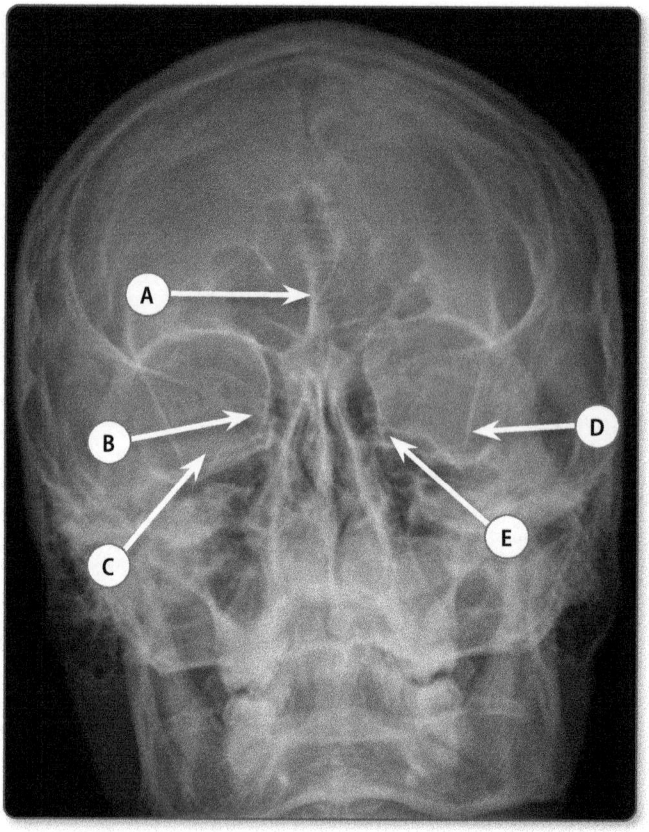

Case 1.59

QUESTION		WRITE YOUR ANSWER HERE
A	Name the structure labelled A.	
B	Name the structure labelled B.	
C	Name the structure labelled C.	
D	Name the structure labelled D.	
E	Name the structure labelled E.	

Case 1.60

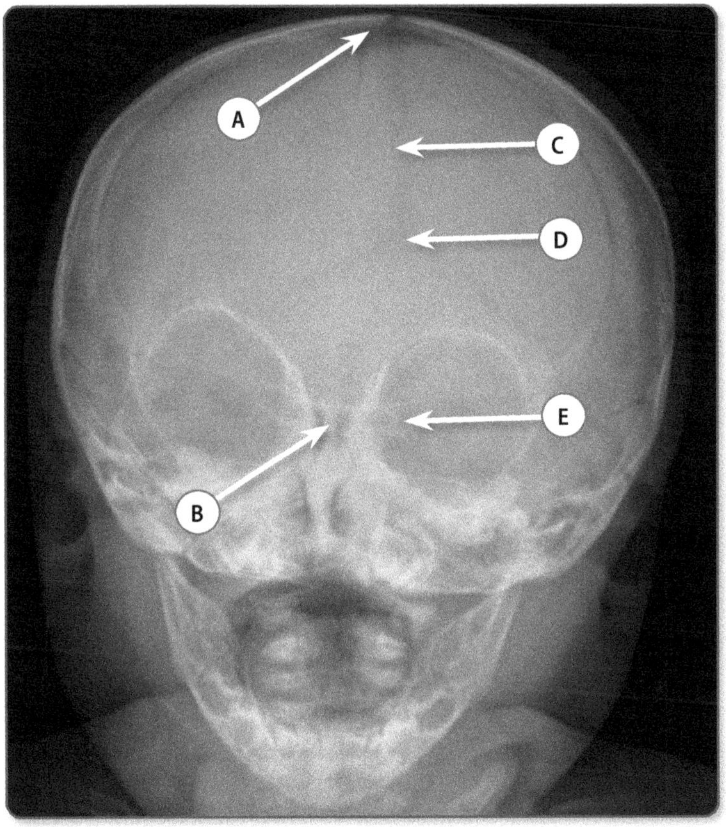

Case 1.60

QUESTION		WRITE YOUR ANSWER HERE
A	Name the structure labelled A.	
B	Name the structure labelled B.	
C	Name the structure labelled C.	
D	Name the structure labelled D.	
E	Name the structure labelled E.	

Case 1.61

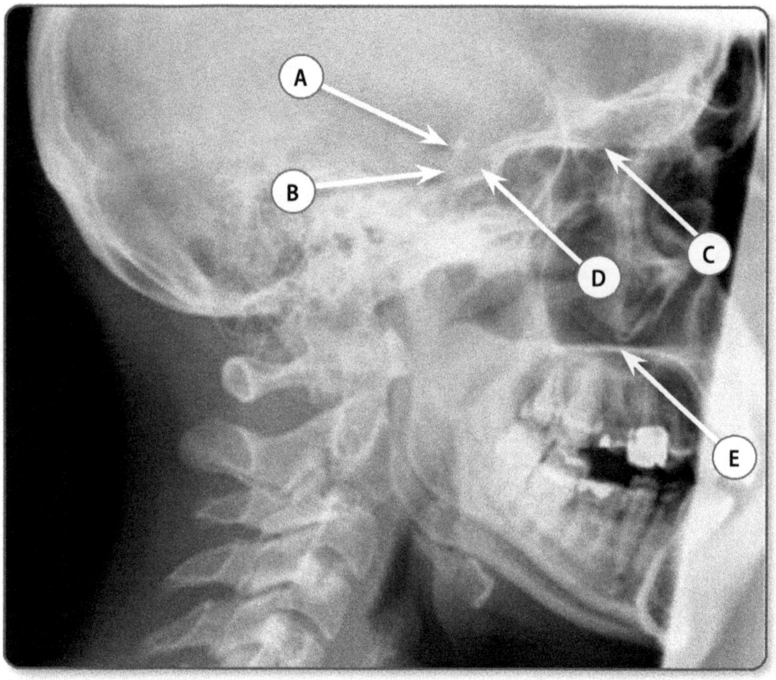

Case 1.61

QUESTION		WRITE YOUR ANSWER HERE
A	Name the structure labelled A.	
B	Name the structure labelled B.	
C	Name the structure labelled C.	
D	Name the structure labelled D.	
E	Name the structure labelled E.	

Case 1.62

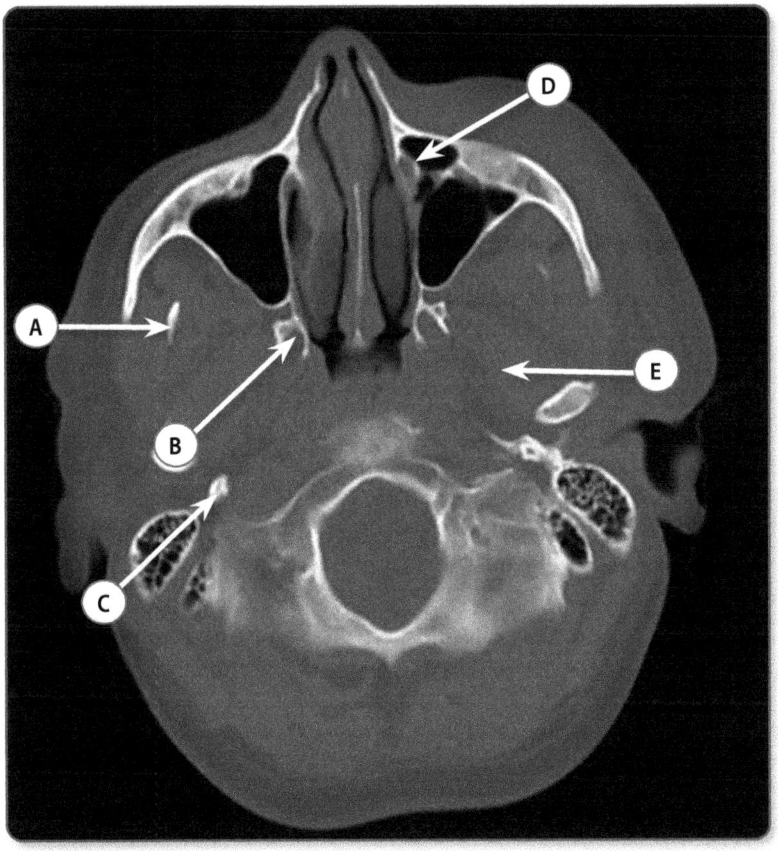

Case 1.62

QUESTION		WRITE YOUR ANSWER HERE
A	Name the structure labelled A.	
B	Name the structure labelled B.	
C	Name the structure labelled C.	
D	Name the structure labelled D.	
E	Name the structure labelled E.	

Answers

Case 1.1

A Rostrum of the corpus callosum

B Genu of the corpus callosum

C Body of the fornix

D Splenium of the corpus callosum

E Mamillary body of the hypothalamus

Midline sagittal MRI of the brain.

The corpus callosum lies in the depths of the great longitudinal fissure (interhemispheric fissure). It is composed of commissural fibres that unite corresponding regions of the two cerebral hemispheres. In this image, we can identify the major parts of the corpus callosum. From rostral to caudal these are: rostrum, genu, body and splenium.

The fornix is a C-shaped fascicle of fibres that links the hippocampus with the mamillary body of the hypothalamus. The horizontal bundles of fibres that come together in the midline form the body of the fornix. The upper surface of this structure provides attachments to the septum pellucidum, a membrane that separates the anterior horns of the lateral ventricles.

Weir J, Abrahams P. Imaging Atlas of Human Anatomy, 6th edition. Edinburgh: Mosby, 2021:11.

Ryan S, McNicholas M, Eustace SJ. Anatomy for Diagnostic Imaging, 3rd edition. Edinburgh: Saunders, 2010:57.

Butler P, Mitchell AM, Ellis H. Applied Radiological Anatomy. Cambridge: Cambridge University Press, 1999:36.

Case 1.2

A Anterior pituitary (adenohypophysis)

B Infundibulum

C Interpeduncular cistern

D Body of corpus callosum

E Pineal gland

Midline sagittal MRI of the brain.

The pituitary gland is a pea-sized structure that sits in the sella turcica of the sphenoid bone. It consists of the posterior pituitary (neurohypophysis) and the anterior pituitary (adenohypophysis). The posterior pituitary is a neuronal structure and can be considered as an expansion of the distal part of the infundibulum (pituitary stalk). On a T1-weighted MRI such as this one, the posterior pituitary is bright (high signal). This helps to identify it with confidence. The anterior pituitary is larger.

The interpeduncular cistern is located at the base of the brain, spanning the space between the temporal lobes. It is deepest between the cerebral peduncles of the midbrain, hence the name. It contains the optic chiasm where the optic nerves partially cross.

The pineal gland (also called pineal body) lies in the midline immediately rostral to the superior colliculi of the midbrain. It is part of the epithalamus which is one of the four main subdivisions of the diencephalon. The hypothalamus is the most ventral part of the diencephalon and lies inferior to the thalamus and ventromedial to the subthalamus.

Weir J, Abrahams P. Imaging Atlas of Human Anatomy, 6th edition. Edinburgh: Mosby, 2021:11.

Ryan S, McNicholas M, Eustace SJ. Anatomy for Diagnostic Imaging, 3rd edition. Edinburgh: Saunders, 2010:57.

Butler P, Mitchell AM, Ellis H. Applied Radiological Anatomy. Cambridge: Cambridge University Press, 1999:36.

Case 1.3

A Clivus

B Optic chiasm

C Cingulate gyrus

D Massa intermedia of thalami

E Tonsil of cerebellum

Midline sagittal MRI of the brain.

The clivus (Latin for 'slope') is a shallow depression behind the dorsum sellae. It forms a sloping process at the junction of the occipital and sphenoid bones. The optic chiasm is where half of the fibres of the optic nerve cross to the other side. A mass in the pituitary or the suprasellar fossa can compress this structure. The cingulate gyrus lies above the corpus callosum. It is considered as part of the limbic system and it is thus separate to the frontal and parietal lobes. The thalamus resembles a small hen's egg. Together with the hypothalamus, it forms the lateral wall of the third ventricle. The cerebellar tonsils are the most antero-inferior part of the cerebellar hemispheres. They lie close to the midline and therefore can be seen in a midline sagittal image.

Weir J, Abrahams P. Imaging Atlas of Human Anatomy, 6th edition. Edinburgh: Mosby, 2021:11.

Case 1.4

A Pons

B Ventral midbrain (tegmentum)

C Quadrigeminal plate (tectum)

D 4th ventricle

E Medulla oblongata

Midline sagittal MRI of the brain.

The brainstem connects the cerebral hemispheres with the spinal cord. It consists of three parts: (1) the midbrain, (2) the pons and (3) the medulla.

The midbrain is the most superior part of the brainstem. The quadrigeminal plate is the dorsal part of the midbrain. It is also referred to as tectum (Latin for 'roof'). It is separated from the ventral midbrain (tegmentum) by the cerebral aqueduct (aqueduct of Sylvius), which connects the 3rd and 4th ventricles.

The pons is the widest part of the brainstem. It has a bulbous anterior part. Its posterior part forms the upper part of the floor of the 4th ventricle. The lower part of the floor of the 4th ventricle is formed by the posterior surface of the medulla.

Weir J, Abrahams P. Imaging Atlas of Human Anatomy, 6th edition. Edinburgh: Mosby, 2021:11.

Ryan S, McNicholas M, Eustace SJ. Anatomy for Diagnostic Imaging, 3rd edition. Edinburgh: Saunders, 2010:57.

Butler P, Mitchell AM, Ellis H. Applied Radiological Anatomy. Cambridge: Cambridge University Press, 1999:36.

Case 1.5

A Cisterna magna

B Pontine cistern

C Suprasellar cistern

D Straight sinus

E Quadrigeminal cistern

Midline sagittal MRI of the brain.

The subarachnoid space is deep in several places, particularly around the base of the brain. These spaces are referred to as subarachnoid cisterns and are named according to nearby structures. The cistern magna lies below the cerebellar hemispheres and behind the medulla. The pontine cistern lies between the pons and the clivus. The interpeduncular cistern lies between the temporal lobes and is widest between the cerebral peduncles of the midbrain.

The quadrigeminal cistern lies posterior to the quadrigeminal plate, between the splenium of the corpus callosum and the vermis of the cerebellum. The suprasellar cistern lies above the pituitary fossa. It is continuous posteriorly with the quadrigeminal cistern.

The straight sinus appears as a flow void on this T1-weighted image.

Weir J, Abrahams P. Imaging Atlas of Human Anatomy, 6th edition. Edinburgh: Mosby, 2021:11.

Ryan S, McNicholas M, Eustace SJ. Anatomy for Diagnostic Imaging, 3rd edition. Edinburgh: Saunders, 2010:74.

Case 1.6

A Right central sulcus

B Right precentral gyrus

C Right superior frontal sulcus

D Left postcentral gyrus

E Superior sagittal sinus

Axial MRI through the central sulcus.

The central sulcus (or Rolandic fissure) separates the frontal from the parietal lobe in each hemisphere. It runs in the near coronal plane. Anterior to the central sulcus lies the precentral gyrus which contains the primary motor cortex. Posterior to the central sulcus lies the postcentral gyrus or primary somatosensory cortex.

The superior frontal sulcus runs in the sagittal plane and separates the superior and middle frontal gyri. The posterior end of the superior frontal sulcus forms at right angles with the precentral sulcus. Identifying the precentral sulcus allows us to identify the central sulcus as it is the sulcus immediately posterior to it.

Weir J, Abrahams P. Imaging Atlas of Human Anatomy, 6th edition. Edinburgh: Mosby, 2021:9.

Butler P, Mitchell AM, Ellis H. Applied Radiological Anatomy. Cambridge, United Kingdom: Cambridge University Press, 1999:43.

Case 1.7

A Right putamen

B Head of the right caudate nucleus

C Anterior horn of the right lateral ventricle

D Interhemispheric fissure

E Anterior limb of the left internal capsule

Axial MRI of the brain at the level of the lateral ventricles.

This axial section and the midline sagittal MRI must be studied in detail. They contain key anatomical structures and are always likely to feature in the examination. These structures should be studied in sagittal and coronal images to begin to form a three-dimensional understanding of brain anatomy.

Within the cerebral hemispheres, there lie a number of nuclear masses collectively known as basal ganglia. The major components are the caudate nucleus, the putamen and the globus pallidus. For anatomical purposes, the putamen and globus pallidus are together called lentiform or lenticular nucleus. The putamen lies lateral to the globus pallidus.

The anterior limb of the internal capsule separates the lentiform nucleus from the head of the caudate nucleus.

Weir J, Abrahams P. Imaging Atlas of Human Anatomy, 6th edition. Edinburgh: Mosby, 2021:8–9.

Ryan S, McNicholas M, Eustace SJ. Anatomy for Diagnostic Imaging, 3rd edition. Edinburgh: Saunders, 2010:56.

Case 1.8

A Interhemispheric fissure

B Right insular cortex

C Splenium of corpus callosum

D Left tapetum

E Posterior limb of the internal capsule (right)

Axial MRI of the brain at the level of the lateral ventricles.

The sylvian fissure (or lateral sulcus) separates the frontal from the temporal lobes.

Lateral to the putamen, there is a thin sheet of grey matter known as the claustrum. It is sandwiched between two layers of white matter: the external capsule medially and the extreme capsule laterally. Lateral to the extreme capsule and in the floor of the lateral sulcus, lies the cortex referred to as the insula (of Reil).

The left and right cerebral hemispheres fill the cranial vault above the tentorium cerebelli. They are connected in the midline by the corpus callosum which lies deep in the interhemispheric fissure (median longitudinal fissure). The corpus callosum is a large mass of commissural fibres. The genu is its most anterior part. Fibres extending laterally from the body of the corpus callosum are called the tapetum. They form part of the roof and lateral wall of the lateral ventricle.

Weir J, Abrahams P. Imaging Atlas of Human Anatomy, 6th edition. Edinburgh: Mosby, 2021:8–9.

Ryan S, McNicholas M, Eustace SJ. Anatomy for Diagnostic Imaging, 3rd edition. Edinburgh: Saunders, 2010:56.

Case 1.9

A Right thalamus

B Posterior limb of the internal capsule (right)

C Anterior horn of the right lateral ventricle

D Septum pellucidum

E Choroid plexus (left)

Axial CT of the brain at the level of the basal ganglia.

This axial image is at the same level as the image in the previous case. It is, however, a different modality. T1-weighted MRIs can show the anatomy very clearly but CTs of the brain may be used in the examination. Make sure that you are comfortable with both modalities.

The windowing in this image has been set to optimise the appearance of brain parenchyma. The cortical and deep grey matter appears brighter than the white matter.

The thalamus is separated from the lentiform nucleus by the posterior limb of the internal capsule.

The septum pellucidum is a thin triangular membrane that separates the anterior horn of the lateral ventricles. Anatomical variants are common in this structure and you should be familiar with them.

Weir J, Abrahams P. Imaging Atlas of Human Anatomy, 6th edition. Edinburgh: Mosby, 2021:8–9.

Ryan S, McNicholas M, Eustace SJ. Anatomy for Diagnostic Imaging, 3rd edition. Edinburgh: Saunders, 2010:56.

Case 1.10

A Fourth ventricle

B Right flocculus

C Right middle cerebellar peduncle

D Right cerebellar hemisphere

E Left cerebellopontine angle cistern

Axial MRI at the level of the fourth ventricle.

On axial imaging, the lower pons is dominated by the posterolaterally directed middle cerebellar peduncles. Lateral to these structures lie the cerebellopontine angle cisterns which are limited posteriorly by the flocculi, a pair of small cerebellar lobes.

The fourth ventricle has a 'roof' dorsally and a 'floor' ventrally. The roof is formed by the cerebellum and the floor by the pons and medulla. The lateral walls are formed by the cerebellar peduncles. Study these structures in the midline sagittal images to form a three-dimensional understanding.

Weir J, Abrahams P. Imaging Atlas of Human Anatomy, 6th edition. Edinburgh: Mosby, 2021:7.

Ryan S, McNicholas M, Eustace SJ. Anatomy for Diagnostic Imaging, 3rd edition. Edinburgh: Saunders, 2010:55.

Butler P, Mitchell AM, Ellis H. Applied Radiological Anatomy. Cambridge: Cambridge University Press, 1999:32.

Case 1.11

A Right cingulate gyrus

B Optic chiasm

C Left cavernous internal carotid artery

D Left sylvian fissure

E Sphenoidal sinus

Coronal MRI of the brain.

In this image, we see the internal carotid artery in the cavernous sinus. Note that on T1- and T2-weighted MRI, rapidly flowing blood is displayed as black signal voids. The internal carotid artery is a branch of the common carotid artery and receives 70% of its blood flow. It arises approximately at the level of the C3 vertebral body and enters the skull through the carotid canal. This marks the onset of the petrous segment. It passes through the foramen lacerum where the laceral segment begins.

It is a short segment and it ends at the petrolingual ligament, where the cavernous segment begins. The cavernous segment ends at the proximal dura ring.

The optic chiasm is where the optic nerves partially cross. It lies anterior to the pituitary stalk and superomedially to the cavernous sinuses. The body of the sphenoid bone contains the sphenoidal sinuses which provide a route for surgical access to the pituitary gland via the nose.

By reviewing the coronal images, we can appreciate the sylvian fissure separates the superior surface of the temporal lobe from the anterior surface of the frontal lobe and the anterior surface of the parietal lobe.

Weir J, Abrahams P. Imaging Atlas of Human Anatomy, 6th edition. Edinburgh: Mosby, 2021:13.

Ryan S, McNicholas M, Eustace SJ. Anatomy for Diagnostic Imaging, 3rd edition. Edinburgh: Saunders, 2010:59.

Butler P, Mitchell AM, Ellis H. Applied Radiological Anatomy. Cambridge: Cambridge University Press, 1999:45.

Case 1.12

A Right hippocampus

B Left fornix

C Third ventricle

D Pons

E Left parahippocampal gyrus

Coronal T2-weighted MRI of the brain.

The limbic system is composed of functionally related structures which surround the corpus callosum at the medial surface of the cerebral hemispheres. You may be asked to identify parts of the limbic system such as the cingulate, splenial and parahippocampal gyri, the hippocampus, the dentate gyrus and the fornix. It is worth spending some time studying diagrams of the limbic system and reviewing its appearance on coronal and parasagittal MRIs.

The thalami are bodies of grey matter that lie in the lateral walls of the third ventricle.

Weir J, Abrahams P. Imaging Atlas of Human Anatomy, 6th edition. Edinburgh: Mosby, 2021:13.

Ryan S, McNicholas M, Eustace SJ. Anatomy for Diagnostic Imaging, 3rd edition. Edinburgh: Saunders, 2010:59.

Butler P, Mitchell AM, Ellis H. Applied Radiological Anatomy. Cambridge: Cambridge University Press, 1999:45.

Case 1.13

A Right internal carotid artery (cervical segment)

B Right internal carotid artery (petrous segment)

C Right internal carotid artery (cavernous segment)

D Right middle cerebral artery

E Right anterior cerebral artery

Magnetic resonance angiography – coronal view.

The internal carotid artery arises from the common carotid artery and lies posterolateral to the external carotid artery. No branches arise from the common carotid artery or the cervical segment of the internal carotid artery.

The internal carotid artery enters the skull through the carotid canal. That is where the petrous segment begins. The course here is anteromedial and horizontal as it can be seen in this image. The artery then turns superiorly and enters the cavernous sinus. At this point the cavernous segment begins. Note the siphon shape that the artery assumes in this segment. Emerging from the cavernous sinus the artery divides into its terminal branches: the anterior cerebral artery and the middle cerebral artery.

Weir J, Abrahams P. Imaging Atlas of Human Anatomy, 6th edition. Edinburgh: Mosby, 2021:1–4.

Ryan S, McNicholas M, Eustace SJ. Anatomy for Diagnostic Imaging, 3rd edition. Edinburgh: Saunders, 2010:80–87.

Butler P, Mitchell AM, Ellis H. Applied Radiological Anatomy. Cambridge: Cambridge University Press, 1999:50–57.

Case 1.14

A Right anterior cerebral artery

B Left vertebral artery

C Right middle cerebral artery

D Left internal carotid artery

E Left posterior cerebral artery

Magnetic resonance angiography – axial view.

The circle of Willis lies in the suprasellar cistern. It is formed by links between the internal carotid arteries and the vertebrobasilar system. The single anterior communicating artery links the two anterior cerebral arteries. There are two posterior communicating arteries, one on each side in conventional anatomy, that link the internal carotid artery with the vertebrobasilar system. The circle of Willis is not circular in shape but rather is star-shaped (**Figure 1.1**). It is complete in only a minority of individuals so do not be thrown by a missing branch.

Weir J, Abrahams P. Imaging Atlas of Human Anatomy, 6th edition. Edinburgh: Mosby, 2021:1–4.

Ryan S, McNicholas M, Eustace SJ. Anatomy for Diagnostic Imaging, 3rd edition. Edinburgh: Saunders, 2010:80–87.

Butler P, Mitchell AM, Ellis H. Applied Radiological Anatomy. Cambridge: Cambridge University Press, 1999:50–57.

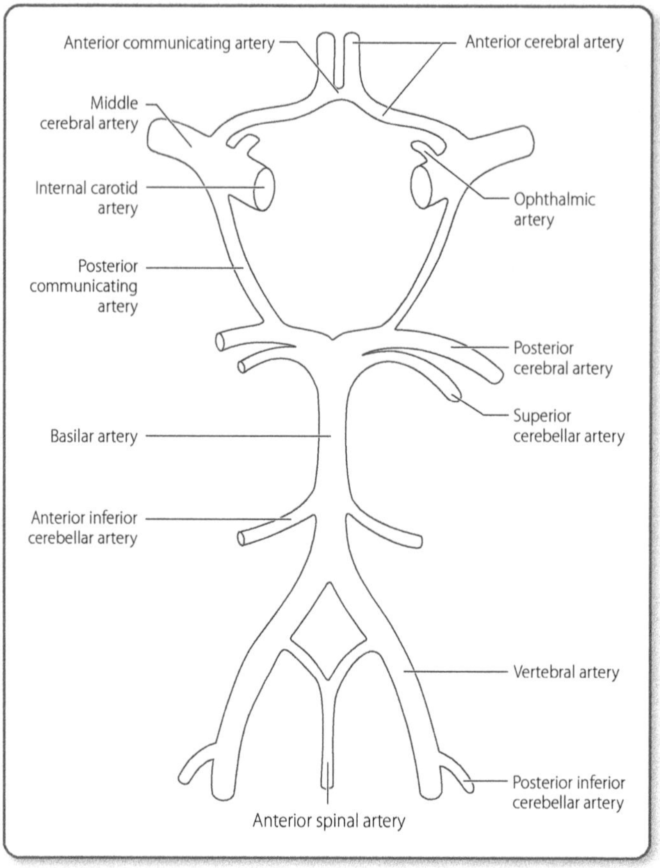

Figure 1.1 The circle of Willis.

Case 1.15

A Basilar artery

B Internal carotid artery

C Posterior cerebral artery

D Posterior communicating artery

E Frontopolar artery

Magnetic resonance angiography – lateral view.

In this image, we see the same vessels as in the previous two images but from the side. On lateral images such as this one and on some catheter angiograms, it is not possible to accurately determine laterality. If that is the case, simply name the vessel rather than guessing the side.

The frontopolar artery is a branch of the anterior cerebral artery that extends to the anterior pole of the brain.

The ophthalmic artery is the first branch of the internal carotid artery distal to the cavernous sinus.

Weir J, Abrahams P. Imaging Atlas of Human Anatomy, 6th edition. Edinburgh: Mosby, 2021:1–4.

Ryan S, McNicholas M, Eustace SJ. Anatomy for Diagnostic Imaging, 3rd edition. Edinburgh: Saunders, 2010:80–87.

Butler P, Mitchell AM, Ellis H. Applied Radiological Anatomy. Cambridge: Cambridge University Press, 1999:50–57.

Case 1.16

A Petrous part of the left internal carotid artery

B Cavernous part of the left internal carotid artery

C Left middle cerebral artery (M1 segment)

D Left anterior cerebral artery (A1 segment)

E Left pericallosal artery (A3 segment)

Catheter angiogram of the carotid artery.

Catheter angiography is used for diagnosis and treatment of vascular problems in the brain. This is an image from an angiogram of the carotid artery.

The internal carotid artery is the biggest vessel and has a characteristic shape. The different segments of the artery are seen in this image, including the terminal branches of the internal carotid artery: the anterior and middle cerebral arteries. The anterior cerebral artery arises from the internal carotid artery at the anterior perforated substance. It is divided into segments:

- A1 is the first segment and it extends from the origin to the level of the anterior communicating artery
- A2 begins after the anterior communicating artery and continues to the bifurcation of the artery into its terminal branches

Two branches are given off in A2:

- The orbital frontal artery is the first branch after the anterior communicating artery
- The frontopolar artery arises distal to the orbital frontal, close to where the artery loops over the genu

After the artery loops over the genu, it passes posteriorly on the superior surface of the corpus callosum. At this point it bifurcates into the callosal marginal and the pericallosal artery (which forms the A3 segment).

Weir J, Abrahams P. Imaging Atlas of Human Anatomy, 6th edition. Edinburgh: Mosby, 2021:1–4.

Ryan S, McNicholas M, Eustace SJ. Anatomy for Diagnostic Imaging, 3rd edition. Edinburgh: Saunders, 2010:80–87.

Butler P, Mitchell AM, Ellis H. Applied Radiological Anatomy. Cambridge: Cambridge University Press, 1999:50–57.

Case 1.17

A Right vertebral artery

B Basilar artery

C Posterior communicating artery

D Posterior cerebral artery

E Superior cerebellar artery

Catheter angiogram of the vertebral artery.

The vertebral arteries are the first branches of the subclavian arteries on each side. They ascend the neck within the foramina transversaria. They pass through the foramen magnum to enter the skull. At that point they pierce the dura and enter the subarachnoid space. The left and right vertebral arteries join to form the basilar artery at the level of the pontomedullary junction. The posterior inferior cerebellar arteries (PICA) arise from the vertebral arteries just before they join. The anterior inferior cerebellar arteries (AICA) and the superior cerebellar arteries arise from the basilar artery.

In this image, we see the right vertebral artery filled with contrast, suggesting it is the vessel which has been catheterised. It then enters the skull and to continue as the basilar artery after joining with the left vertebral artery. Some retrograde filling of the smaller left vertebral artery is also seen. The terminal branches are labelled: the posterior cerebral arteries and the posterior communicating arteries. Just before the basilar artery splits into the terminal branches, it gives off the superior cerebellar artery.

Weir J, Abrahams P. Imaging Atlas of Human Anatomy, 6th edition. Edinburgh: Mosby, 2021:1–4.

Ryan S, McNicholas M, Eustace SJ. Anatomy for Diagnostic Imaging, 3rd edition. Edinburgh: Saunders, 2010:80–87.

Butler P, Mitchell AM, Ellis H. Applied Radiological Anatomy. Cambridge: Cambridge University Press, 1999:50–57.

Case 1.18

A Superior sagittal sinus

B Straight sinus

C Vein of Galen

D Transverse sinus

E Inferior sagittal sinus

Catheter angiogram in venous phase – lateral view.

The venous drainage of the brain (**Figure 1.2**) does not follow the arterial supply. The venous sinuses are low pressure veins within folds of dura. The superior sagittal sinus begins anteriorly and runs to the back in the midline to the internal occipital protuberance. Posteriorly the sinus turns to one dominant side (usually the right) and continues as the transverse sinus.

The internal cerebral veins run in the roof of the third ventricle on each side and unite under the splenium of the corpus callosum, to form the great cerebral vein of Galen. This is a short vein that passes posterosuperiorly behind the splenium to drain in the anterior end of the straight sinus where it unites with the inferior sagittal sinus.

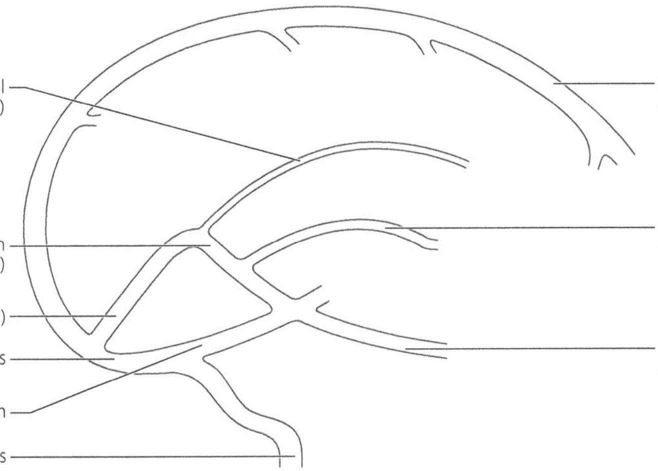

Figure 1.2 Venous drainage of the brain – lateral view.

The basal veins of Rosenthal begin at the anterior perforated substance by the union of the anterior cerebral vein, the deep middle cerebral vein and the striate veins. The basal veins of Rosenthal pass around the midbrain on each side to join the great cerebral vein of Galen (**Figure 1.2**).

Weir J, Abrahams P. Imaging Atlas of Human Anatomy, 6th edition. Edinburgh: Mosby, 2021:5–6.

Ryan S, McNicholas M, Eustace SJ. Anatomy for Diagnostic Imaging, 3rd edition. Edinburgh: Saunders, 2010:87–90.

Butler P, Mitchell AM, Ellis H. Applied Radiological Anatomy. Cambridge: Cambridge University Press, 1999:57–58.

Case 1.19

A Superior sagittal sinus

B Confluence of sinuses (torcular herophili)

C Right transverse sinus

D Right sigmoid sinus

E Right jugular vein

Catheter angiogram in venous phase – anteroposterior view.

The inferior sagittal sinus runs in the lower free edge of the falx cerebri. Posteriorly, it joins the great cerebral vein to become the straight sinus. The straight sinus then runs posteriorly to meet the sagittal sinus at the confluence of sinuses (torcular herophili). The transverse sinuses run on either side to the mastoid bone where they turn inferiorly and become the sigmoid sinuses. There is often asymmetry in the size of the transverse sinuses, with one side being dominant. The transverse and sigmoid sinuses together are known as the lateral sinus. The sigmoid sinus continues through the jugular foramen as the internal jugular vein.

Weir J, Abrahams P. Imaging Atlas of Human Anatomy, 6th edition. Edinburgh: Mosby, 2021:5–6.

Ryan S, McNicholas M, Eustace SJ. Anatomy for Diagnostic Imaging, 3rd edition. Edinburgh: Saunders, 2010:87–90.

Butler P, Mitchell AM, Ellis H. Applied Radiological Anatomy. Cambridge: Cambridge University Press, 1999:57–58.

Case 1.20

A Right superior rectus

B Right optic nerve

C Left superior oblique

D Left medial rectus

E Vomer

Coronal soft tissue CT through the orbits.

Six extrinsic ocular muscles insert into the sclera. The four rectus muscles arise from a common tendinous ring (annulus of Zinn) that surrounds the optic canal and part of the superior orbit fissure. They insert onto the globe anterior to the equator and have the following functions:

- Medial rectus rotates the pupil medially.
- Lateral rectus rotates the pupil laterally.
- Superior rectus rotates the pupil superiorly.
- Inferior rectus rotates the pupil inferiorly.

The superior oblique arises from the sphenoidal bone superomedial to the optic foramen. It passes through the trochlea to insert onto the upper outer surface posterior to the equator, directing the pupil inferiorly and laterally.

The inferior oblique arises from the orbital floor to insert onto the lower outer part posterior to the equator, directing the pupil laterally and superiorly.

The vomer forms the bony part of the nasal septum and separates the choanae.

Weir J, Abrahams P. Imaging Atlas of Human Anatomy, 6th edition. Edinburgh: Mosby, 2021:37.

Ryan S, McNicholas M, Eustace SJ. Anatomy for Diagnostic Imaging, 3rd edition. Edinburgh: Saunders, 2010:27.

Case 1.21

A Frontal sinus

B Hard palate

C Anterior arch of atlas

D Clivus

E Pituitary fossa

Lateral skull radiograph.

The frontal sinuses are often asymmetrical and lie between the inner and outer tables of the frontal bone above the nose and medial orbits. They are lined by mucous-secreting epithelium, and drain through the frontonasal duct into the infundibulum, which opens into the semilunar hiatus of the middle meatus.

The palate forms the floor of the nasal cavities and the roof of the mouth. The hard (bony) palate is concave and formed from the palatine processes of the maxillae and the horizontal plates of the palatine bones.

The pituitary fossa is a depression in the sella turcica of the upper surface of the sphenoid bone in which the pituitary gland sits. The sella turcica is surrounded by the anterior and posterior clinoid processes (clinoid meaning 'bedpost') like the posts of a four poster bed. The posterior part of the sella turcica is the dorsum sellae, which is continuous with the clivus.

Weir J, Abrahams P. Imaging Atlas of Human Anatomy, 6th edition. Edinburgh: Mosby, 2021:23–27.

Ryan S, McNicholas M, Eustace SJ. Anatomy for Diagnostic Imaging, 3rd edition. Edinburgh: Saunders, 2010:4.

Case 1.22

A Sagittal suture

B Right lambdoid suture

C Right frontal sinus

D Left maxillary sinus

E Ramus of right mandible

Occipitofrontal skull projection.

The sagittal suture is in the midline between the two parietal bones. The two parietal bones are joined to the occipital bone by the lambdoid suture, which is often visible on an occipitofrontal projection. The frontal bones join the parietal bones at the coronal suture. The bregma is the junction between the coronal and sagittal sutures, and the lambda is the junction between the lambdoid and sagittal sutures (**Figure 1.3**).

Ryan S, McNicholas M, Eustace SJ. Anatomy for Diagnostic Imaging, 3rd edition. Edinburgh: Saunders, 2010:2–6.

Weir J, Abrahams P. Imaging Atlas of Human Anatomy, 6th edition. Edinburgh: Mosby, 2021:23–27.

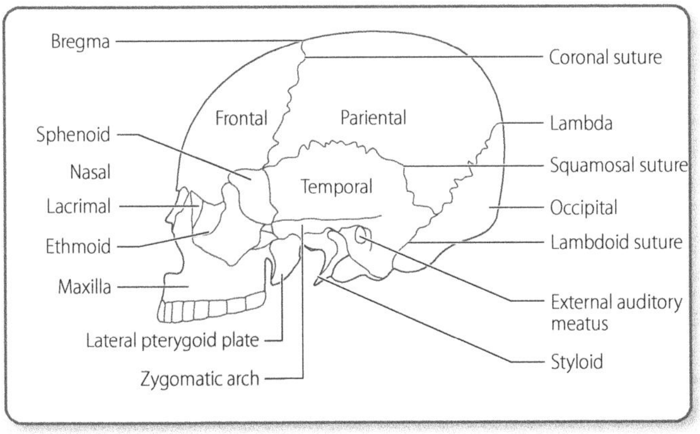

Figure 1.3 The cranial bones and sutures.

Case 1.23

A Right temporomandibular fossa

B Left mandibular notch

C Right angle of mandible

D Right coronoid process

E Right external acoustic meatus

Radiographs of both temporomandibular joints.

These are closed and open mouth plain radiographs of the temporomandibular joints.

On opening the mouth, the mandibular condyle translates anteriorly. The next question explains the temporomandibular joints in more detail.

Case 1.24

A External auditory meatus

B Articular disc

C Condyle of mandible

D Temporal lobe

E Lateral pterygoid muscle

MRI of the temporomandibular joint (TMJ).

The TMJ is a synovial joint, of which the articular surfaces are the articular tubercle of the temporal bone, the mandibular fossa, and the condyle of the mandible (**Figure 1.4**). These articular surfaces are covered in fibrous cartilage.

The joint is separated into superior and inferior compartments (both have a separate synovial membrane) by the fibrocartilaginous disc. Translational movements occur

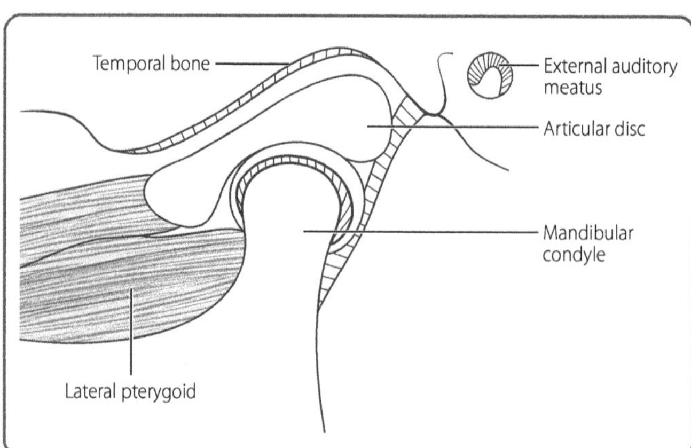

Figure 1.4 The temporomandibular joint.

Table 1.1 The types of mandibular movement at the temporomandibular joint and the muscles that control each one.

Mandibular movement	Muscles involved
Depression (open mouth)	• Suprahyoid • Infrahyoid • Lateral pterygoid
Protrusion	• Lateral pterygoid • Masseter • Medial pterygoid
Elevation (close mouth)	• Temporalis • Masseter • Medial pterygoid
Retrusion	• Temporalis • Masseter
Lateral movement	• Retractors of same • Protrudes of opposite

in the superior compartment, rotational in the inferior compartment. The condyle of the mandible sits in the fossa at rest and slides anteriorly on to the articular tubercle when open.

Muscles producing mandibular movements at the temporomandibular joints are given in **Table 1.1**.

Weir J, Abrahams P. Imaging Atlas of Human Anatomy, 6th edition. Edinburgh: Mosby, 2021:28.

Ryan S, McNicholas M, Eustace SJ. Anatomy for Diagnostic Imaging, 3rd edition. Edinburgh: Saunders, 2010:17–18.

Case 1.25

A Right lower second molar

B Left upper central incisor

C Floor of left maxillary sinus

D Left lower canine

E Hyoid bone

Orthopantomogram (OPG).

An OPG is a panoramic radiograph of the mandible and maxilla in order to image the dentition. It is acquired by rotating a horizontal arm from ear to ear. This means that the central hyoid bone is projected into both edges of the film.

One must not neglect to learn the teeth. OPGs are common examinations.

Case 1.26

A Upper left lateral incisor

B Lower left second premolar

C Lower right second molar

D Lower right third molar (wisdom tooth)

E Lower right canine

Orthopantomogram (OPG).

There are 20 deciduous or milk teeth which usually begin erupting by 6 months of age. The symphysis menti fuses at 2 years of age. The permanent teeth develop in the maxilla and mandible during childhood, and are calcified by 3 years of age.

As the permanent teeth erupt, the roots of the deciduous teeth are resorbed. The medial teeth begin erupting before the lateral teeth, and the lower before the upper. The permanent teeth are present by 12–13 years of age, except the wisdom teeth (third molars) which erupt in early adulthood.

There are 20 deciduous teeth, and 32 permanent teeth. In each quadrant:

- Child: Two incisors, one canine, two molars.
- Adult: Two incisors, one canine, two premolars, three molars.

Supernumerary teeth can be seen on an OPG, and they characteristically occur lateral to the last tooth in each series.

At the centre of each tooth sits the radiolucent highly vascular pulp tissue, which is surrounded by a layer of dentine. Dentine comprises an organic and calcified structure, arranged in porous tubules, and has a radiographic density similar to compact bone. The exposed intraoral portion of each tooth (the crown) has an outer layer of enamel which comprises calcium hydroxyapatite crystals. This is densely radio-opaque. At the cementoenamel junction, which sits at the level of the alveolar ridge, the tooth is no longer covered with enamel, but with cementum. This cementum provides the surround to the root system.

The root and neck of the tooth are surrounded by the radiolucent periodontal membrane. The lamina dura is a dense line of bone which surrounds this and each root, and is continuous with the lamina dura of adjacent teeth (**Figures 1.5** and **1.6**).

Ryan S, McNicholas M, Eustace SJ. Anatomy for Diagnostic Imaging, 3rd edition. Edinburgh: Saunders, 2010:19.

Weir J, Abrahams P. Imaging Atlas of Human Anatomy, 6th edition. Edinburgh: Mosby, 2021:50.

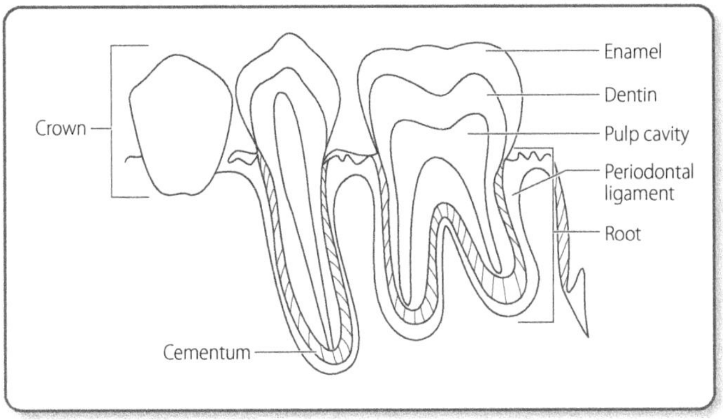

Figure 1.5 The anatomy of the tooth.

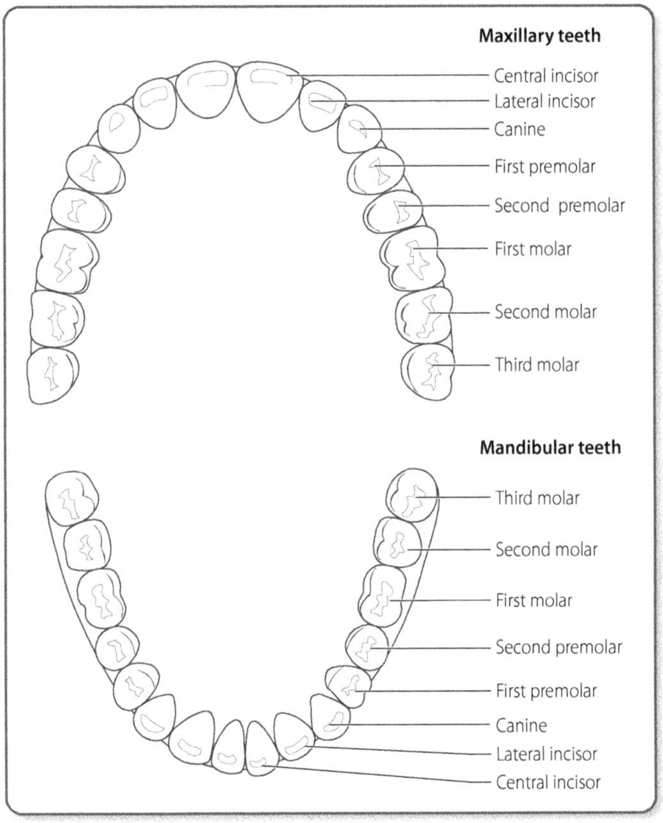

Figure 1.6 The distribution of adult teeth.

Case 1.27

A Right zygomaticofrontal suture

B Frontal process of right zygoma

C Left lamina papyracea

D Nasal septum

E Left zygomatic arch

Occipitofrontal projection of facial bones.

The zygomatic/malar bone forms the prominence of the cheek, and articulates with the frontal, maxillary and temporal bones at the zygomaticofrontal, zygomaticomaxillary and zygomaticotemporal sutures respectively. It forms the boundary of the temporal fossa superiorly and the infratemporal fossa inferiorly.

The medial orbit of the wall is formed mainly from ethmoid bone, with contributions from maxillary, lacrimal and sphenoid bones. The paper-thin bone separating the orbit from the ethmoid air cells is the lamina papyracea.

The nasal septum is part bony and part cartilaginous and divides the nasal cavity in two in the sagittal plane. The main contributors are:

- Perpendicular plate of ethmoid – descends from the cribriform plate to form the superior part of the septum
- Vomer – is thin and flat, and forms the posterior and inferior septum
- Septal cartilage – joins with the bony septum.

Weir J, Abrahams P. Imaging Atlas of Human Anatomy, 6th edition. Edinburgh: Mosby, 2021:23–27.

Ryan S, McNicholas M, Eustace SJ. Anatomy for Diagnostic Imaging, 3rd edition. Edinburgh: Saunders, 2010:12.

Case 1.28

A Right infraorbital foramen

B Left lamina papyracea

C Lateral wall of right maxillary sinus

D Right frontal sinus

E Left maxillary sinus

Radiograph of the orbits.

The maxillary sinuses, or antra, are the largest paranasal sinuses. They are pyramidal in shape and are situated in the bodies of the maxillae.

- The zygomatic bone forms the apex.
- The lateral wall of the nasal cavity forms the base/medial wall of maxillary sinus. This is continued superiorly as a bony projection called the uncinate process.

- The floor of the orbit forms the roof.
- The alveolar part of the maxilla forms the floor. There are often elevations on the floor of the maxillary sinus formed from the roots of the maxillary teeth below.

The superior alveolar branches of the maxillary artery supply the majority of the maxillary sinus, with the greatest palatine artery supplying the floor. The anterior, middle and posterior superior alveolar nerves – branches of the maxillary nerve – innervate the maxillary sinus.

The infraorbital foramen transmits the terminal branch of the maxillary (cranial nerve V2): the infraorbital nerve. This supplies the skin of the cheek, lower eye lid, lateral side of nose, inferior septum and upper lip, upper premolars, incisors and canines, and the mucosa of the upper lip and maxillary sinus.

Weir J, Abrahams P. Imaging Atlas of Human Anatomy, 6th edition. Edinburgh: Mosby, 2021:23–27.

Ryan S, McNicholas M, Eustace SJ. Anatomy for Diagnostic Imaging, 3rd edition. Edinburgh: Saunders, 2010:15.

Case 1.29

A Right foramen rotundum

B Left superior orbital fissure

C Right greater wing of sphenoid

D Right body of sphenoid

E Left ethmoidal air cells

Detail of occipitofrontal projection.

The sphenoid bone forms part of the middle cranial fossa and contributes to the bony orbit. It consists of a body, greater and lesser wings and pterygoid processes. The wings spread laterally, and the pterygoid processes (lateral and medial pterygoid plates) project inferiorly. The body contains the sphenoid sinuses.

The superior orbital fissure is adjacent to the optic foramen medially. It is a slit between the greater and lesser wings of sphenoid. It transmits V1, III, IV and VI cranial nerves, superior ophthalmic veins, and a branch of the middle meningeal artery. The ophthalmic artery may communicate with the middle meningeal, therefore forming an anastomotic connection between the internal and external carotid systems.

The foramen rotundum is often visible on facial plain films. It is in the greater wing of sphenoid, posterior to the superior orbital fissure. It travels from the middle cranial fossa to the pterygopalatine fossa and transmits the maxillary (V2) nerve (**Figure 1.7**).

Weir J, Abrahams P. Imaging Atlas of Human Anatomy, 6th edition. Edinburgh: Mosby, 2021:23–27.

Ryan S, McNicholas M, Eustace SJ. Anatomy for Diagnostic Imaging, 3rd edition. Edinburgh: Saunders, 2010:5.

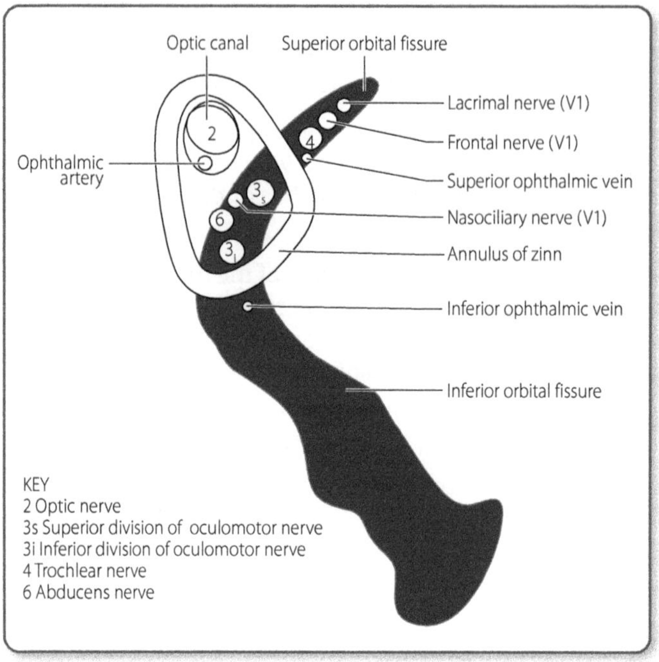

Figure 1.7 The structures of the superior orbital fissure.

Case 1.30

A Parotid (Stensen's) duct

B Epiglottis

C Secondary ductules

D Hyoid

E Body of C4 vertebra

Parotid sialogram.

In this investigation, the parotid duct is cannulated and radio-opaque contrast injected to outline the ductal system. The parotid is the largest of the three salivary glands. It is irregularly shaped as it occupies the space between the ramus of the mandible and the styloid process of the temporal bone. There is a large superficial part and a smaller deeper part, which are continuous around the ramus of the mandible via the isthmus.

The parotid (Stenson's) duct arches over the masseter muscle before turning medially to pierce the buccinator muscle where it drains into the mouth opposite the second upper molar tooth.

The serous secretions have digestive functions and wash particles of food into the oral cavity. The gland is supplied by branches from the external carotid (which travels through the isthmus) and superficial temporal arteries, and is drained by the retromandibular veins. The facial nerve exits the stylomastoid foramen, runs through the deep parotid and into the superficial parotid where it lies superficial to the external carotid. Here, it divides into its five terminal branches.

Weir J, Abrahams P. Imaging Atlas of Human Anatomy, 6th edition. Edinburgh: Mosby, 2021:51.

Ryan S, McNicholas M, Eustace SJ. Anatomy for Diagnostic Imaging, 3rd edition. Edinburgh: Saunders, 2010:22.

Case 1.31

A Right superior canaliculus

B Right inferior canaliculus

C Right lacrimal sac

D Right nasolacrimal duct

E Right mastoid air cells

A macrodacryocystogram.

The canaliculi are injected with radio-opaque contrast media to outline the drainage and ducts of the lacrimal apparatus.

The lacrimal gland lies in the superolateral aspect of the orbit in its own fossa. It lies lateral to levator palpebrae superioris which grooves it, dividing it into superior and inferior parts.

The gland secretes tears, which collect in the lacrimal lake at the medial angle of the eye. The tears drain through lacrimal puncta, and into superior and inferior lacrimal canaliculi. The canaliculi drain into the lacrimal sac, and from here into the nasolacrimal duct, which runs in a bony canal to the inferior meatus of the nasal cavity. The valve of Hasner is a mucosal fold at the distal end which prevents reflux into the duct (**Figure 1.8**).

Weir J, Abrahams P. Imaging Atlas of Human Anatomy, 6th edition. Edinburgh: Mosby, 2021:40.

Ryan S, McNicholas M, Eustace SJ. Anatomy for Diagnostic Imaging, 3rd edition. Edinburgh: Saunders, 2010:28.

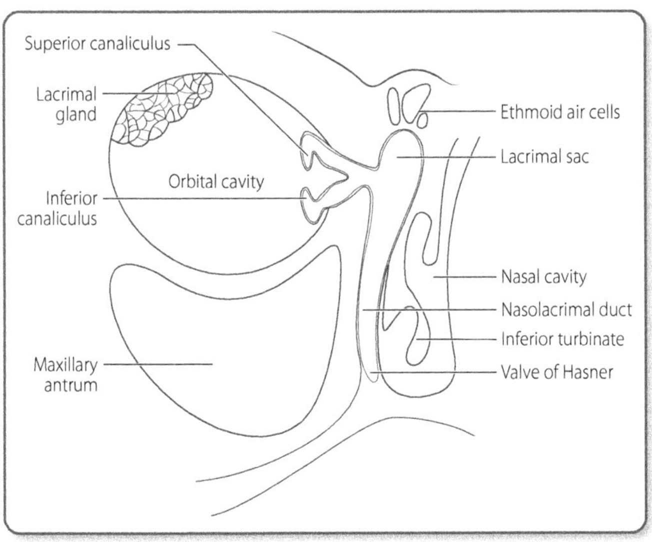

Figure 1.8 The lacrimal apparatus.

Case 1.32

A Incisive canal

B Right alveolar rim

C Right ramus of mandible

D Left medial pterygoid muscle

E Left masseter muscle

Axial CT of facial bones.

The incisive canals transmit the descending palatine artery and the nasopalatine nerve.

The lateral pterygoid muscle originates from the most lateral aspect of the lateral pterygoid plate. It inserts onto the neck of the mandible and disc of the temporomandibular joint where its main action is to protrude the jaw forward.

The medial pterygoid muscle originates from the most medial aspect of the lateral pterygoid plate to insert onto the ramus of the mandible. Its main action is to elevate the mandible.

The masseter muscle originates the zygomatic process of the maxilla and the zygomatic arch to insert onto the coronoid process and ramus of mandible. Its action is to elevate the mandible and occlude the teeth for chewing and biting (**Table 1.1**). Gravity also has a role in the depression (i.e. opening) of the mandible and protrusion occurs as a direct consequence of the opening of the mandible.

Weir J, Abrahams P. Imaging Atlas of Human Anatomy, 6th edition. Edinburgh: Mosby, 2021:29–31.

Case 1.33

A Vomer

B Right infratemporal fossa

C Left medial pterygoid plate

D Right styloid process

E Right lateral pterygoid muscle

Axial CT of nares.

The infratemporal fossa is a space posterior to the maxilla, deep to the ramus of the mandible, and deep and inferior to the zygomatic arch. It contains the lateral and medial pterygoid muscles, the inferior part of the temporal muscle, the maxillary artery and the pterygoid venous plexus. It contains many nerves: mandibular, inferior alveolar, lingual, buccal and chorda tympani, as well as the otic ganglion.

The temporal styloid process is a projection from the inferior aspect of the temporal bone. It serves as an anchor point for many of the muscles of the tongue and larynx.

Weir J, Abrahams P. Imaging Atlas of Human Anatomy, 6th edition. Edinburgh: Mosby, 2021:29–31.

Ryan S, McNicholas M, Eustace SJ. Anatomy for Diagnostic Imaging, 3rd edition. Edinburgh: Saunders, 2010:34.

Case 1.34

A Ostium of left maxillary antrum

B Right pterygopalatine fossa

C Left sphenopalatine foramen

D Right nasolacrimal duct

E Right middle turbinate (concha)

Axial CT of base of skull.

The maxillary antrum drains into the middle meatus of the nasal cavity via the maxillary ostium. The nasolacrimal duct conveys tears from the lacrimal apparatus into the inferior meatus of the nasal cavity.

The middle cranial fossa communicates with the pterygopalatine fossa via the foramen rotundum, which opens into it superiorly. The pterygopalatine fossa contains the V2 cranial nerve which enters the orbit through the inferior orbital fissure. It also contains the maxillary artery, the maxillary nerve, the nerve of the pterygoid canal and the pterygopalatine ganglion.

The sphenopalatine foramen is a communication between the pterygopalatine fossa and the nasal cavity through the perpendicular plate of the palatine bone.

Weir J, Abrahams P. Imaging Atlas of Human Anatomy, 6th edition. Edinburgh: Mosby, 2021:29–34.

Ryan S, McNicholas M, Eustace SJ. Anatomy for Diagnostic Imaging, 3rd edition. Edinburgh: Saunders, 2010:35.

Case 1.35

A Nasal bone

B Perpendicular plate of ethmoid bone

C Left superior orbital fissure

D Right posterior ethmoid air cell

E Right medial rectus

Axial CT at level of ethmoid sinus.

The perpendicular plate of the ethmoid bone descends from the cribriform plate to form the superior part of the bony nasal septum. Above the cribriform plate, it continues as the crista galli.

The ethmoid air cells sit between the lateral walls of the nasal cavity and the medial walls of the orbits. Haller cells are infraorbital extensions of ethmoid air cells. Agger nasi cells are enlarged air cells located anteriorly towards the frontal bones.

Weir J, Abrahams P. Imaging Atlas of Human Anatomy, 6th edition. Edinburgh: Mosby, 2021:29–34.

Ryan S, McNicholas M, Eustace SJ. Anatomy for Diagnostic Imaging, 3rd edition. Edinburgh: Saunders, 2010:36.

Case 1.36

A Crista galli

B Left frontozygomatic suture

C Right frontal bone

D Left lamina papyracea

E Cribriform plate

Coronal CT of the paranasal sinuses.

The cribriform plate of the ethmoid is 'sieve-like' to allow the olfactory nerves to access the nasal cavity from the olfactory bulbs of the brain. The crista galli is the superior continuation of the perpendicular plate of ethmoid above the cribriform plate.

The frontozygomatic suture is the suture between the frontal and zygomatic bones.

Weir J, Abrahams P. Imaging Atlas of Human Anatomy, 6th edition. Edinburgh: Mosby, 2021:29–34.

Moore KL, Dalley AF, Agur AMR. Clinically Oriented Anatomy, 6th edition. Philadelphia: Lippincott Williams & Wilkins, 2009:868.

Case 1.37

A Right maxillary sinus

B Hard palate

C Ethmoid air cell

D Left middle turbinate (concha)

E Left inferior turbinate (concha)

Coronal CT of the paranasal sinuses.

The superior, middle and inferior nasal turbinates (conchae) divide the nasal cavity into four passages:

1. Sphenoethmoidal recess into which the sphenoidal sinus drains
2. Superior meatus into which the posterior ethmoidal air cells drain
3. Middle meatus, where the frontal sinus drains into the anterior opening; the anterior ethmoid air cells and maxillary sinus drain into the middle meatus at the hiatus semilunaris, below the ethmoid bulla
4. Inferior meatus into which the nasolacrimal duct drains tears from the lacrimal sac.

The greater palatine, superior labial branch of the facial and ethmoidal branches of the ophthalmic artery supply the nasal cavity. Little's area is a vascular area of mucosa prone to epistaxis in the anterior and inferior septum.

Weir J, Abrahams P. Imaging Atlas of Human Anatomy, 6th edition. Edinburgh: Mosby, 2021:29–34.

Ryan S, McNicholas M, Eustace SJ. Anatomy for Diagnostic Imaging, 3rd edition. Edinburgh: Saunders, 2010:28.

Case 1.38

A Left anterior clinoid process

B Planum sphenoidale

C Right infratemporal fossa

D Left greater wing of sphenoid

E Right sphenoidal sinus

Coronal CT at the level of the sphenoid sinus.

The clinoid processes are the bony prominences surrounding the sella turcica. The planum sphenoidale forms the roof of the sphenoid sinus.

The sphenoid sinuses are in the body of the sphenoid and are separated by a bony septum. They may extend into the wings of the sphenoid. The sella turcica and optic chiasm are superior. The cavernous sinus runs adjacent to the lateral walls of the sphenoid sinuses; the roof of the nasopharynx is formed by its floor.

Weir J, Abrahams P. Imaging Atlas of Human Anatomy, 6th edition. Edinburgh: Mosby, 2021:29–34.

Ryan S, McNicholas M, Eustace SJ. Anatomy for Diagnostic Imaging, 3rd edition. Edinburgh: Saunders, 2010:28.

Case 1.39

A Right common carotid artery

B Right sternocleidomastoid

C Right strap muscle

D Thyroid isthmus

E Left lobe of thyroid

Transverse ultrasound section of the thyroid gland.

The thyroid gland is derived from the first and second pharyngeal pouches and lies deep to the sternohyoid and sternothyroid muscles. The central isthmus lies anterior to the trachea and joins the two lateral lobes. On ultrasound, the strap muscles and sternomastoid muscle are usually visible anteriorly, along with the common carotid artery and internal jugular vein running adjacent to it in the carotid sheath (**Figure 1.9**).

Weir J, Abrahams P. Imaging Atlas of Human Anatomy, 6th edition. Edinburgh: Mosby, 2021:45.

Ryan S, McNicholas M, Eustace SJ. Anatomy for Diagnostic Imaging, 3rd edition. Edinburgh: Saunders, 2010:42.

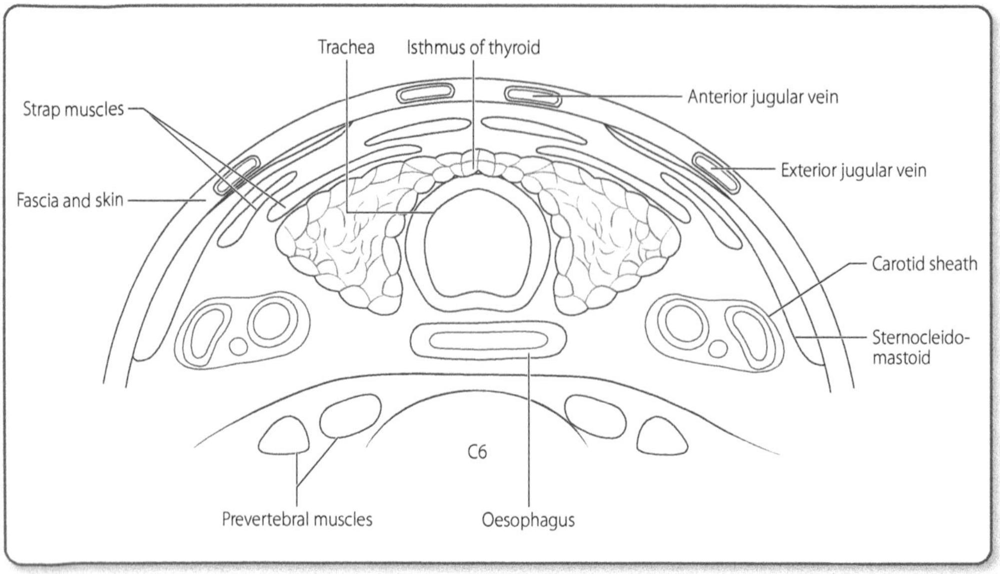

Figure 1.9 The thyroid and its associated structures.

Case 1.40

A Left external carotid artery

B Left internal maxillary artery

C Left facial artery

D Left occipital artery

E Left superficial temporal artery

External carotid angiogram.

The common carotids bifurcate into the internal and external carotids at the level of C4. The internal carotids have no branches in the neck. The external carotid arteries supply much of the face and neck. They travel posterior and superiorly in the neck, through the substance of the parotid gland, before terminating into the maxillary and superficial temporal arteries. The other branches are the ascending pharyngeal, superior thyroid, lingual, facial, occipital and posterior auricular arteries (**Figure 1.10**).

Weir J, Abrahams P. Imaging Atlas of Human Anatomy, 6th edition. Edinburgh: Mosby, 2021:1–6.

Ryan S, McNicholas M, Eustace SJ. Anatomy for Diagnostic Imaging, 3rd edition. Edinburgh: Saunders, 2010:44.

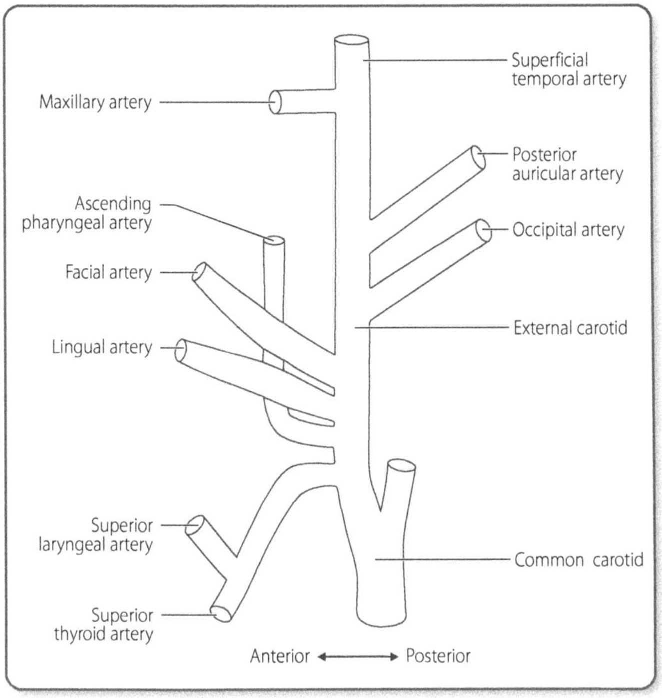

Figure 1.10 The external carotid artery and its branches.

Case 1.41

A Odontoid peg

B Right inferior facet of atlas

C Left occipital condyle

D Left petro-occipital suture

E Pinna of right ear

Coronal CT section of the bones of the neck.

The cervical vertebrae have the foramen transversarium which transmit the vertebral arteries. The C1 vertebral body, the atlas (atlas, in Greek mythology, supported the weight of the earth on his shoulders) supports the weight of the skull. The occipital condyles of the foramen magnum rest on the superior articular facets of C1 to transmit the weight of the skull to the vertebral column. The atlas has anterior and posterior arches, and not a spinous process or body. The body is fused with that of the axis to become the odontoid process.

The C2 vertebral body, the axis, has two large superior articular facets which allow the atlas to rotate on it. The dens, or odontoid process, projects superiorly from the body, and acts as the pivot around which the axis rotates.

Weir J, Abrahams P. Imaging Atlas of Human Anatomy, 6th edition. Edinburgh: Mosby, 2021:42–45.

Ryan S, McNicholas M, Eustace SJ. Anatomy for Diagnostic Imaging, 3rd edition. Edinburgh: Saunders, 2010:91–92.

Case 1.42

A Left masseter

B Left medial pterygoid

C Right parotid gland

D Right semispinalis capitis

E Left sternocleidomastoid

Axial CT of soft tissues of the neck.

Sternocleidomastoid has two heads originating from the mastoid process of the temporal bone and the superior nuchal line of the occipital bone. The sternal head attaches to the manubriosternum, and the clavicular head attaches to the medial third of the clavicle. Acting together, they flex the neck. Acting individually, they rotate the head and neck. The two heads of the sternocleidomastoid divide the neck into the anterior and posterior triangles (**Table 1.2**).

The transversospinal muscle group is one of the deep or intrinsic layers of back muscles, along with splenius and erector spinae muscles. Semispinalis is the most superficial of the transversospinal group, with the semispinalis capitis having the most superior attachment. It travels from the occipital bone to the cervical and transverse processes. It aids in maintaining posture and controlling movements of the vertebral column.

Weir J, Abrahams P. Imaging Atlas of Human Anatomy, 6th edition. Edinburgh: Mosby, 2021:42–45.

Ryan S, McNicholas M, Eustace SJ. Anatomy for Diagnostic Imaging, 3rd edition. Edinburgh: Saunders,2010:22.

Table 1.2 The muscles of the neck

Muscle type	Muscles
Lateral	• Platysma • Sternocleidomastoid • Trapezius
Suprahyoid	• Mylohyoid • Geniohyoid • Stylohyoid • Digastric
Infrahyoid	• Sternohyoid • Omohyoid • Sternothyroid • Thyrohyoid

Case 1.43

A Right malleus

B Right incus

C Right vestibule

D Right internal auditory meatus

E Left mastoid air cells

High-resolution axial CT of the temporal bone.

The ear has two functions: hearing and equilibrium. The function of the external ear is to collect and conduct sound to the tympanic membrane.

The tympanic membrane is the border between the external and middle ear. The middle ear is a cavity in the petrous temporal bone, consisting of the tympanic cavity just internal to the tympanic membrane, and an epitympanic recess/attic just superior to the membrane. The tympanic membrane is attached to the external auditory canal by a small spur of bone called the scutum.

Weir J, Abrahams P. Imaging Atlas of Human Anatomy, 6th edition. Edinburgh: Mosby, 2021:35–36.

Ryan S, McNicholas M, Eustace SJ. Anatomy for Diagnostic Imaging, 3rd edition. Edinburgh: Saunders, 2010:28–32.

Case 1.44

A Left Eustachian tube

B Left oval window

C Right aditus ad antrum

D Right epitympanic recess/attic

E Right petrous temporal bone

High-resolution axial CT of the temporal bone.

The tegmen tympani is a thin plate of bone forming the roof of the tympanic cavity and separating it from the middle cranial fossa and temporal lobe. A narrow posterior opening in the attic, the aditus to the mastoid antrum, communicates with the mastoid air cells, therefore acting as a route for the spread of infection.

The floor of the cavity is a thin plate of bone separating it from the bulb of the jugular vein, and is continuous with the Eustachian tube, which runs into the lateral wall of the nasopharynx.

The medial wall is the lateral wall of the inner ear. There are prominences from the lateral semicircular canal (the arcuate eminence), and the initial/basal turn of the cochlea (the promontory).

Weir J, Abrahams P. Imaging Atlas of Human Anatomy, 6th edition. Edinburgh: Mosby, 2021:35–36.

Ryan S, McNicholas M, Eustace SJ. Anatomy for Diagnostic Imaging, 3rd edition. Edinburgh: Saunders, 2010:28–32.

Case 1.45

A Right cochlea

B Left malleus

C Left incus

D Right carotid canal

E Left hypotympanum

High-resolution CT (coronal reformat) of the temporal bone.

There are three ossicles which transmit vibrations from the tympanic membrane to the oval window. The malleus is attached to the tympanic membrane and articulates with the incus at the incudomalleolar joint. The incus articulates with the stapes, which is attached to the oval window. The round window is inferior and allows pressure equalisation within the vestibule.

Tensor tympani, supplied by the mandibular nerve, inserts onto the malleus to tense the tympanic membrane in the presence of loud sounds.

The inner ear lies medial to the middle ear (**Figure 1.11**). The bony labyrinth consists of a vestibule, which is a communication between the anterior cochlea, and the posterior semicircular canals. The vestibular duct opens into the posterior fossa.

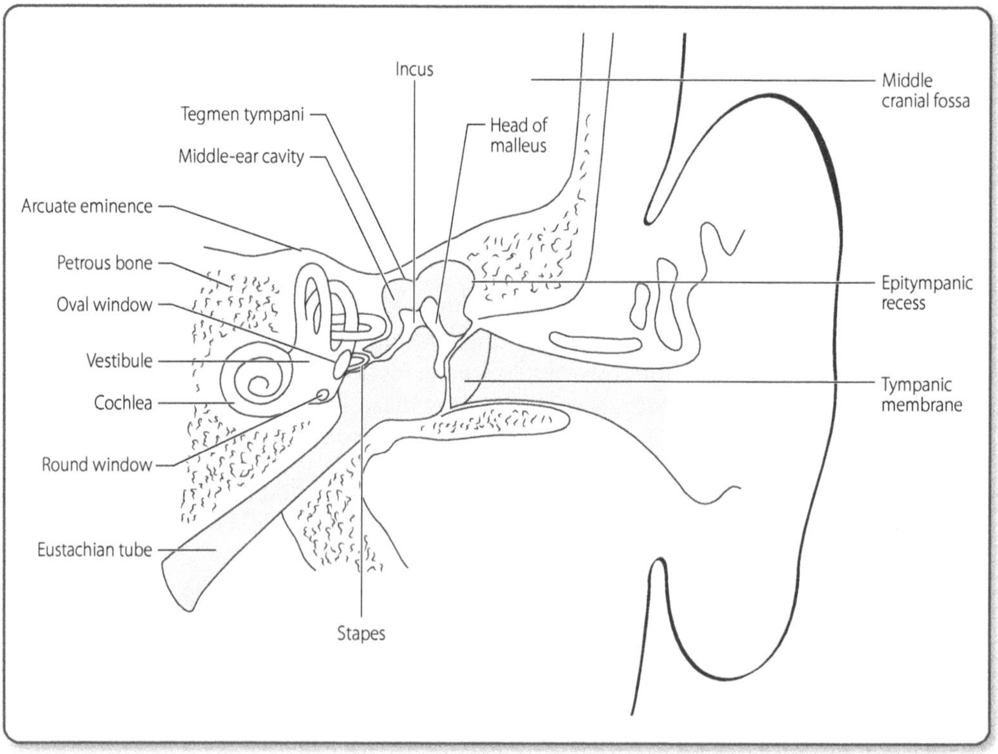

Figure 1.11 The inner ear.

The cochlea is spiral, consisting of 2.5–2.75 turns, and is the hearing apparatus. The cochlear duct passes parallel to the internal auditory meatus to open in the posterior fossa.

The three semicircular canals (anterior, posterior and lateral) are the balance apparatus.

The internal auditory meatus transmits the facial (anteriorly) and vestibulocochlear nerves (posteriorly) from the posterior fossa.

Weir J, Abrahams P. Imaging Atlas of Human Anatomy, 6th edition. Edinburgh: Mosby, 2021:35–36.

Ryan S, McNicholas M, Eustace SJ. Anatomy for Diagnostic Imaging, 3rd edition. Edinburgh: Saunders, 2010:28–32.

Case 1.46

A Left lobe of the thyroid

B Right internal jugular vein

C Oesophagus

D Left prevertebral muscles

E Right sternocleidomastoid

Soft-tissue axial CT through the neck at the level of the thyroid.

The thyroid is relatively high-attenuating on CT due to its high iodine content. The sternocleidomastoid is seen as a large muscular structure anteriorly. The internal jugular vein is posterior to the thyroid, and wider and more irregular than the most medial common carotid artery. The oesophagus is usually collapsed behind the trachea. The prevertebral muscles lie in the floor of the anterior and posterior triangles of the neck. They lie deep to the prevertebral fascia, and anterior to the vertebral bodies. They can be split into anterior and lateral groups (**Table 1.3**).

Weir J, Abrahams P. Imaging Atlas of Human Anatomy, 6th edition. Edinburgh: Mosby, 2021:42–44.

Ryan S, McNicholas M, Eustace SJ. Anatomy for Diagnostic Imaging, 3rd edition. Edinburgh: Saunders, 2010:42–43.

Table 1.3 The prevertebral muscles

Muscle type	Muscles
Anterior	• Longus colli • Longus capitis • Rectus capitis • Rectus capitis lateralis
Lateral	• Splenius capitis • Levator scapulae • Posterior scalene • Middle scalene • Anterior scalene

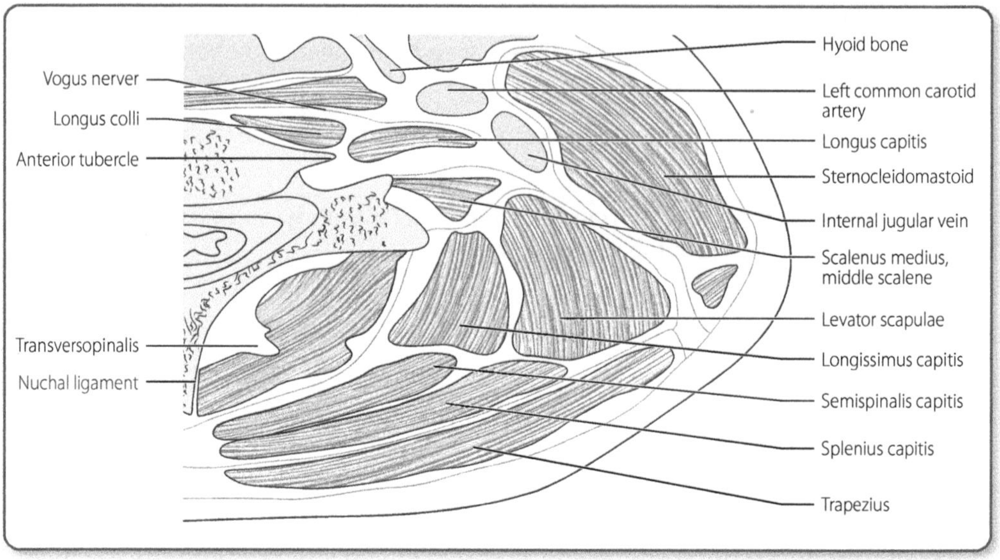

Figure 1.12 The deep muscles of the neck.

Case 1.47

A Right sternocleidomastoid muscle

B Left ramus of the mandible

C Left inferior oblique muscle

D Right splenius capitis

E Left semispinalis

Axial T1-weighted MRI at the level of the pharynx.

The orientation of the deep muscles of the neck is complex and best described diagrammatically (**Figure 1.12**).

Weir J, Abrahams P. Imaging Atlas of Human Anatomy, 6th edition. Edinburgh: Mosby, 2021:46–48.

Case 1.48

A Uvula

B Right medial pterygoid

C Left lateral pterygoid

D Right submandibular gland

E Palatal constrictor muscles

Coronal MRI of the neck.

The uvula is a soft-tissue projection from the middle of the soft palate. It aids in articulation of speech, particularly in guttural, uvular consonant and clicking sounds not found in English. The palatal constrictor muscles (palatoglossus and palatopharyngeus) run from the base of the uvula to the tongue and pharynx. They form the anterior and posterior fauces, between which the palatine tonsils sit.

The submandibular gland sits in the submandibular or digastric triangle, which is a space between the inferior border of the mandible and the anterior and posterior bellies of the digastric muscle. The submandibular (Wharton's) duct opens in the floor of the mouth adjacent to the frenulum of the tongue.

Weir J, Abrahams P. Imaging Atlas of Human Anatomy, 6th edition. Edinburgh: Mosby, 2021:35–36.

Ryan S, McNicholas M, Eustace SJ. Anatomy for Diagnostic Imaging, 3rd edition. Edinburgh: Saunders, 2010:17, 41.

Case 1.49

A Sphenoid sinus

B Intrinsic muscle of tongue

C Soft palate

D Hard palate

E Mandible

Midline sagittal T2-weighted MRI of the head and neck.

The nasopharynx is the space between the posterior choanae and the soft palate. It communicates with the oropharynx and the nasal cavity.

Weir J, Abrahams P. Imaging Atlas of Human Anatomy, 6th edition. Edinburgh: Mosby, 2021:35–36.

Ryan S, McNicholas M, Eustace SJ. Anatomy for Diagnostic Imaging, 3rd edition. Edinburgh: Saunders, 2010:33.

Case 1.50

A Nasopharynx

B Genioglossus

C Epiglottis

D Intrinsic muscle

E Mylohyoid

Midline sagittal MRI of the head and neck.

The muscles of the tongue work synergistically in order to perform movement. The tongue is formed from two groups of muscles which are split down the middle by the fibrous lingual septum. Extrinsic muscles alter the position of the tongue; they originate outside the tongue and attach to it. They are the:

- Genioglossus
- Hyoglossus
- Styloglossus
- Palatoglossus

Intrinsic muscles alter the shape of the tongue; they are confined to the tongue.

The tongue is also supported by the muscles of the floor of the mouth (**Figures 1.13** and **1.14**):

- Mylohyoid forms the floor of the mouth. A muscular sling from the mylohyoid line on the inner aspect of the mandible to the hyoid bone.
- Geniohyoid, superior to mylohyoid, reinforces the floor of the mouth.
- Digastricus has two bellies. The anterior runs from the mastoid process to the hyoid bone. The posterior from the anterior mandible to the hyoid bone.
- Stylohyoid runs parallel and lateral to the poster digastric, from the styloid process to the hyoid bone.

The epiglottis is attached to the posterior aspect of the thyroid cartilage and protects the larynx by directing swallowed matter laterally into the piriform fossa.

Weir J, Abrahams P. Imaging Atlas of Human Anatomy, 6th edition. Edinburgh: Mosby, 2021:44–45.

Ryan S, McNicholas M, Eustace SJ. Anatomy for Diagnostic Imaging, 3rd edition. Edinburgh: Saunders, 2010:33.

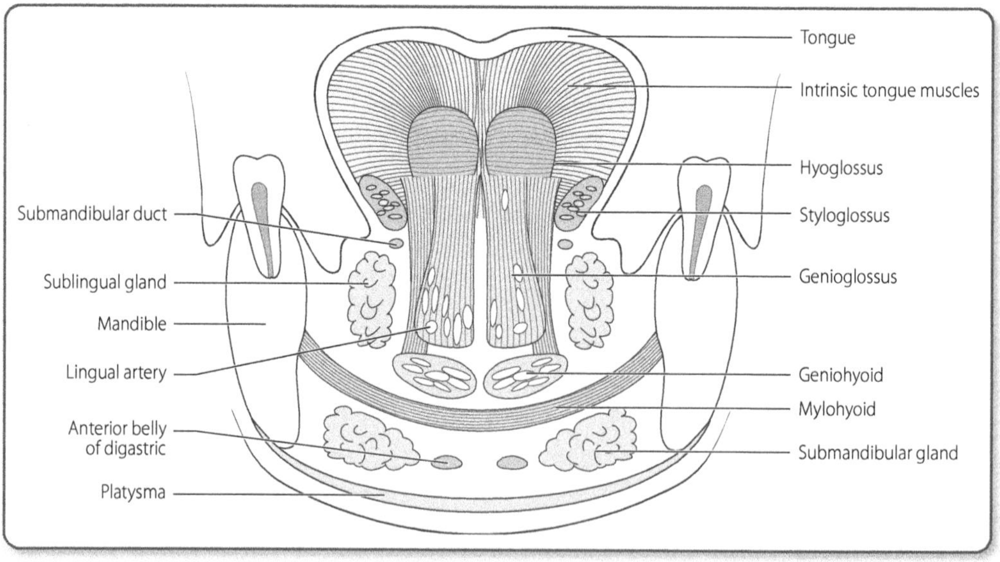

Figure 1.13 Coronal anatomy of the tongue and floor of mouth.

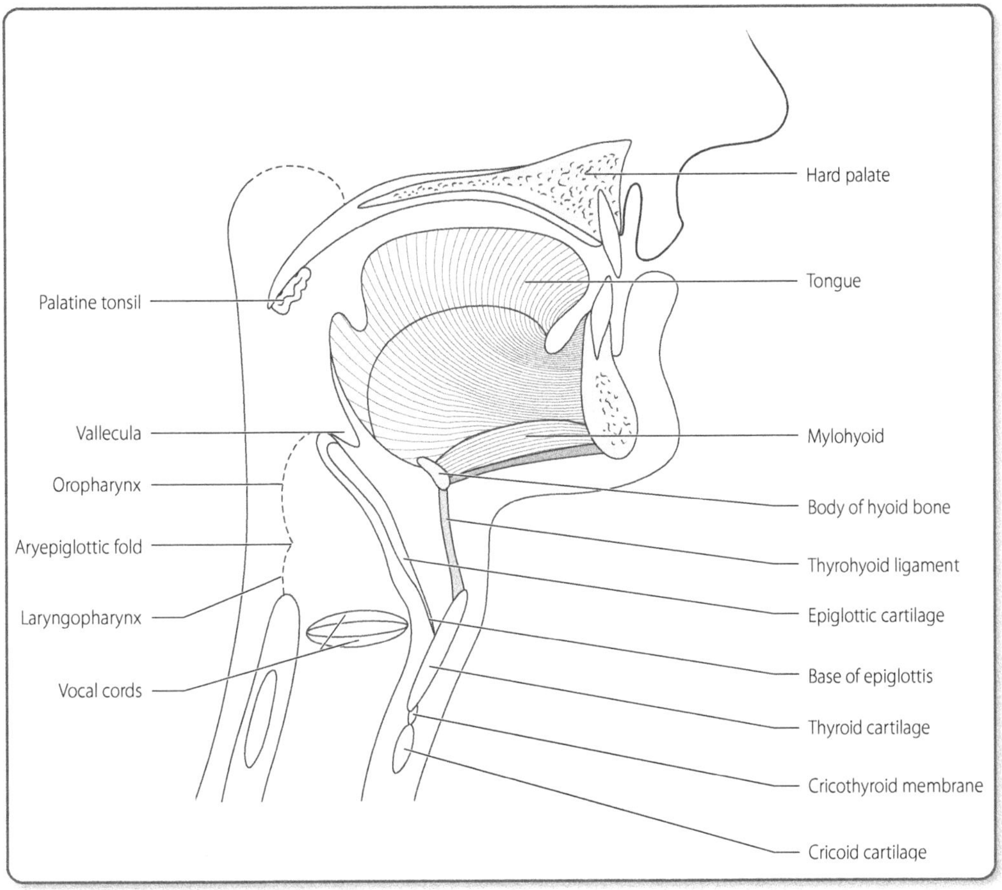

Figure 1.14 Sagittal anatomy of the tongue and pharynx.

Case 1.51

A Posterior pituitary

B Anterior pituitary

C Optic tract

D Suprasellar cistern

E Mammillary body

Coronal T1-weighted MRI through the pituitary fossa.

The optic chiasm can be seen just superior to the pituitary gland.

The suprasellar cistern is the subarachnoid cistern just superior to the pituitary, between the third ventricle and the diaphragma sellae. It is continuous with the sylvian cistern laterally and the interpeduncular cistern posteriorly. Part of the anterior circle of Willis and optic chiasm sit in the suprasellar cistern.

Weir J, Abrahams P. Imaging Atlas of Human Anatomy, 6th edition. Edinburgh: Mosby, 2021:10–12.

Moore KL, Dalley AF, Agur AMR. Clinically Oriented Anatomy, 6th edition. Philadelphia: Lippincott Williams & Wilkins, 2009:887.

Ryan S, McNicholas M, Eustace SJ. Anatomy for Diagnostic Imaging, 3rd edition. Edinburgh: Saunders, 2010:66.

Case 1.52

A Right internal carotid artery

B Pituitary gland

C Third ventricle

D Optic chiasm

E Pituitary stalk

Coronal MRI through the pituitary fossa.

The pituitary gland sits in the pituitary fossa of the sella turcica. It is connected to cell bodies of the hypothalamus by a stalk or infundibulum, which arises from the tuber cinereum in the floor of the third ventricle (**Figures 1.15** and **1.16**).

The posterior lobe produces the hormones oxytocin and vasopressin, and their presence gives a high signal on T1-weighted MRI. They are released in response to nervous stimulation from the hypothalamus.

The anterior lobe is of lower signal and secretes adrenocorticotropic hormone, thyroid-stimulating hormone, luteinising hormone, follicle-stimulating hormone, growth hormone and prolactin in response to factors carried down from the hypothalamus by the hypophyseal veins.

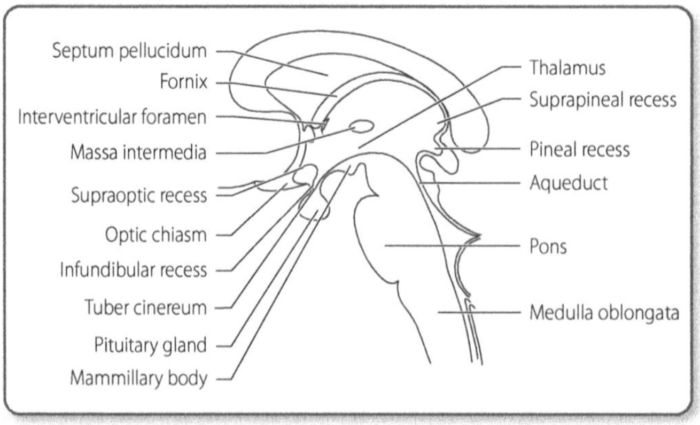

Figure 1.15 Sagittal anatomy of the third and fourth ventricles.

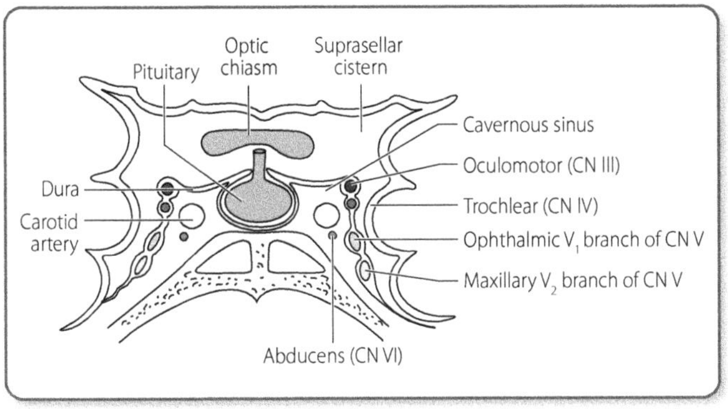

Figure 1.16 Coronal anatomy of the cavernous sinus. C, carotid artery; SS, sphenoid sinus.

The third ventricle is the slit-thin midline ventricle which lies between the thalami.

Weir J, Abrahams P. Imaging Atlas of Human Anatomy, 6th edition. Edinburgh: Mosby, 2021:10–12.

Ryan S, McNicholas M, Eustace SJ. Anatomy for Diagnostic Imaging, 3rd edition. Edinburgh: Saunders, 2010:66.

Case 1.53

A Right infraorbital foramen

B Right temporomandibular joint

C Right angle of mandible

D Odontoid peg

E Left zygomatic arch

Plain radiograph of the facial bones in an occipitomental projection.

Each half of the mandible is made up of a horizontal body, and vertical ramus, which meet at the angle of the mandible. The two halves of the mandible meet at the symphysis menti in the midline. The ramus has two bony projections at its superior margin – the coronoid process anteriorly, and the condylar process posteriorly, which articulates with the temporal bone at the temporomandibular joint.

The zygoma articulates with the temporal, frontal, and maxillary bones. These sutures are known as:

- Zygomaticotemporal suture
- Zygomaticofrontal suture
- Zygomaticomaxillary suture

Its anterior end acts to reinforce the orbit at its inferolateral margin. The zygoma can be assessed on an occipitomental projection, or a modified Towne's view (PA with mouth open).

Ryan S, McNicholas M, Eustace SJ. Anatomy for Diagnostic Imaging, 3rd edition. Edinburgh: Saunders, 2011:11, 16.

Weir J, Abrahams P. Imaging Atlas of Human Anatomy, 6th edition. Edinburgh: Mosby, 2021:23–27.

Case 1.54

A Right mandibular condyle

B Right foramen spinosum

C Right jugular foramen

D Left foramen ovale

E Clivus

Axial CT of the head.

The foramen spinosum is a small foramen in the skull base. It is found posterolaterally to the foramen rotundum, and contains the middle meningeal artery on its path from the infratemporal fossa towards the middle cranial fossa.

The foramen ovale is a larger foramen, found in the greater wing of sphenoid, posterolateral to the foramen rotundum. It contains the third division of the fifth cranial nerve and the accessory meningeal artery as they pass between the middle cranial fossa and the infratemporal fossa.

At the junction of the occipital and petrous bones, posteriorly is found the jugular foramen. It has a course which runs inferomedially from the posterior cranial fossa, and it has a somewhat irregular, often asymmetrical shape. The jugular foramen can be divided into two compartments by a fibrocartilaginous band – the smallest anteromedial compartment is known as the pars nervosa, and the largest posteromedial compartment, the pars vascularis. The pars nervosa contains the inferior petrosal sinus (which drains into the internal jugular vein) and the 9th cranial nerve. The pars vascularis contains the jugular bulb, as well as the ascending occipital and pharyngeal arteries. The 10th and 11th cranial nerves are also found within the pars vascularis.

Ryan S, McNicholas M, Eustace SJ. Anatomy for Diagnostic Imaging, 3rd edition. Edinburgh: Saunders, 2011:8.

Weir J, Abrahams P. Imaging Atlas of Human Anatomy, 6th edition. Edinburgh: Mosby, 2021:29–30.

Butler P, Mitchell AM, Ellis H. Applied Radiological Anatomy. Cambridge: Cambridge University Press, 1999:94.

Case 1.55

A Frontal bone (outer table of skull vault)

B Coronal suture

C Tongue

D Soft palate

E Lambdoid suture

Lateral radiograph of an infant's skull.

The skull vault is made up of an inner and outer table (or diploe), between which is found the diploic space. This space is filled with marrow and is traversed by the diploic veins.

The frontal bone develops in two halves in children, separated vertically by the metopic suture. This usually fuses by the age of 5, however, in some individuals it does not fuse. A persistent metopic suture is found in approximately 5–10% of the population. The floor of the anterior cranial fossa is largely made up of the orbital plates of the frontal bone, with the cribriform plate located between them.

The coronal suture marks the interface between the frontal and parietal bones. The parietal bones are separated from each other by the sagittal suture, which runs perpendicularly from the coronal suture, until it meets the lambdoid suture posteriorly. The lambdoid sutures run at an oblique angle, separating the parietal and occipital bones. The parietal bone also articulates with the greater wing of sphenoid anteriorly, and inferiorly it meets the temporal bone.

The side of the skull vault below the parietal and frontal bones is formed by the greater wing of sphenoid and the squamous part of the temporal bone. The point at which the sutures between the frontal, parietal, sphenoidal and temporal bones meet is known as the pterion. These sutures are as follows:

- Sphenosquamosal: Between the sphenoid and temporal bones
- Sphenofrontal: Between the greater wing of sphenoid and frontal bones
- Sphenoparietal: Between the greater wing of sphenoid and parietal bones
- Squamosal: Between the temporal and parietal bones

Ryan S, McNicholas M, Eustace SJ. Anatomy for Diagnostic Imaging, 3rd edition. Edinburgh: Saunders, 2011:1–3.

Weir J, Abrahams P. Imaging Atlas of Human Anatomy, 6th edition. Edinburgh: Mosby, 2021:23–27.

Case 1.56

A Right Eustachian tube

B Right external acoustic canal

C Sphenoid sinus

D Left carotid canal

E Left internal acoustic canal

Axial CT of the head.

The carotid canal transmits the internal carotid artery on its course through the petrous bone. It is a circular opening, found just anterior to the jugular fossa, separated from it by a bony crest. It is separated from the inner ear, laterally, by the tympanic plate. The internal carotid takes a tortuous course, and the carotid canal has a vertical course at first, before turning at right angles to continue in a horizontal and medial direction, with the artery then entering the foramen lacerum.

The Eustachian or pharyngotympanic tube connects the lower part of the middle ear with the lateral wall of the nasopharynx. It provides a mechanism for equalising pressure across the tympanic membrane. At its proximal end, the Eustachian tube is bony, but as it continues over approximately 3.5 cm, it becomes cartilaginous.

The internal auditory canal transmits the 7th (facial) and 8th (vestibulocochlear) cranial nerves as well as the labyrinthine artery from the posterior fossa. It is approximately 1 cm in length and runs a roughly horizontal course in the coronal plane. At the lateral end of the canal both nerves pass through the lamina cribrosa, after which the facial nerve continues through the facial canal and the vestibulocochlear nerve gives off branches to supply the cochlea and vestibule. The canal itself is divided into four quadrants by the crista falciformis, which runs horizontally, and the vertical crests. The posterior quadrants are occupied by the superior and inferior vestibular branches of the vestibulocochlear nerve. The anterosuperior compartment of the canal is occupied by the facial and intermediate nerves. The anteroinferior compartment is occupied by the cochlear branch of the vestibulocochlear nerve.

Weir J, Abrahams P. Imaging Atlas of Human Anatomy, 6th edition. Edinburgh: Mosby, 2021:30.

Ryan S, McNicholas M, Eustace SJ. Anatomy for Diagnostic Imaging, 3rd edition. Edinburgh: Saunders, 2011:8, 29.

Cunningham DJ, Robinson A. Cunningham's textbook of anatomy. New York: William Wood and Company, 1898:129.

Case 1.57

A Right infratemporal fossa

B Nasopharynx

C Left anterior clinoid process

D Left greater wing of sphenoid

E Left lateral pterygoid plate

Coronal CT of the head.

The sphenoid bone is made up of a body (the basisphenoid), greater and lesser wings, as well as the pterygoid plates, which extend inferiorly behind the maxilla. The lesser wing of the sphenoid bone makes up the posterior part of the floor of the anterior cranial fossa, while the greater wing forms the floor of the middle cranial fossa. The posterior border of the lesser wing is demarcated by the sphenoid ridge, while the posterior border of the greater wing is found where it meets the petrous ridge. Below the greater wing of sphenoid is found the infratemporal fossa, into which open the foramen ovale and spinosum.

The sphenoid sinuses are contained within the body of sphenoid. These are paired, usually asymmetric structures.

The infratemporal fossa is found below the floor of the middle cranial fossa, lateral to the nasopharynx and posterior to the maxilla. Behind it is found the styloid process, the carotid artery, jugular vein, and the deep part of the parotid gland. Laterally, this space extends to the zygomatic arch, mandibular ramus and the temporalis muscle. There is no separation between the temporal fossa superiorly and the infratemporal fossa below – they communicate via the space between the zygomatic arch and the skull.

The medial extent of the infratemporal fossa is bounded by the lateral pterygoid plate, and the pterygoid muscles are contained within it. The pterygomaxillary fissure separates the pterygoid plates from the maxilla superiorly.

There is a small medial depression of the pterygomaxillary fissure, called the pterygopalatine fossa, which is found between the pterygoid process and the posterior maxilla. This fossa has several spaces which open into it. Superiorly, it communicates with the orbit via the inferior orbital fissure, and the middle cranial fossa via the foramen rotundum. Through the sphenopalatine foramen, it communicates with the nasal cavity, and through the greater palatine canal, the mouth. Laterally, this space opens out into the infratemporal fossa. From the foramen rotundum, the maxillary division of the 5th cranial nerve crosses this space before passing through the inferior orbital fissure. It also contains the pterygopalatine segment of the maxillary artery.

Ryan S, McNicholas M, Eustace SJ. Anatomy for Diagnostic Imaging, 3rd edition. Edinburgh: Saunders, 2011:35.

Weir J, Abrahams P. Imaging Atlas of Human Anatomy, 6th edition. Edinburgh: Mosby, 2021:31.

Butler P, Mitchell AM, Ellis H. Applied Radiological Anatomy. Cambridge: Cambridge University Press, 1999:22.

Case 1.58

A Right foramen lacerum

B Right lambdoid suture

C Left petro-occipital fissure

D Left carotid canal

E Internal occipital protuberance

Axial CT of the head.

The temporal bone is made up of four parts:

1. Squamous: Forms part of the skull base and the lateral vault.
2. Petrous: Forms part of the skull base and contains the middle and inner ears.
3. Mastoid: Contains mastoid air cells within the mastoid process behind the ear.
4. Styloid process: Inferior projection.

The occipital bone makes up the posterior aspect of the skull vault and continues anteriorly to form part of the skull base. It contains the foramen magnum, anterior to which it forms the clivus. This portion, anterior to the foramen magnum, is known as the basiocciput, and articulates with the sphenoid bone anteriorly, and the petrous temporal bone laterally. The petro-occipital fissure is found at the base of the petrous temporal bone and the clivus, and is continuous with the jugular foramen posteriorly.

The internal occipital protuberance is a bony prominence on the internal surface of the posterior cranial fossa in the midline and marks a point of attachment of the tentorium cerebelli.

The foramen lacerum is a jagged bony canal found posteriorly and medial to the foramen ovale, between the petrous apex, the body of sphenoid and the basiocciput. The internal carotid artery traverses the superior part of the foramen lacerum; it contains only small veins and nerves.

Ryan S, McNicholas M, Eustace SJ. Anatomy for Diagnostic Imaging, 3rd edition. Edinburgh: Saunders, 2011:3.

Weir J, Abrahams P. Imaging Atlas of Human Anatomy, 6th edition. Edinburgh: Mosby, 2021:7.

Butler P, Mitchell AM, Ellis H. Applied Radiological Anatomy. Cambridge: Cambridge University Press, 1999:23.

Case 1.59

A Crista galli

B Right superior orbital fissure

C Right greater wing of sphenoid

D Left innominate line

E Left foramen rotundum

Frontal skull radiograph.

The crista galli is a bony protrusion from the internal surface of the floor of the anterior cranial fossa in the midline. It marks a point of attachment of the falx cerebri, which is a dural septum that runs in the sagittal plane between the two hemispheres.

The superior orbital fissure is triangular in shape and is found between the greater and lesser wings of the sphenoid bone. The structures which pass through this fissure are:

- 3rd cranial nerve
- 4th cranial nerve
- First division (orbital) of 5th cranial nerve
- 6th cranial nerve
- Superior orbital vein
- Middle meningeal artery branch vessel

The foramen rotundum passes from Meckel's cave in the middle cranial fossa to the pterygopalatine fossa, with the second division (maxillary) of the 5th cranial nerve running through it. It is circular in shape and is found posteriorly to the superior orbital fissure in the greater wing of the sphenoid bone. It is best seen on an angled occipitofrontal view (20° caudal), or an occipitomental view.

The innominate line is seen on occipitomental views of the orbits as a straight line running obliquely from the upper outer part of the orbit, inferiorly and medially. It is caused by the beam hitting the curve of the greater wing of sphenoid at a tangent.

Weir J, Abrahams P. Imaging Atlas of Human Anatomy, 6th edition. Edinburgh: Mosby, 2021:23.

Butler P, Mitchell AM, Ellis H. Applied Radiological Anatomy. Cambridge: Cambridge University Press, 1999:64, 98.

Ryan S, McNicholas M, Eustace SJ. Anatomy for Diagnostic Imaging, 3rd edition. Edinburgh: Saunders, 2011:8, 11–13.

Case 1.60

A Anterior fontanelle

B Planum sphenoidale

C Sagittal suture

D Lambda

E Left lesser wing of sphenoid

Frontal skull radiograph from an infant.

The sutures have quite a different appearance in the neonate/infant compared to an adult. They begin as straight lines, with open fontanelles at the points where they meet, and there may be wormian bones visible. In the first few days of life, some overlapping of the bones may be seen. As the skull grows and matures, the sutures begin to fuse, and change from having a straight appearance to an interlocking pattern. This appearance develops in the first year, and by 2 years of age the sutures have a more adult, serrated pattern. The anterior fontanelle forms a diamond shape between the coronal, metopic and sagittal sutures. It usually closes by the age of 18 months, at which point the junction between the coronal and sagittal sutures becomes known as the bregma. The posterior fontanelle forms a triangular shape between the sagittal and lambdoid sutures. It usually closes by 6–8 months, and the junction of these sutures is then known as the lambda.

Ryan S, McNicholas M, Eustace SJ. Anatomy for Diagnostic Imaging, 3rd edition. Edinburgh: Saunders, 2011:1, 10.

Weir J, Abrahams P. Imaging Atlas of Human Anatomy, 6th edition. Edinburgh: Mosby, 2021:23–25.

Case 1.61

A Posterior clinoid process

B Dorsum sellae

C Greater wing of sphenoid

D Pituitary fossa (sella turcica)

E Hard palate

Lateral skull radiograph.

The pituitary fossa, or sella turcica, is found on the superior surface of the body of sphenoid. The posterior part of the pituitary fossa is known as the dorsum sellae – this is continuous with the clivus behind. The posterior clinoid processes form two lateral projections, which extend from the dorsum sellae. Anteriorly is the tuberculum sellae, which is a bony prominence on the anterior surface of the sella. There are two bony projections from the anterior aspect of the sella, which are called the anterior clinoid processes – these are part of the lesser wing of sphenoid. Anterior to the tuberculum sellae, between the anterior clinoid processes, is a depression which is known as the sulcus chiasmaticus; the optic chiasm lies over it, and the optic canals are found to each side of it.

The planum sphenoidale is a horizontal portion of the lesser wing of sphenoid, anterior to the sulcus chiasmaticus. It articulates with the cribriform plate anteriorly.

Ryan S, McNicholas M, Eustace SJ. Anatomy for Diagnostic Imaging, 3rd edition. Edinburgh: Saunders, 2011:3.

Weir J, Abrahams P. Imaging Atlas of Human Anatomy, 6th edition. Edinburgh: Mosby, 2021:24.

Butler P, Mitchell AM, Ellis H. Applied Radiological Anatomy. Cambridge: Cambridge University Press, 1999:22.

Case 1.62

A Right coronoid process of mandible

B Right pterygoid fossa

C Right styloid process

D Left nasolacrimal duct

E Left lateral pterygoid muscle

Axial CT of the head.

The lacrimal gland produces tears to lubricate the eye. These drain via the lacrimal punctae in the medial margins of each eyelid. They then pass through the superior and inferior lacrimal canaliculae. The canaliculae drain into the lacrimal sac, located in a depression in the medial wall of the bony orbit. From here, the lacrimal sac empties into the nasolacrimal duct. This duct passes through a bony canal to the inferior meatus in the nasal cavity.

The styloid process extends inferiorly from the base of the petrous temporal bone. The stylomastoid foramen is found posterior to the styloid process, with the facial nerve passing through it. The styloid process and the styloid muscles separate the nasopharynx anteromedially from the carotid sheath which is found posterolaterally.

Stylopharyngeus contributes to the inner layer of the pharyngeal muscles, and styloglossus runs anteriorly to act as an extrinsic muscle of the tongue. The stylohyoid ligament extends from the styloid process to the superior surface of the hyoid bone, and may sometimes be identified on lateral radiographs if it is calcified.

Ryan S, McNicholas M, Eustace SJ. Anatomy for Diagnostic Imaging, 3rd edition. Edinburgh: Saunders, 2011:20, 28.

Weir J, Abrahams P. Imaging Atlas of Human Anatomy, 6th edition. Edinburgh: Mosby, 2021:30.

Butler P, Mitchell AM, Ellis H. Applied Radiological Anatomy. Cambridge: Cambridge University Press, 1999:23, 30, 107.

Case 2.2

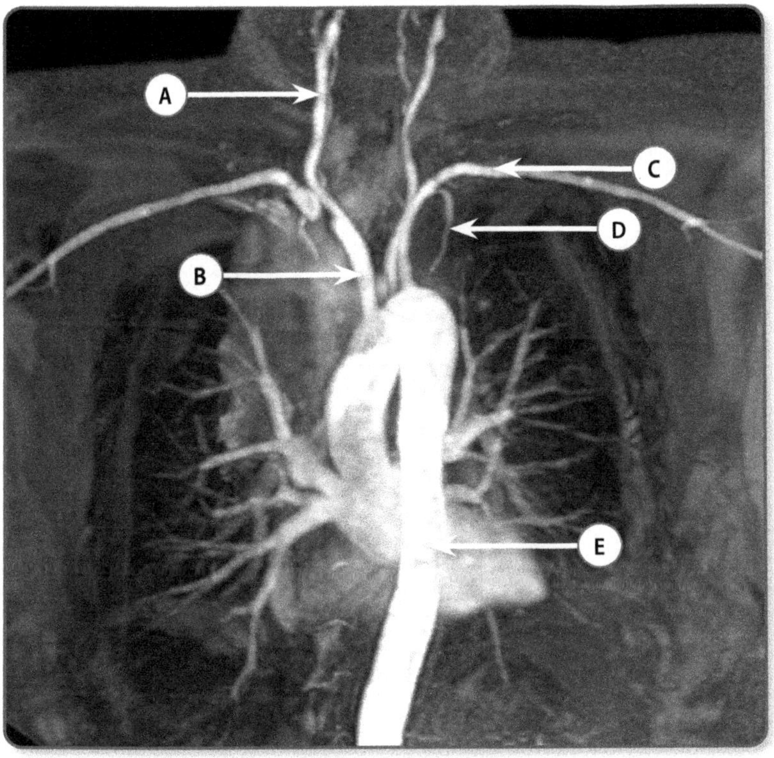

Case 2.2

QUESTION		WRITE YOUR ANSWER HERE
A	Name the structure labelled A.	
B	Name the structure labelled B.	
C	Name the structure labelled C.	
D	Name the structure labelled D.	
E	Name the structure labelled E.	

Case 2.3

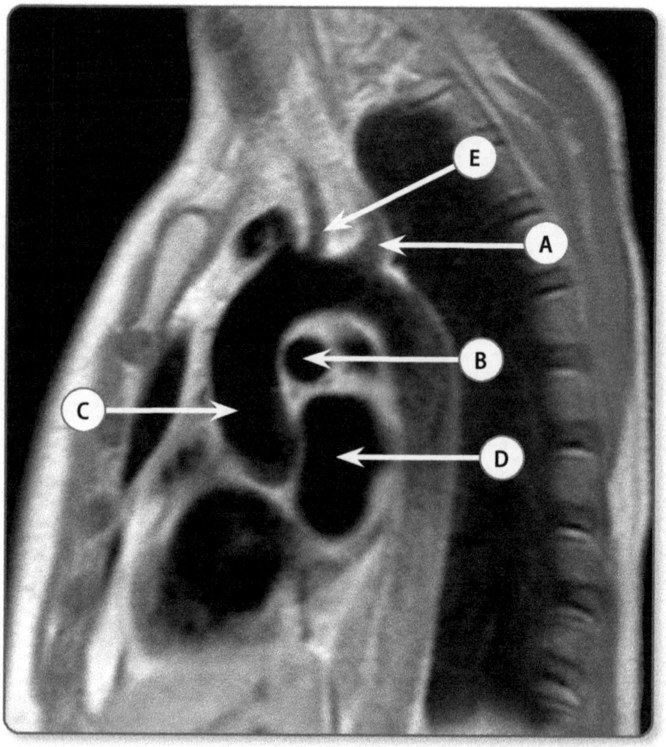

Case 2.3

QUESTION		WRITE YOUR ANSWER HERE
A	Name the structure labelled A.	
B	Name the structure labelled B.	
C	Name the structure labelled C.	
D	Name the structure labelled D.	
E	Name the structure labelled E.	

Cardiac and vascular

Case 2.1

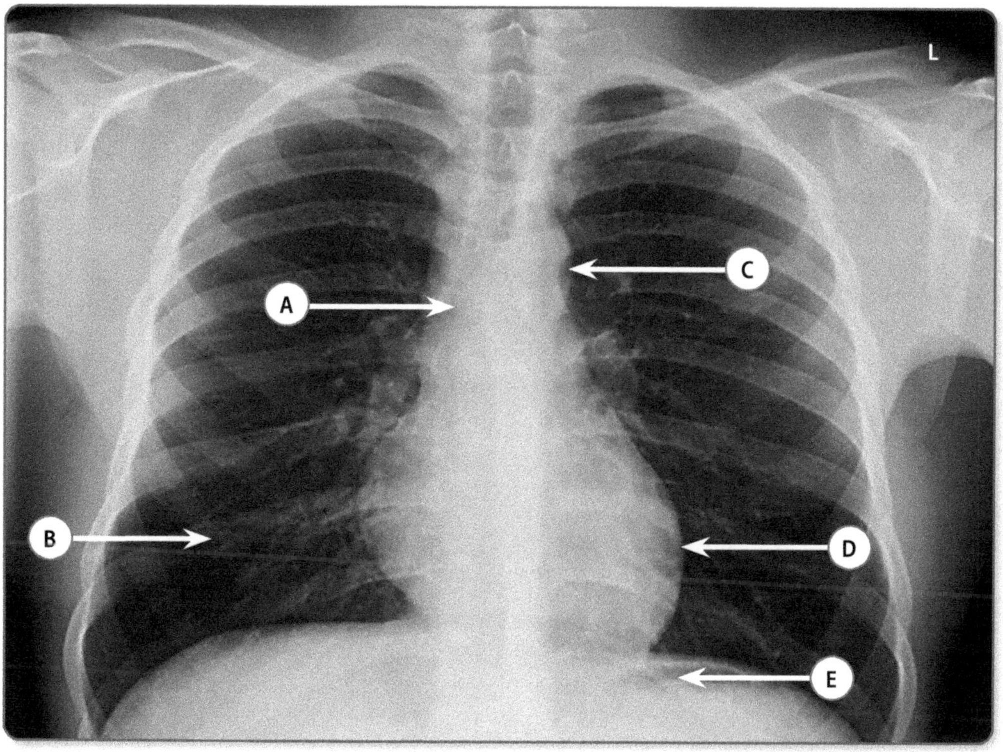

Case 2.1

QUESTION		WRITE YOUR ANSWER HERE
A	Name the structure labelled A.	
B	Name the structure labelled B.	
C	Name the structure labelled C.	
D	Name the structure labelled D.	
E	Name the structure labelled E.	

Chapter 2

Chest

Case 2.4

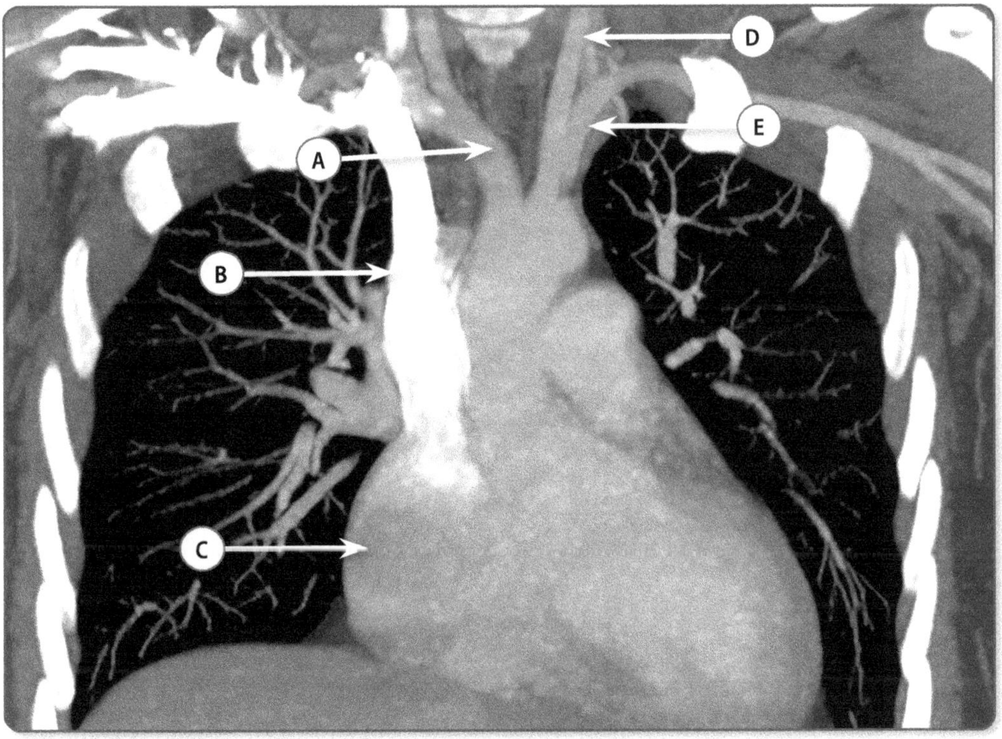

Case 2.4

QUESTION		WRITE YOUR ANSWER HERE
A	Name the structure labelled A.	
B	Name the structure labelled B.	
C	Name the structure labelled C.	
D	Name the structure labelled D.	
E	Name the structure labelled E.	

Case 2.5

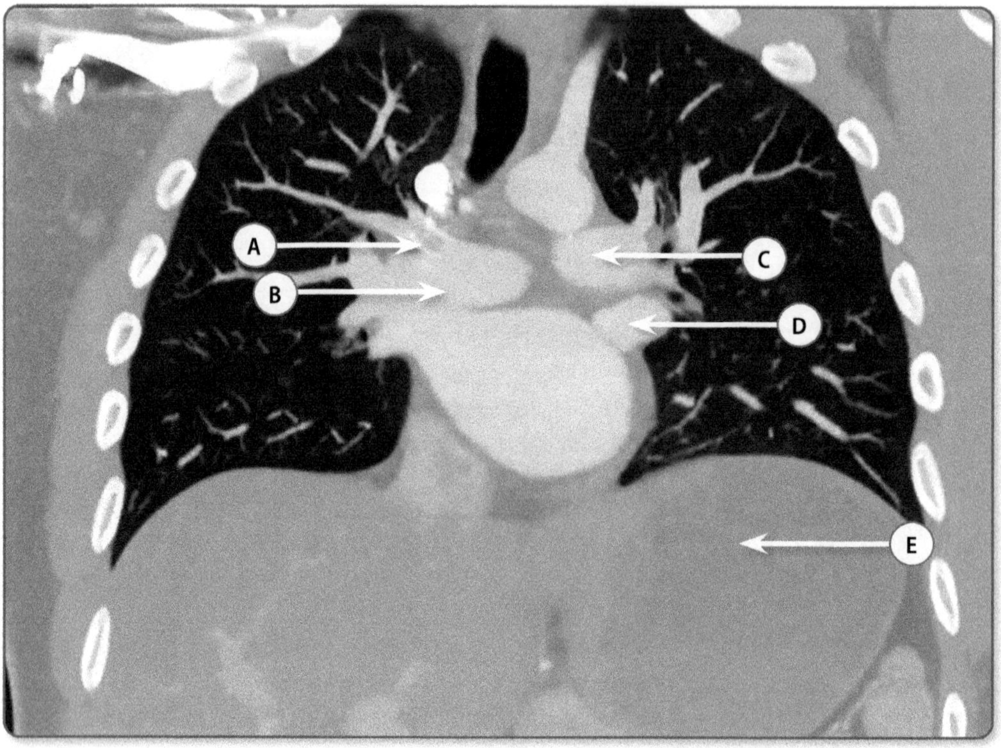

Case 2.5

QUESTION		WRITE YOUR ANSWER HERE
A	Name the structure labelled A.	
B	Name the structure labelled B.	
C	Name the structure labelled C.	
D	Name the structure labelled D.	
E	Name the structure labelled E.	

Case 2.6

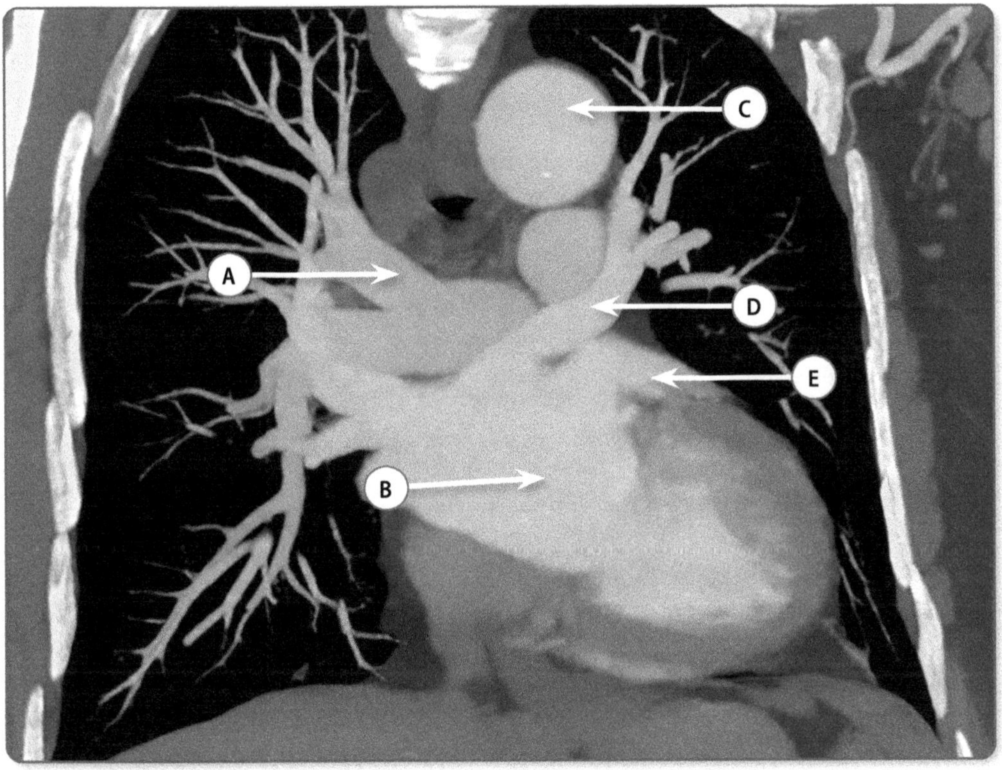

Case 2.6

QUESTION		WRITE YOUR ANSWER HERE
A	Name the structure labelled A.	
B	Name the structure labelled B.	
C	Name the structure labelled C.	
D	Name the structure labelled D.	
E	Name the structure labelled E.	

Case 2.7

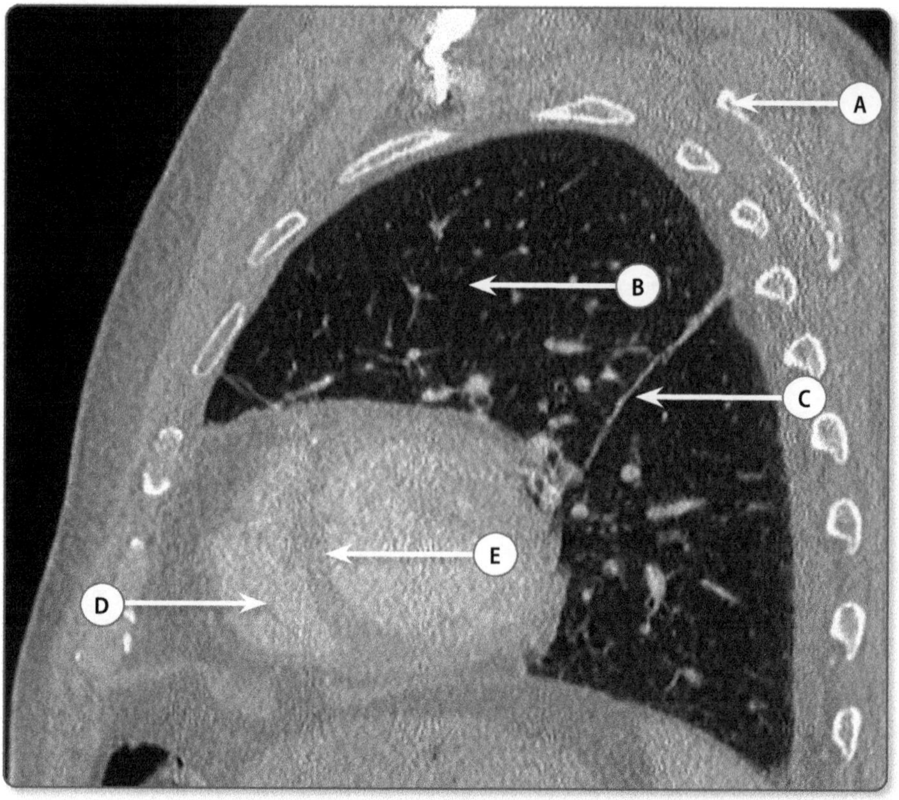

Case 2.7

QUESTION		WRITE YOUR ANSWER HERE
A	Name the structure labelled A.	
B	Name the structure labelled B.	
C	Name the structure labelled C.	
D	Name the structure labelled D.	
E	Name the structure labelled E.	

Case 2.8

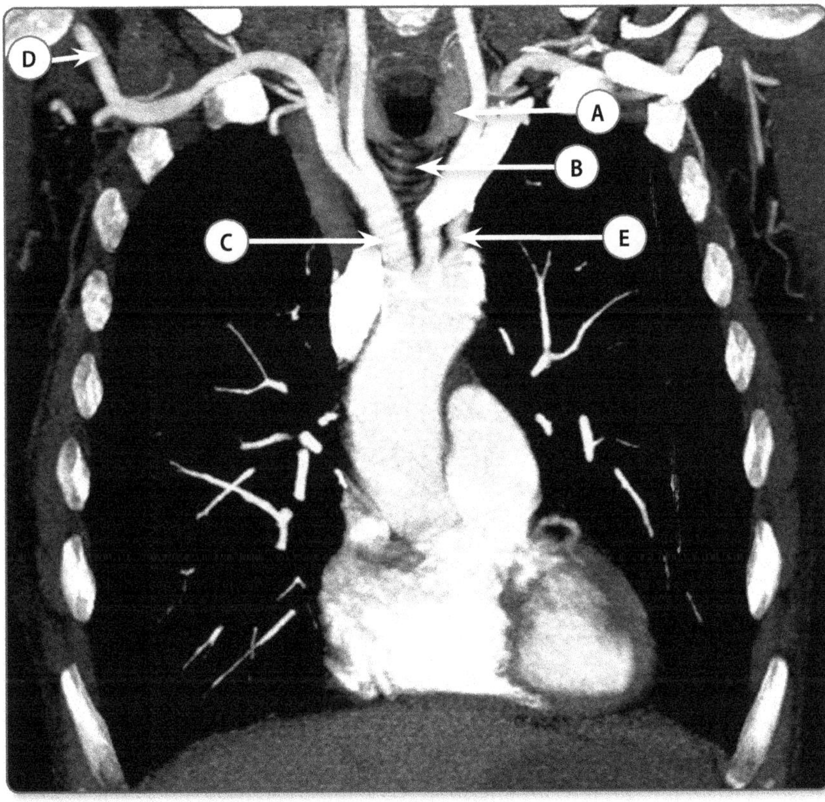

Case 2.8

QUESTION		WRITE YOUR ANSWER HERE
A	Name the structure labelled A.	
B	Name the structure labelled B.	
C	Name the structure labelled C.	
D	Name the structure labelled D.	
E	Name the structure labelled E.	

Case 2.9

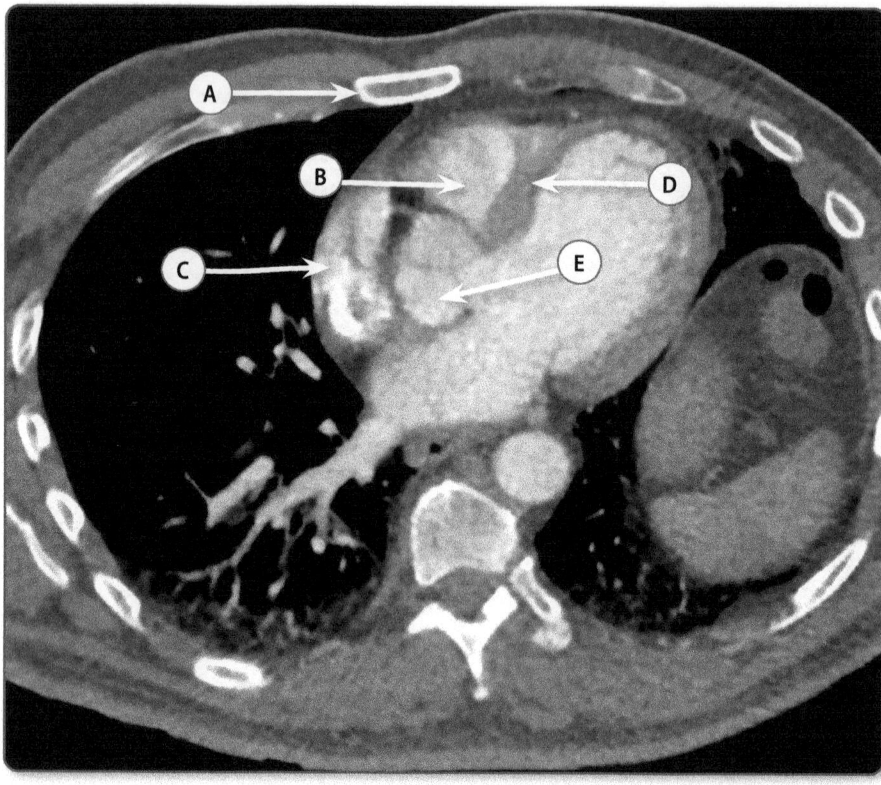

Case 2.9

QUESTION		WRITE YOUR ANSWER HERE
A	Name the structure labelled A.	
B	Name the structure labelled B.	
C	Name the structure labelled C.	
D	Name the structure labelled D.	
E	Name the structure labelled E.	

Case 2.10

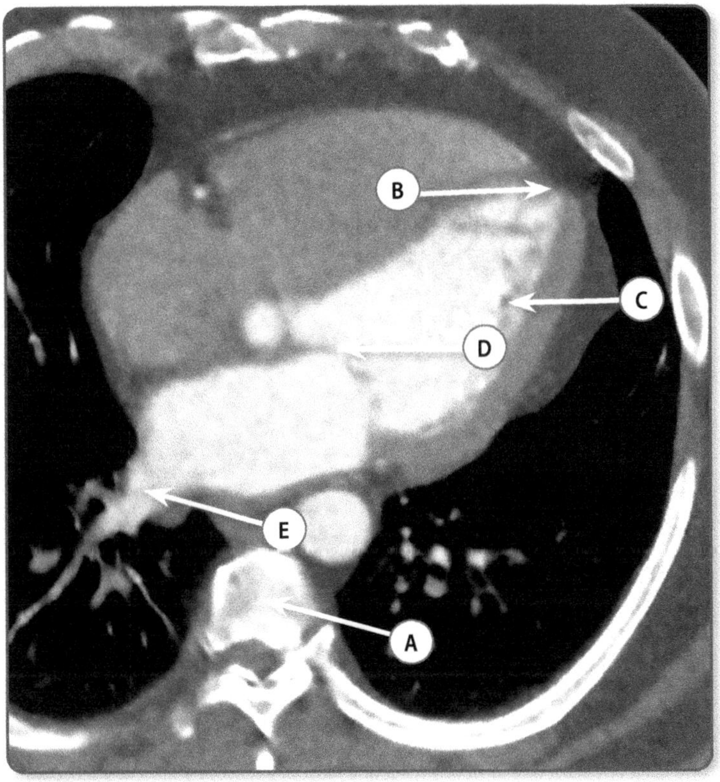

Case 2.10

QUESTION		WRITE YOUR ANSWER HERE
A	Name the structure labelled A.	
B	Name the structure labelled B.	
C	Name the structure labelled C.	
D	Name the structure labelled D.	
E	Name the structure labelled E.	

Case 2.11

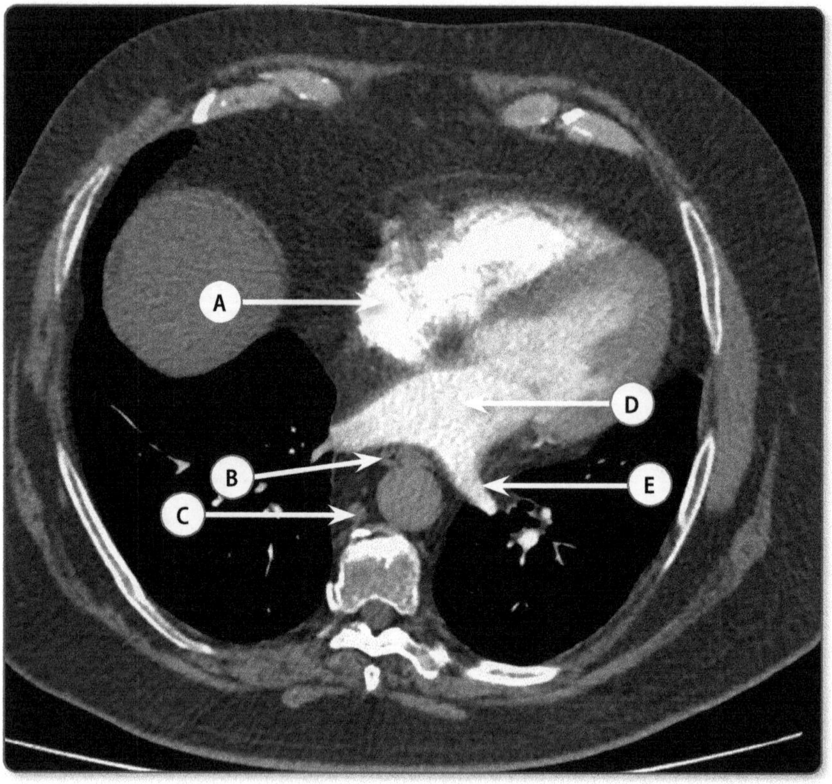

Case 2.11

QUESTION		WRITE YOUR ANSWER HERE
A	Name the structure labelled A.	
B	Name the structure labelled B.	
C	Name the structure labelled C.	
D	Name the structure labelled D.	
E	Name the structure labelled E.	

Case 2.12

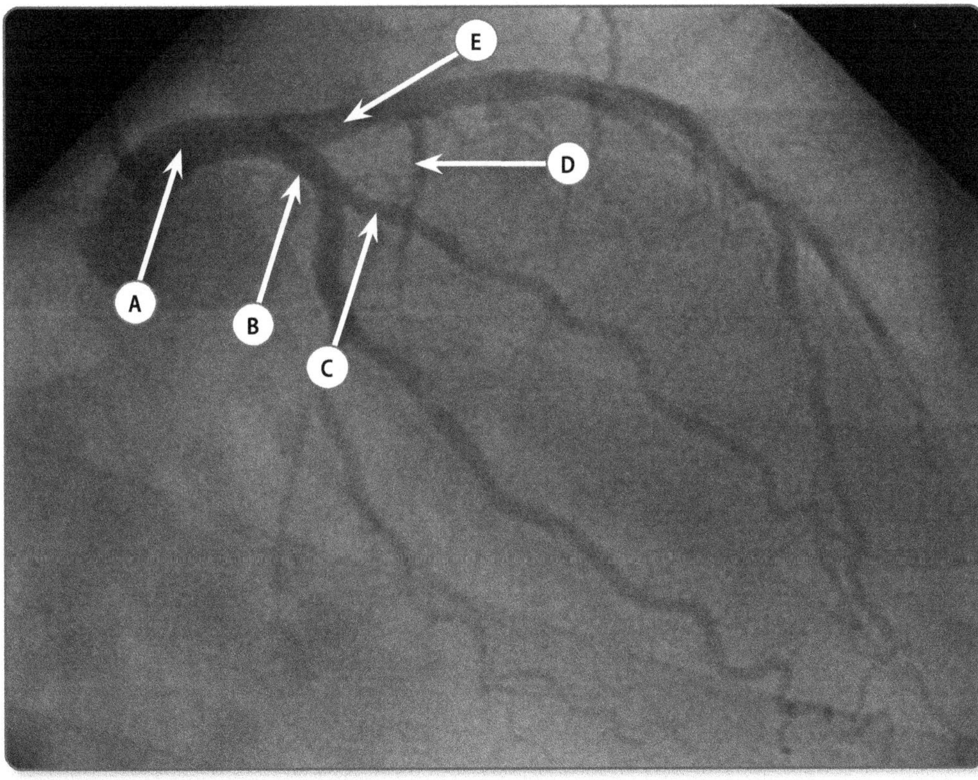

Case 2.12

QUESTION		WRITE YOUR ANSWER HERE
A	Name the structure labelled A.	
B	Name the structure labelled B.	
C	Name the structure labelled C.	
D	Name the structure labelled D.	
E	Name the structure labelled E.	

Case 2.13

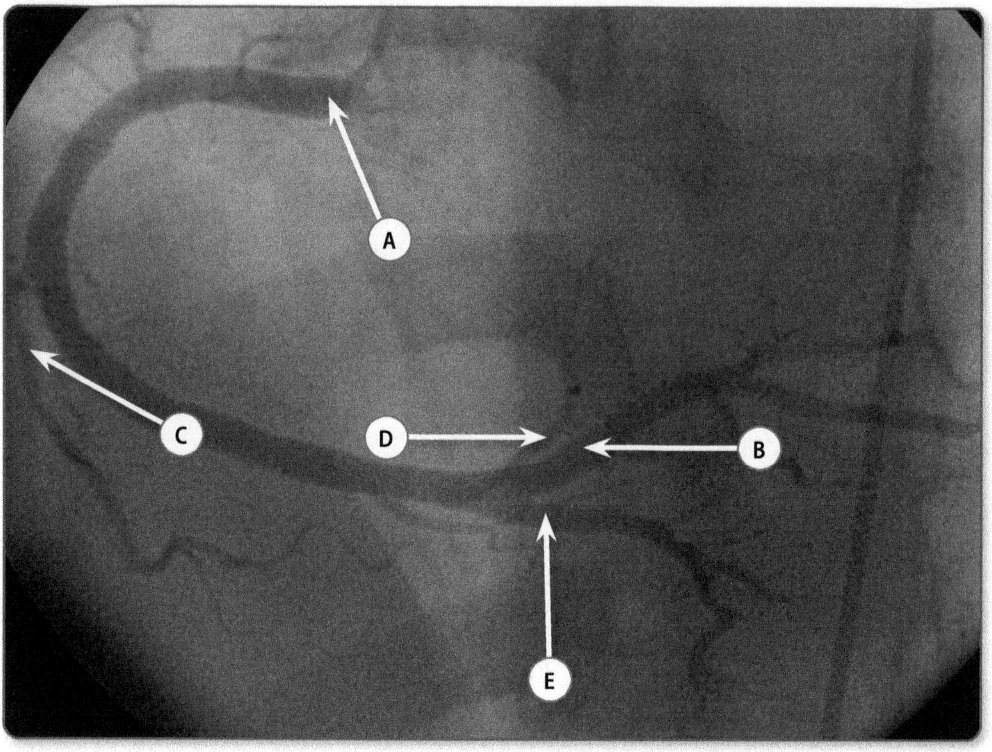

Case 2.13

QUESTION		WRITE YOUR ANSWER HERE
A	Name the structure labelled A.	
B	Name the structure labelled B.	
C	Name the structure labelled C.	
D	Name the structure labelled D.	
E	Name the structure labelled E.	

Case 2.14

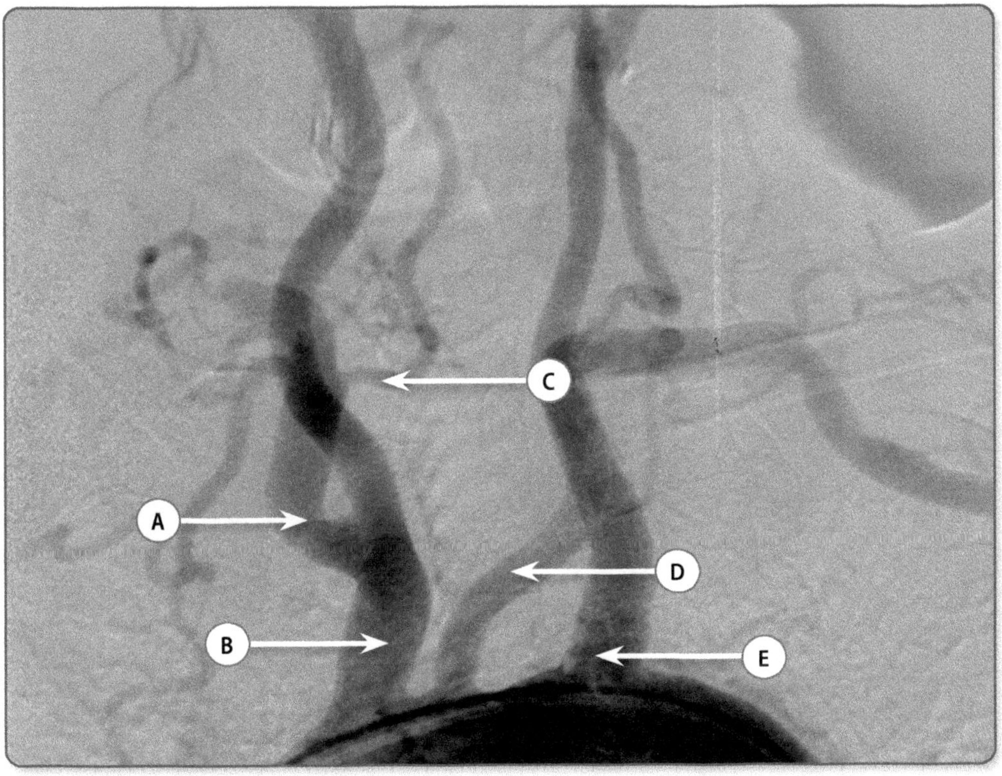

Case 2.14

QUESTION		WRITE YOUR ANSWER HERE
A	Name the structure labelled A.	
B	Name the structure labelled B.	
C	Name the structure labelled C.	
D	Name the structure labelled D.	
E	Name the structure labelled E.	

Case 2.15

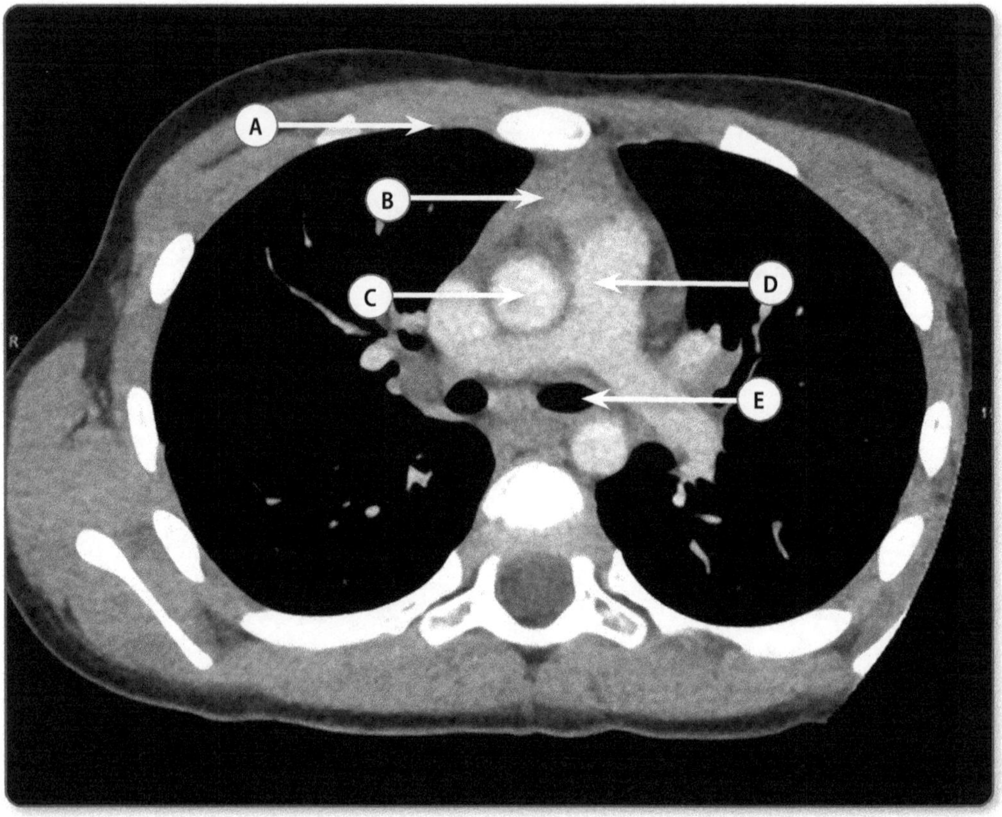

Case 2.15

QUESTION		WRITE YOUR ANSWER HERE
A	Name the structure labelled A.	
B	Name the structure labelled B.	
C	Name the structure labelled C.	
D	Name the structure labelled D.	
E	Name the structure labelled E.	

Case 2.16

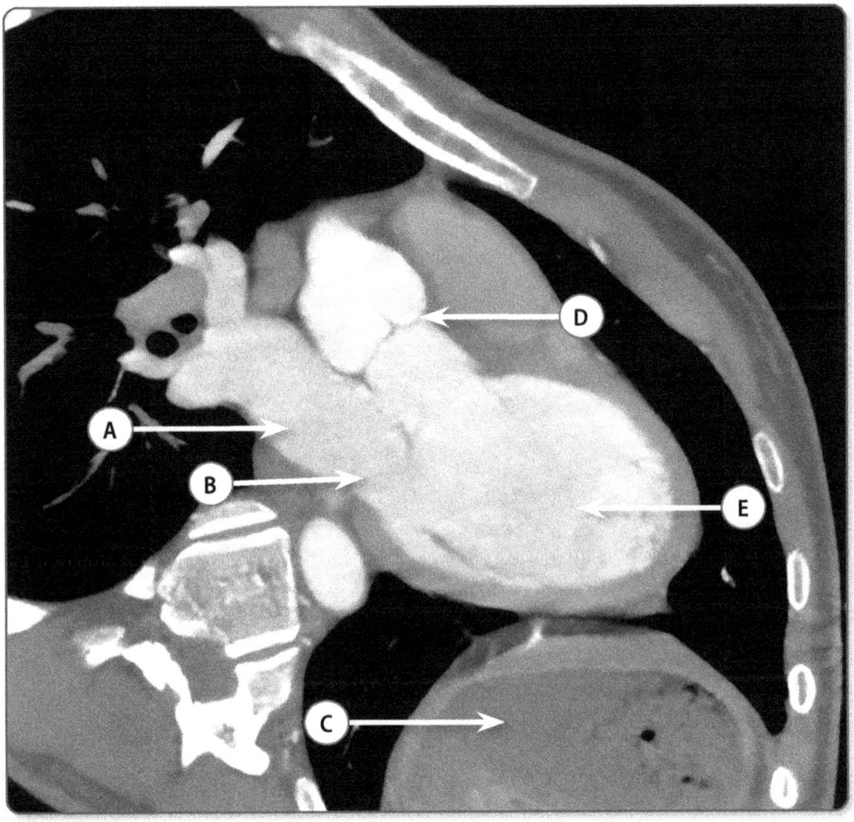

Case 2.16

QUESTION		WRITE YOUR ANSWER HERE
A	Name the structure labelled A.	
B	Name the structure labelled B.	
C	Name the structure labelled C.	
D	Name the structure labelled D.	
E	Name the structure labelled E.	

Case 2.17

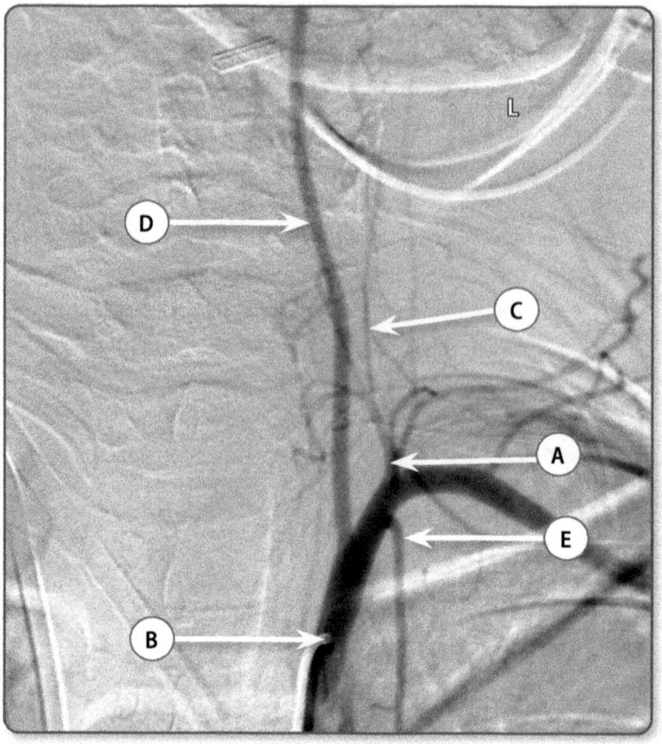

Case 2.17

QUESTION		WRITE YOUR ANSWER HERE
A	Name the structure labelled A.	
B	Name the structure labelled B.	
C	Name the structure labelled C.	
D	Name the structure labelled D.	
E	Name the structure labelled E.	

Case 2.18

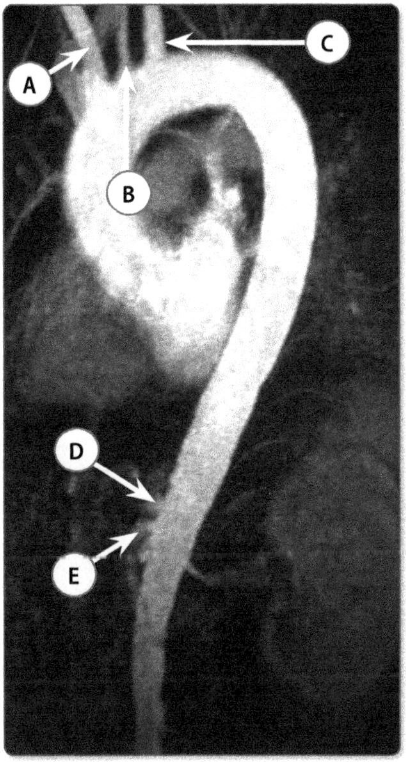

Case 2.18

QUESTION		WRITE YOUR ANSWER HERE
A	Name the structure labelled A.	
B	Name the structure labelled B.	
C	Name the structure labelled C.	
D	Name the structure labelled D.	
E	Name the structure labelled E.	

Case 2.19

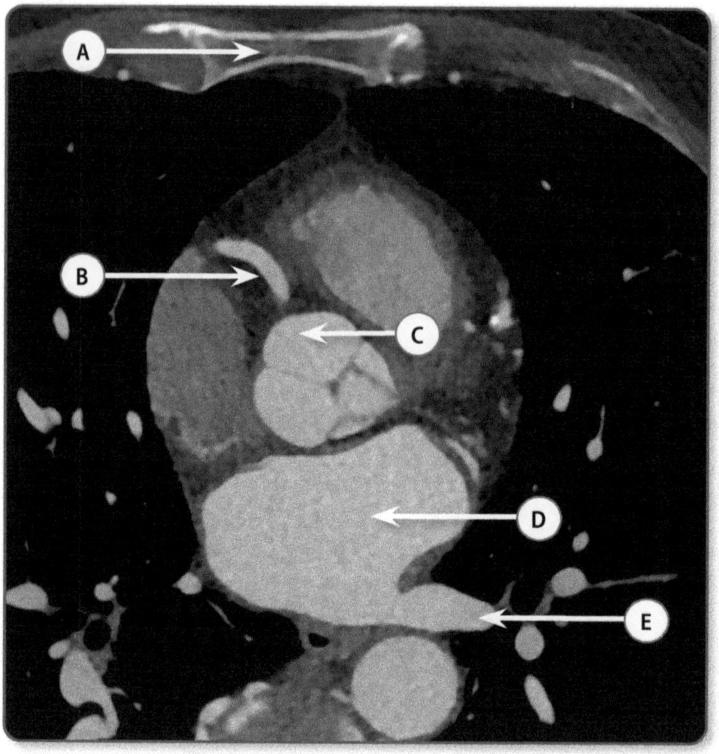

Case 2.19

QUESTION		WRITE YOUR ANSWER HERE
A	Name the structure labelled A.	
B	Name the structure labelled B.	
C	Name the structure labelled C.	
D	Name the structure labelled D.	
E	Name the structure labelled E.	

Case 2.20

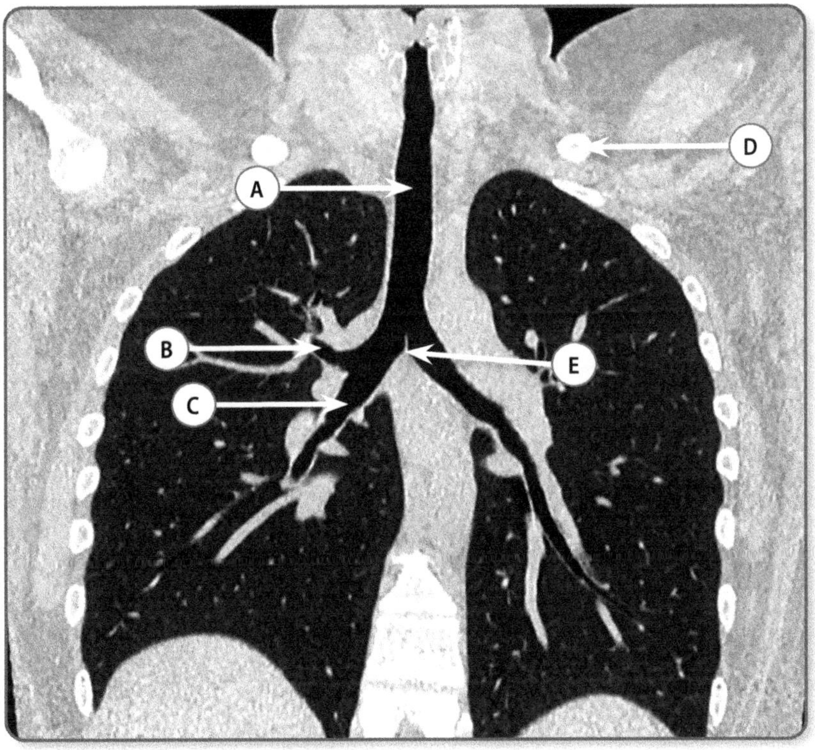

Case 2.20

QUESTION		WRITE YOUR ANSWER HERE
A	Name the structure labelled A.	
B	Name the structure labelled B.	
C	Name the structure labelled C.	
D	Name the structure labelled D.	
E	Name the structure labelled E.	

Case 2.21

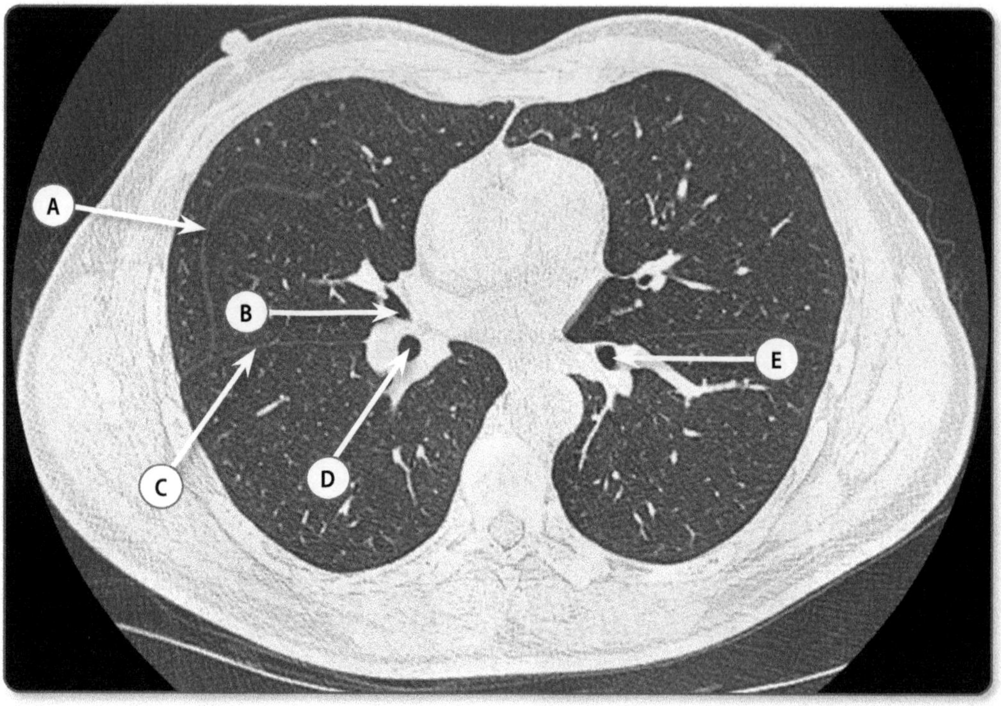

Case 2.21

QUESTION		WRITE YOUR ANSWER HERE
A	Name the structure labelled A.	
B	Name the structure labelled B.	
C	Name the structure labelled C.	
D	Name the structure labelled D.	
E	Name the structure labelled E.	

Case 2.22

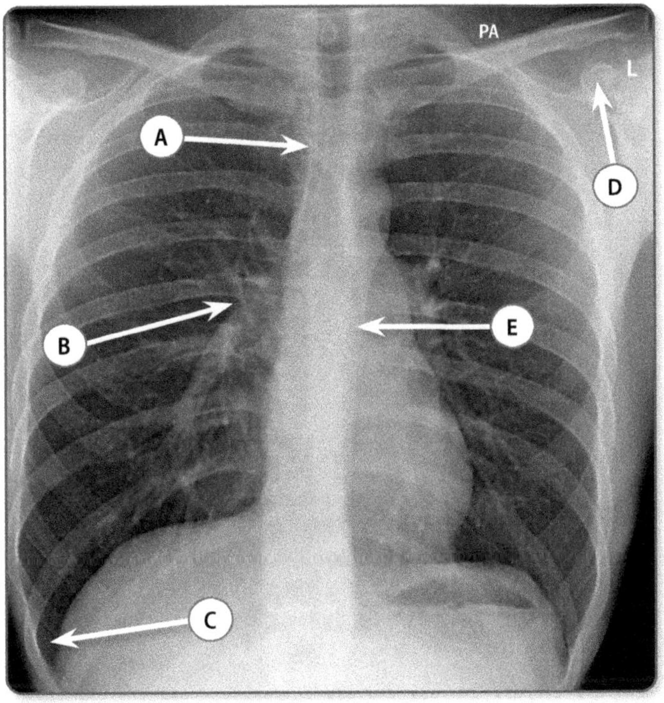

Case 2.22

QUESTION		WRITE YOUR ANSWER HERE
A	Name the structure labelled A.	
B	Name the structure labelled B.	
C	Name the structure labelled C.	
D	Name the structure labelled D.	
E	Name the structure labelled E.	

Case 2.23

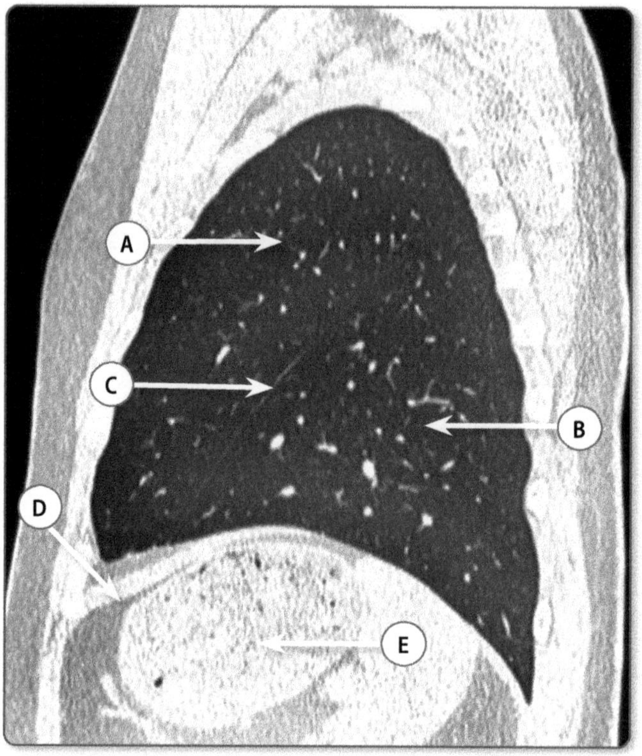

Case 2.23

QUESTION		WRITE YOUR ANSWER HERE
A	Name the structure labelled A.	
B	Name the structure labelled B.	
C	Name the structure labelled C.	
D	Name the structure labelled D.	
E	Name the structure labelled E.	

Case 2.24

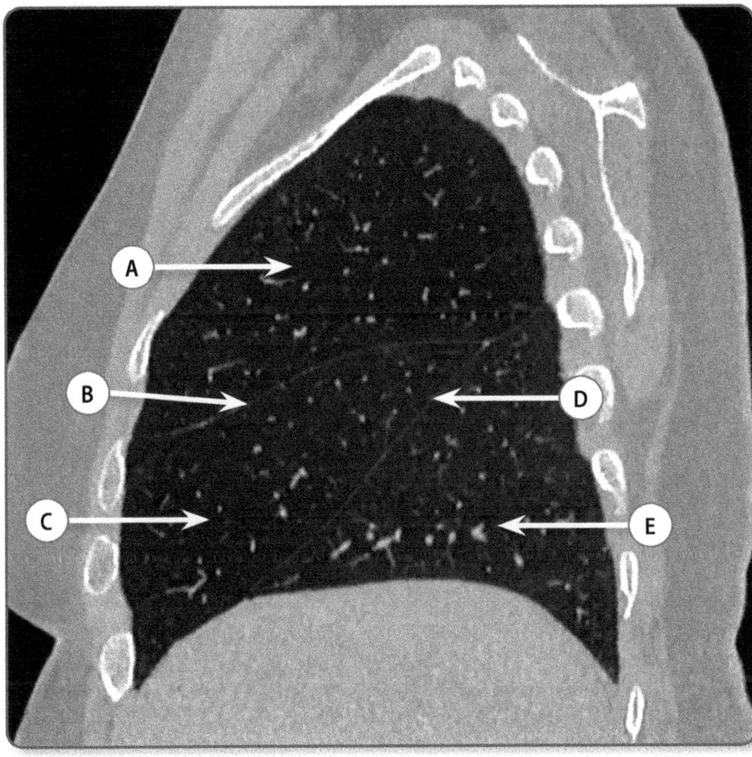

Case 2.24

QUESTION		WRITE YOUR ANSWER HERE
A	Name the structure labelled A.	
B	Name the structure labelled B.	
C	Name the structure labelled C.	
D	Name the structure labelled D.	
E	Name the structure labelled E.	

Case 2.25

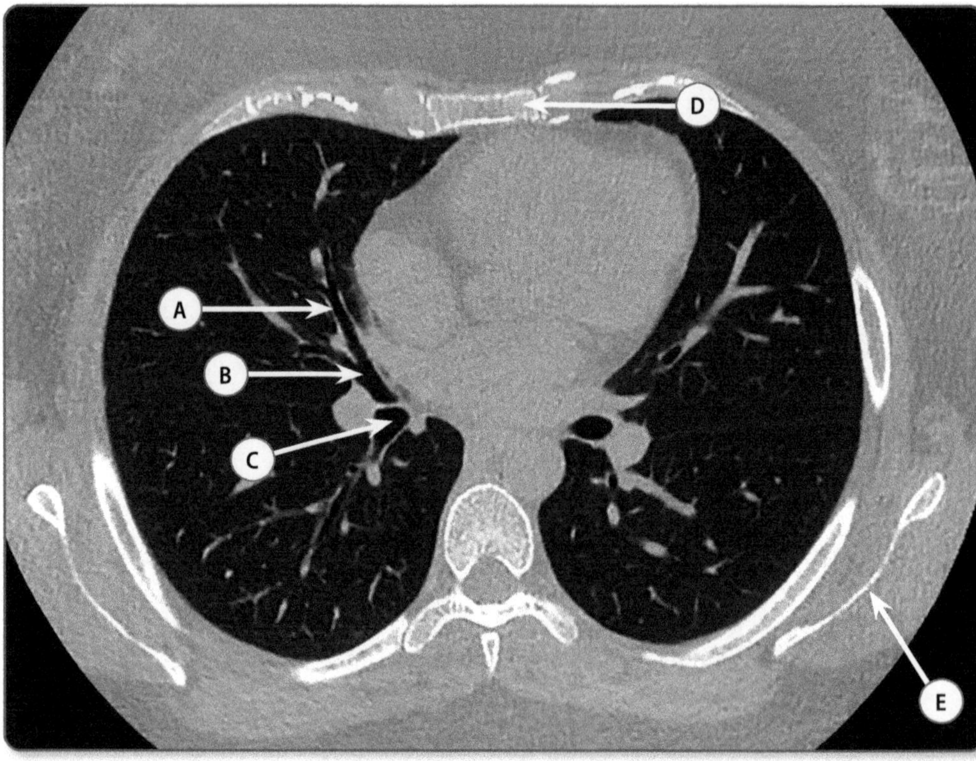

Case 2.25

QUESTION		WRITE YOUR ANSWER HERE
A	Name the structure labelled A.	
B	Name the structure labelled B.	
C	Name the structure labelled C.	
D	Name the structure labelled D.	
E	Name the structure labelled E.	

Chest wall and diaphragm

Case 2.26

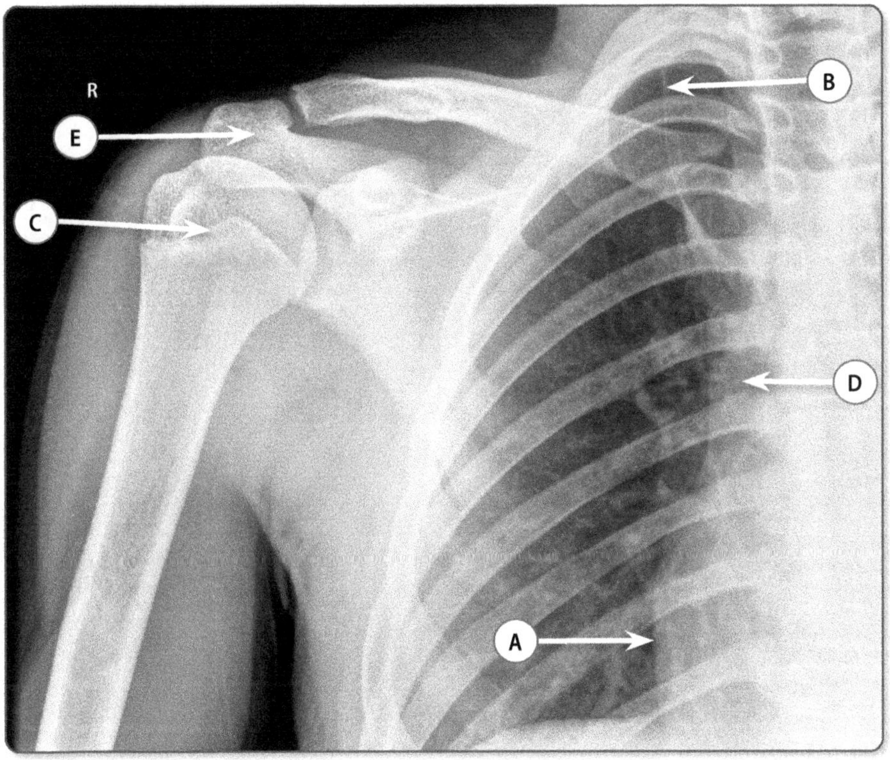

Case 2.26

QUESTION		WRITE YOUR ANSWER HERE
A	Name the structure labelled A.	
B	Name the structure labelled B.	
C	Name the structure labelled C.	
D	Name the structure labelled D.	
E	Name the structure labelled E.	

Case 2.27

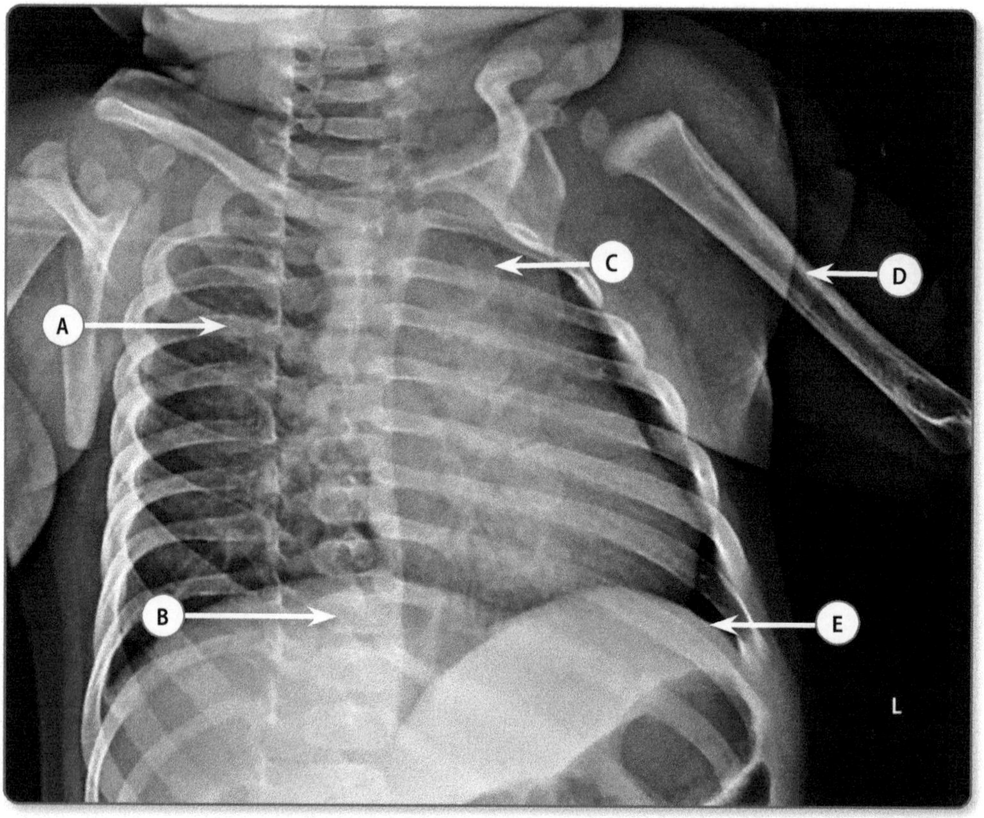

Case 2.27

QUESTION		WRITE YOUR ANSWER HERE
A	Name the structure labelled A.	
B	Name the structure labelled B.	
C	Name the structure labelled C.	
D	Name the structure labelled D.	
E	Name the structure labelled E.	

Case 2.28

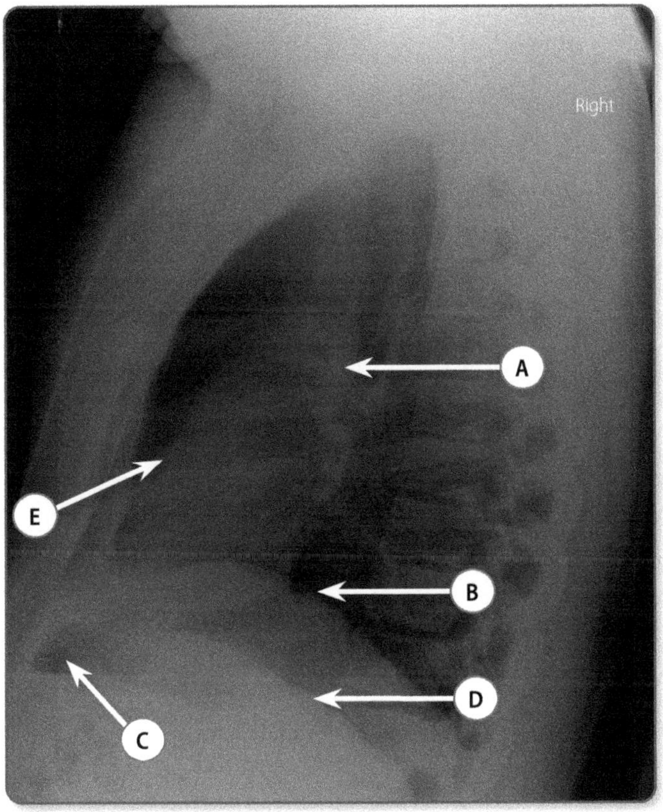

Case 2.28		
QUESTION		WRITE YOUR ANSWER HERE
A	Name the structure labelled A.	
B	Name the structure labelled B.	
C	Name the structure labelled C.	
D	Name the structure labelled D.	
E	Name the structure labelled E.	

Case 2.29

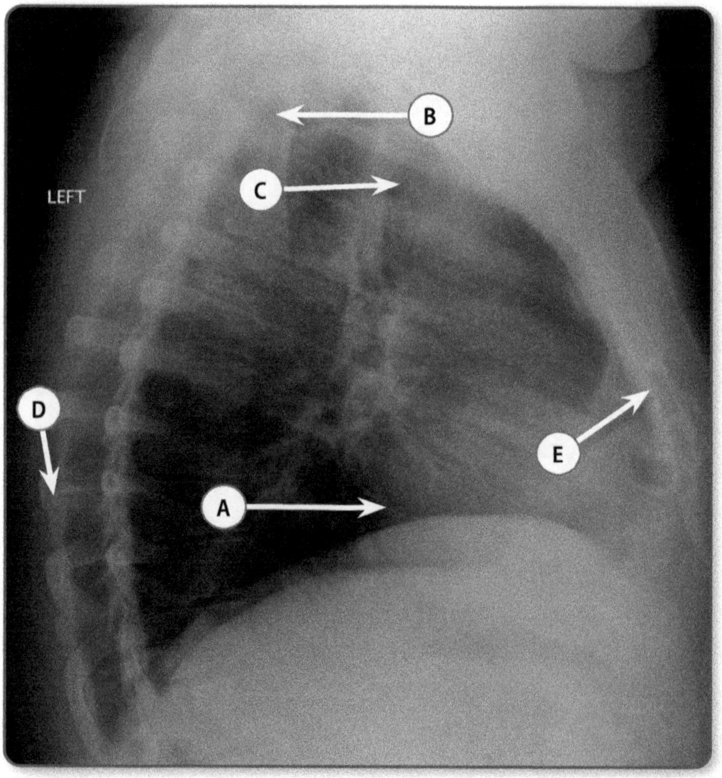

Case 2.29

QUESTION		WRITE YOUR ANSWER HERE
A	Name the structure labelled A.	
B	Name the structure labelled B.	
C	Name the structure labelled C.	
D	Name the structure labelled D.	
E	Name the structure labelled E.	

Case 2.30

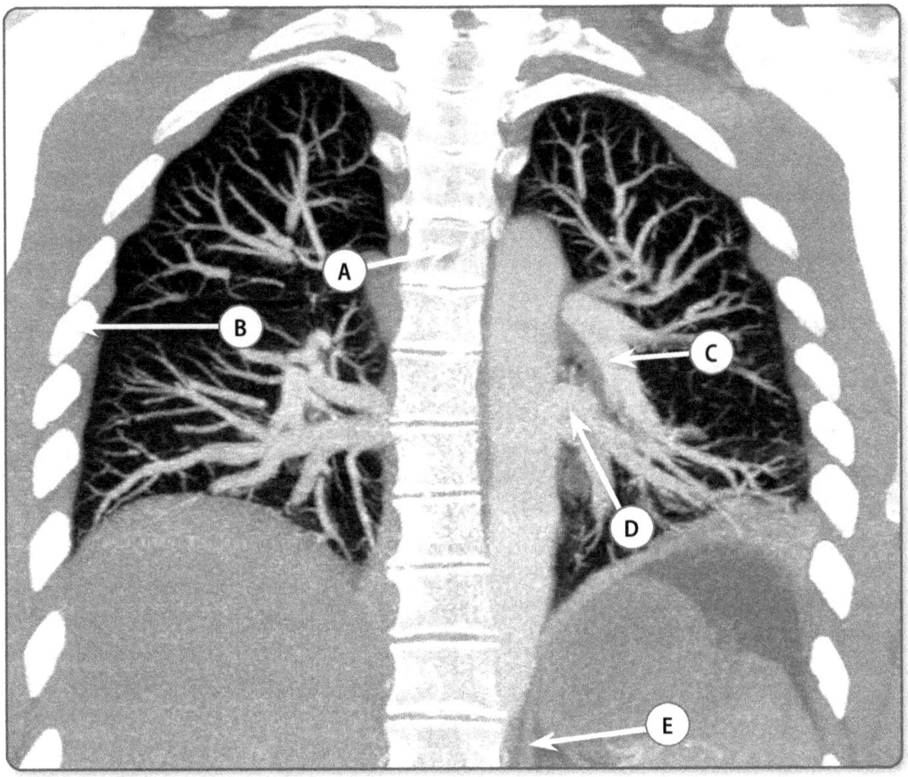

Case 2.30

QUESTION		WRITE YOUR ANSWER HERE
A	Name the structure labelled A.	
B	Name the structure labelled B.	
C	Name the structure labelled C.	
D	Name the structure labelled D.	
E	Name the structure labelled E.	

Case 2.31

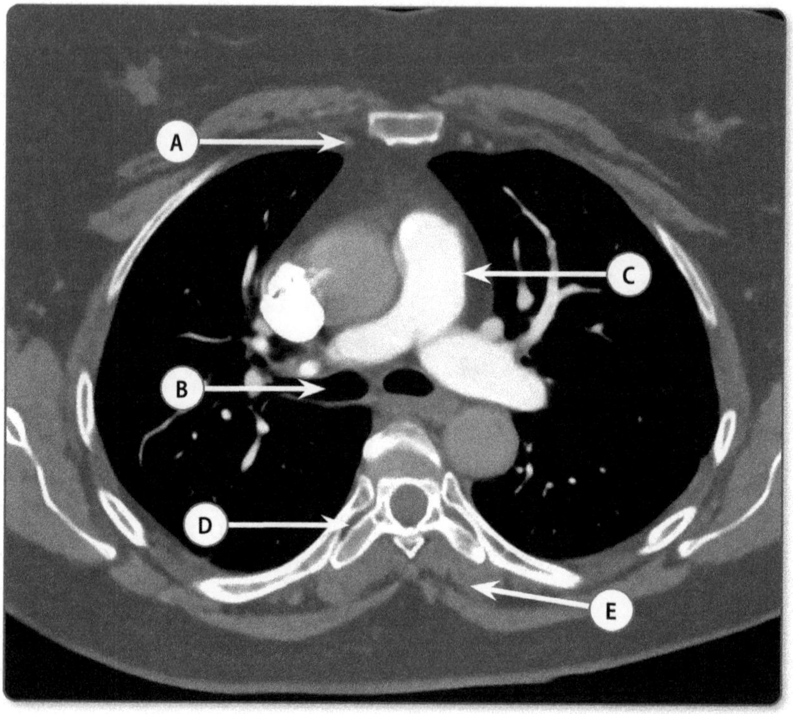

Case 2.31

QUESTION		WRITE YOUR ANSWER HERE
A	Name the structure labelled A.	
B	Name the structure labelled B.	
C	Name the structure labelled C.	
D	Name the structure labelled D.	
E	Name the structure labelled E.	

Case 2.32

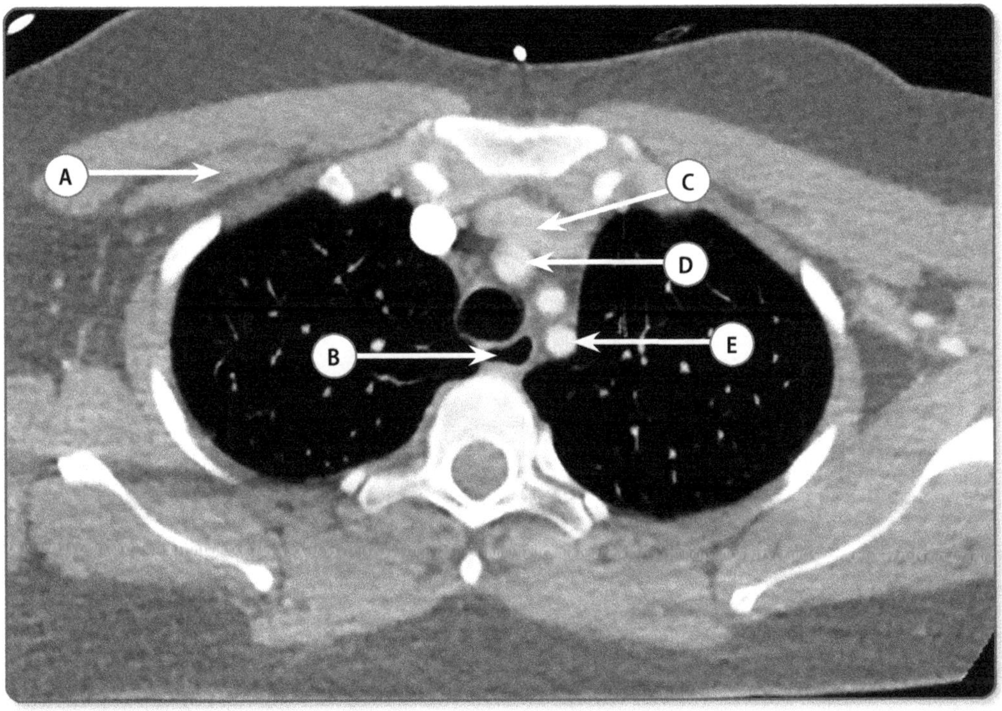

Case 2.32		
QUESTION		WRITE YOUR ANSWER HERE
A	Name the structure labelled A.	
B	Name the structure labelled B.	
C	Name the structure labelled C.	
D	Name the structure labelled D.	
E	Name the structure labelled E.	

Case 2.33

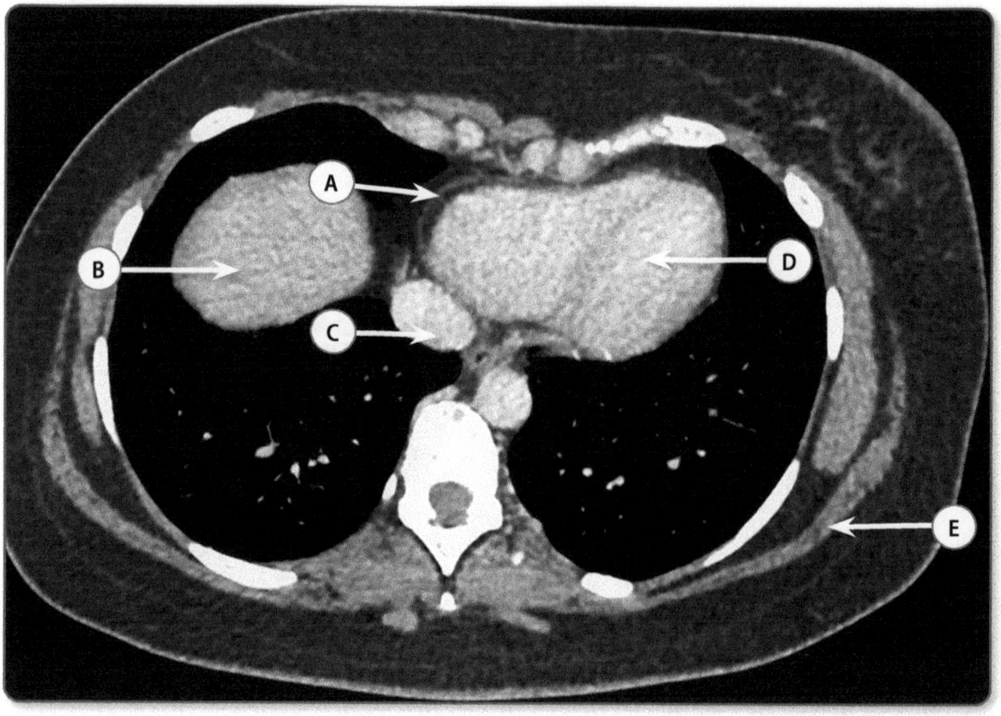

Case 2.33

QUESTION		WRITE YOUR ANSWER HERE
A	Name the structure labelled A.	
B	Name the structure labelled B.	
C	Name the structure labelled C.	
D	Name the structure labelled D.	
E	Name the structure labelled E.	

Case 2.34

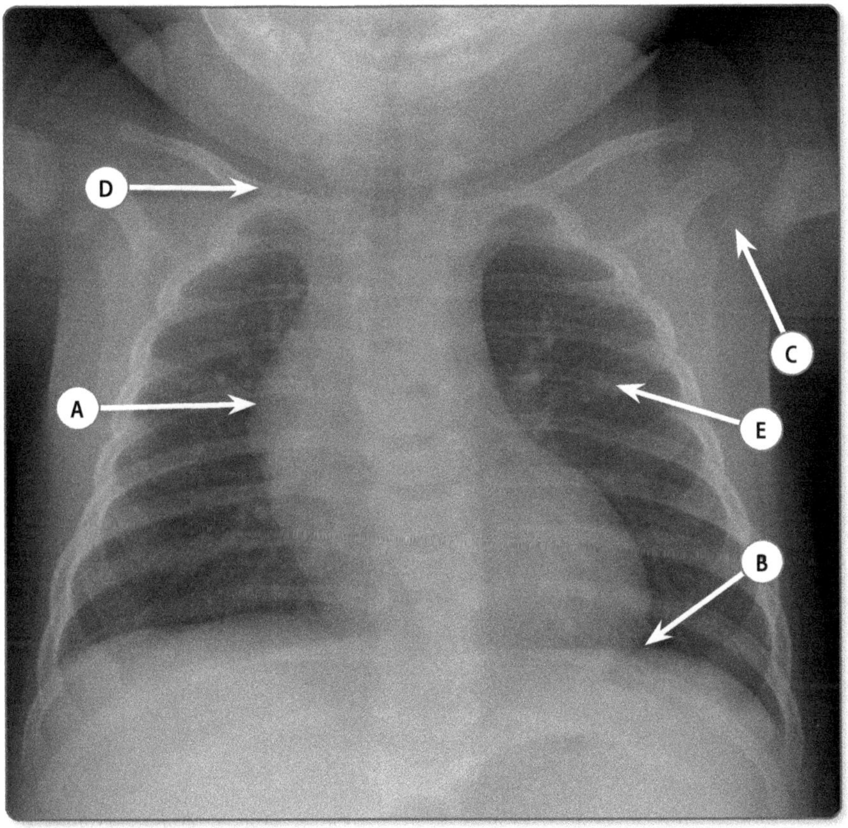

Case 2.34

QUESTION		WRITE YOUR ANSWER HERE
A	Name the structure labelled A.	
B	Name the structure labelled B.	
C	Name the structure labelled C.	
D	Name the structure labelled D.	
E	Name the structure labelled E.	

Breast

Case 2.35

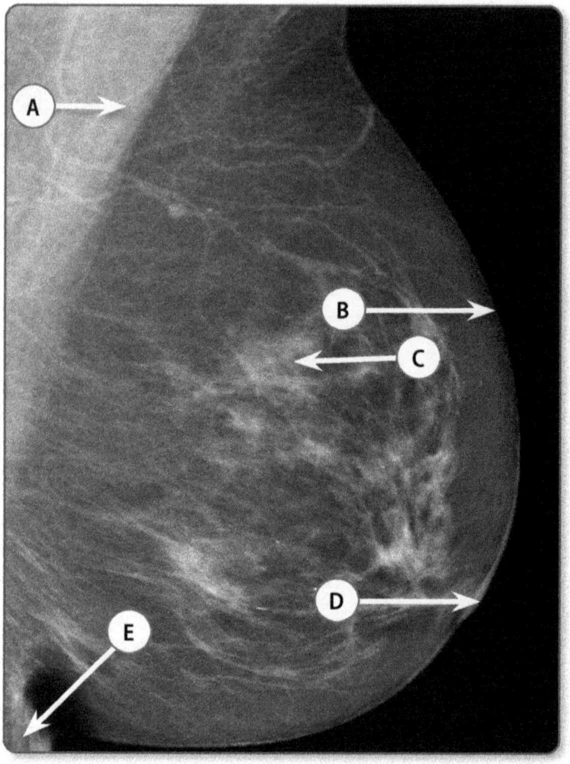

Case 2.35

QUESTION		WRITE YOUR ANSWER HERE
A	Name the structure labelled A.	
B	Name the structure labelled B.	
C	Name the structure labelled C.	
D	Name the structure labelled D.	
E	Name the structure labelled E.	

Answers

Case 2.1

A Right main bronchus

B Right 9th rib

C Aortic arch

D Left ventricle border

E Gastric fundus

Plain frontal chest radiograph.

The trachea bifurcates into the left and right main bronchi at the level of the sternal angle (T5 level; T4 on inspiration, T6 on expiration). The trachea is made of 15–20 incomplete rings of cartilage which are completed posteriorly by the trachealis muscle.

The aortic arch passes posteriorly from right to left to lie just left of T4. It is anterior to the trachea and arches over the left main bronchus and pulmonary artery. Lying to the right are the trachea, oesophagus, thoracic duct and body of T4 from front to back. The ligamentum arteriosum is the fibrous remnant of the ductus arteriosus which is connected to its inferior aspect. The aortic isthmus is the junction of the descending aorta with the arch. This is liable to injury in blunt trauma as it is fixed.

The aortic arch, or aortic knuckle, is seen forming the left upper mediastinal contour and continues as the descending thoracic aorta which can be seen behind the cardiac shadow. The descending aorta is found in the posterior mediastinum. A right-sided aortic arch, or double aortic arch, is sometimes seen as a normal variant. These particular anomalies can create complete vascular rings, and may cause compressive symptoms affecting the trachea and oesophagus.

The right atrium forms the right heart border and the superior and inferior vena cava drain into its superior and inferior parts respectively. The left ventricle forms the left heart border.

In a situs solitus patient, the stomach lies predominantly to the left of the midline, with gastric gas rising to a dependent position in the fundus giving rise to a contained bubble of air below the left hemidiaphragm.

Weir J, Abrahams P. Imaging Atlas of Human Anatomy, 4th edition. Edinburgh: Mosby, 2010:90.

Ryan S, McNicholas M, Eustace SJ. Anatomy for Diagnostic Imaging, 3rd edition. Edinburgh: Saunders, 2010:120.

Weber E, Netter FH, Vilensky JA, Carmichael SW. Netter's Concise Radiologic Anatomy. Philadelphia: Saunders/Elsevier, 2009:183.

Case 2.2

A Right common carotid artery

B Brachiocephalic trunk

C Left subclavian artery

D Left internal thoracic artery/left internal mammary artery

E Descending thoracic aorta

MRI aortic angiogram.

The aortic arch begins at the origin of the brachiocephalic trunk. The branch vessels that arise from the aortic arch are, in order:

- Brachiocephalic trunk
- Left common carotid artery
- Left subclavian artery

The brachiocephalic trunk bifurcates into the right subclavian and right common carotid arteries. From the subclavian arteries arise the internal thoracic or internal mammary arteries.

The most common variation in the anatomy of the aortic arch vessels is a common origin of the brachiocephalic trunk and the left common carotid, or so-called bovine arch (20%). In 6%, the left vertebral artery arises directly from the arch, instead of the left subclavian. An anomalous right subclavian artery is another variant, whereby the right subclavian originates as the last of the arch vessels, and takes a retro-oesophageal course as it traverses from left to right. This can cause symptoms of dysphagia, and can be seen on a barium swallow as a persistent indentation posteriorly.

The aortic arch ends, and the descending thoracic aorta begins immediately distal to the left subclavian artery. At this point, the ligamentum venosum (remnant of the ductus arteriosus) joins the lower border of the arch to the main pulmonary artery. The aorta is fixed at this point.

Weir J, Abrahams P. Imaging Atlas of Human Anatomy, 4th edition. Edinburgh: Mosby, 2010:101–103.

Ryan S, McNicholas M, Eustace SJ. Anatomy for Diagnostic Imaging, 3rd edition. Edinburgh: Saunders, 2010:142.

Layton KF. Bovine aortic arch variant in humans: clarification of a common misnomer. Am J Neuroradiol 2006; 27:1541–1542.

Case 2.3

A Left subclavian artery

B Left pulmonary artery

C Ascending thoracic aorta

D Left atrium

E Left common carotid artery

Sagittal thoracic MRI.

Blood can appear 'black' or 'bright' on MRI, depending on which sequence is used. Standard gradient echo sequences will give a 'bright blood' picture. This is a parasagittal section, on a spin echo MRI sequence, on which blood appears 'black'. Spin echo sequences show 'black blood' because of high velocity signal loss. This occurs due to the 180° pulse. Blood which receives the 90° pulse moves out of the slice before the 180° pulse is applied. This means that the blood produces no signal.

The three main branch vessels can be seen arising from the aortic arch as it passes from anterior to posterior. The brachiocephalic trunk arises first, anteriorly, and the left subclavian last, the most posterior. The descending aorta is located in the posterior mediastinum, to the left of midline.

Posterior to the left main pulmonary artery on this section, is the left main bronchus (which also appears dark, as it is filled with air). As the left main pulmonary artery courses laterally, it comes to lie on top of the left main bronchus, which is why the left hilum is higher than the right on a frontal chest radiograph.

The left atrium is the most posterior of the cardiac chambers, as seen on this parasagittal section.

Kagetsu NJ. Flow. http://www.revisemri.com/questions/pulse_sequences/black_blood_bright_blood. (Last accessed 8 April 2024).

Case 2.4

A Brachiocephalic trunk

B Superior vena cava

C Right atrium

D Left common carotid artery

E Left subclavian artery

Coronal maximum intensity projection of a CT pulmonary angiogram.

Variations in the pattern of branching of the aortic arch are common, such that only 65% of people have a 'normal' branching pattern. 2.7% of people have a common origin of the left subclavian and common carotid arteries, to form a left-sided brachiocephalic trunk. This gives a symmetrical appearance to the aortic branches. The right common carotid is seen to arise in its normal position from a standard right-sided brachiocephalic trunk.

Weir J, Abrahams P. Imaging Atlas of Human Anatomy, 4th edition. Edinburgh: Mosby, 2010:140–144.

Ryan S, McNicholas M, Eustace SJ. Anatomy for Diagnostic Imaging, 3rd edition. Edinburgh: Saunders, 2010:117.

Case 2.5

A Right upper lobe pulmonary artery

B Right main pulmonary artery

C Left main pulmonary artery

D Left superior pulmonary vein

E Gastric fundus

Coronal maximum intensity projection from a thorax CT.

The main pulmonary artery arises from the right ventricle, and travels superiorly and posteriorly. It starts off anterior to the aorta, before coming to lie to its left. At the level of T5, it bifurcates into the left and right main pulmonary arteries.

The left main pulmonary artery runs superoposteriorly, and arches over the left main bronchus before entering the hilum. At this point, it branches into its lobar branches.

The right pulmonary artery branches from the main pulmonary trunk at 90°, and passes behind the superior vena cava and ascending aorta, anterior to the right main bronchus. The right main pulmonary artery divides into upper lobe and interlobar branches.

There are four main pulmonary veins which drain into the left atrium; the right and left, superior and inferior pulmonary veins. In the upper zones, the veins lie inferolateral to the arteries, and in the lower zones the veins have quite a horizontal course, compared to the arteries which are much more vertical.

The pulmonary vasculature makes up the hilar point, which can be seen on a frontal chest radiograph. Remember, the hilar point is where the superior pulmonary vein crosses the interlobar pulmonary artery.

Weir J, Abrahams P. Imaging Atlas of Human Anatomy, 4th edition. Edinburgh: Mosby, 2010:110–111.

Ryan S, McNicholas M, Eustace SJ. Anatomy for Diagnostic Imaging, 3rd edition. Edinburgh: Saunders, 2010:128–130.

Case 2.6

A Right upper lobe pulmonary artery

B Left atrium

C Aorta

D Left superior pulmonary vein

E Left atrial appendage

Coronal CT angiogram aorta MIP through the left atrium.

The right pulmonary artery can be easily identified as it arises from the pulmonary trunk. It passes in front of the right main bronchus and behind the ascending aorta (not seen here). After the origin of the right upper lobe pulmonary artery, it becomes the interlobar artery from which the middle and lower lobe branches arise. The arterial branching follows the segmental branching pattern of the airways.

The left atrial appendage serves to increase the capacity of the left atrium, and may be the source of emboli in atrial fibrillation.

Weir J, Abrahams P. Imaging Atlas of Human Anatomy, 4th edition. Edinburgh: Mosby, 2010:100–103.

Ryan S, McNicholas M, Eustace SJ. Anatomy for Diagnostic Imaging, 3rd edition. Edinburgh: Saunders, 2010:122–125.

Weber E, Netter FH, Vilensky JA, Carmichael SW. Netter's Concise Radiologic Anatomy. Philadelphia: Saunders/Elsevier, 2009:177.

Case 2.7

A Left spine of scapula

B Left upper lobe

C Left oblique fissure

D Right ventricle

E Interventricular septum

A left parasagittal CT of the thorax through the right and left ventricles of the heart.

The left oblique fissure extends from about T4/T5 posteriorly to the diaphragm anteriorly. This is similar in both left and right lungs.

The right ventricle is the most anterior chamber of the heart. It is crescent-shaped, and has a thinner wall than the larger, more muscular left ventricle. The left ventricle is large and under higher pressure, therefore producing a bulge into the right ventricle, giving it this crescent shape. Inflow is from the right atrium via the tricuspid valve (three leaflets). Outflow is into the pulmonary artery via the pulmonary valve.

The muscular interventricular septum lies between the two ventricles and bulges into the right ventricle, giving the right ventricle its crescent shape and the left ventricle its circular shape.

Weir J, Abrahams P. Imaging Atlas of Human Anatomy, 4th edition. Edinburgh: Mosby, 2010:104–107.

Ryan S, McNicholas M, Eustace SJ. Anatomy for Diagnostic Imaging, 3rd edition. Edinburgh: Saunders, 2010:134.

Case 2.8

A Left lobe of the thyroid

B Trachea

C Brachiocephalic trunk

D Right axillary artery

E Left subclavian artery

Coronal CT of the thorax through the arch of the aorta.

The ascending aorta begins at the aortic valve which lies at the level of the 2nd costal cartilage. The arch of the aorta passes posteriorly and from right to left.

The subclavian artery becomes the axillary artery at the lateral margin of the first rib. It becomes the brachial artery at the lower aspect of teres major. It provides branches to the lateral thorax and upper limb.

This configuration is only seen in 65% of people as variation is common:

- In 5%, the vertebral artery arises directly from the arch of the aorta, between the left common carotid and left subclavian artery. This leads to four vessels arising from the aorta instead of three

- In 2.7%, there is a common origin of the left common carotid and subclavian arteries (left brachiocephalic artery)
- In 2.5%, the left common carotid artery arises from the brachiocephalic artery
- In 0.5%, there is an aberrant right subclavian artery which arises distal to the left subclavian. It passes to the right passing behind the oesophagus

You should make sure that you have seen images of these variants prior to the examination.

Weir J, Abrahams P. Imaging Atlas of Human Anatomy, 4th edition. Edinburgh: Mosby, 2010:117.

Ryan S, McNicholas M, Eustace SJ. Anatomy for Diagnostic Imaging, 3rd edition. Edinburgh: Saunders, 2010:140–144.

Weber E, Netter FH, Vilensky JA, Carmichael SW. Netter's Concise Radiologic Anatomy. Philadelphia: Saunders/Elsevier, 2008:183.

Case 2.9

A Sternum

B Right ventricle

C Right atrium

D Interventricular septum

E Non-coronary (or right posterior) sinus of the aorta

Axial CT through the heart and aortic valve.

It is important to be able to identify the chambers of the heart both on coronal and axial images.

The right ventricle forms most of the sternocostal surface of the heart. The cavities of the right and left ventricles are separated by the interventricular septum. The cavity of the right ventricle is crescentic in cross-section because the interventricular septum bulges into it.

The aortic valve has three cusps. Above each cusp is a localised dilatation or sinus (sinuses of Valsalva). The right coronary artery arises from the anterior sinus (also known as the right coronary sinus). The left coronary artery arises from the left posterior sinus (also known as the left coronary sinus). No artery arises from the right posterior sinus (also known as the non-coronary sinus).

A tip to help orientate yourself to the sinuses in the axial place, the non-coronary sinus is the one that lies adjacent to the inter-atrial septum in individuals with normal anatomy.

The interventricular septum is a thick muscular septum separating the left and right ventricles. It bulges into the right ventricle due to the increased pressure in the left ventricle.

Weir J, Abrahams P. Imaging Atlas of Human Anatomy, 4th edition. Edinburgh: Mosby, 2010:99.

Ryan S, McNicholas M, Eustace SJ. Anatomy for Diagnostic Imaging, 3rd edition. Edinburgh: Saunders, 2010:139.

Case 2.10

A Thoracic vertebral body

B Apex of heart/left ventricular apex

C Papillary muscle

D Anterior cusp of mitral/bicuspid valve

E Right inferior pulmonary vein

Axial CT of the heart.

The papillary muscles of the heart can be appreciated on CT, particularly on a cardiac gated image. These muscles are located in the ventricles, and act to tether the atrioventricular valves by the chordae tendinae. The chordae are attached to the valve cusps, and prevent them prolapsing during systole, and preventing regurgitation of blood into the atrium. In the left ventricle, there are two papillary muscles, an anterior and a posterior one. The right ventricle contains three papillary muscles: the anterior, posterior and septal.

The bicuspid mitral valve separates the left atrium and left ventricle. The right pulmonary vein drains oxygenated blood from the lungs into the left atrium.

Weir J, Abrahams P. Imaging Atlas of Human Anatomy, 4th edition. Edinburgh: Mosby, 2010:99.

Ryan S, McNicholas M, Eustace SJ. Anatomy for Diagnostic Imaging, 3rd edition. Edinburgh: Saunders, 2010:139.

Weber E, Netter FH, Vilensky JA, Carmichael SW. Netter's Concise Radiologic Anatomy. Philadelphia: Saunders/Elsevier, 2009:191.

Case 2.11

A Right atrium

B Oesophagus

C Azygous vein

D Left atrium

E Left superior pulmonary vein

Axial CT pulmonary angiogram.

The right atrium receives deoxygenated blood from the superior vena cava (SVC), inferior vena cava (IVC) and coronary sinus through its smooth posterior wall. The SVC drains superiorly at the level of the right third costal cartilage. The IVC drains at the level of the right fifth costal cartilage. The coronary sinus opens in between the right atrioventricular orifice and the IVC opening.

The anterior wall is rough and composed of pectinate muscular ridges. These ridges are continuous with the right atrial appendage/auricle which overlies the aorta and serves to increase the capacity of the right atrium. The interatrial septum has a depression, the fossa ovalis, the remnant of the foramen ovale which allows a right to left shunt during fetal circulation.

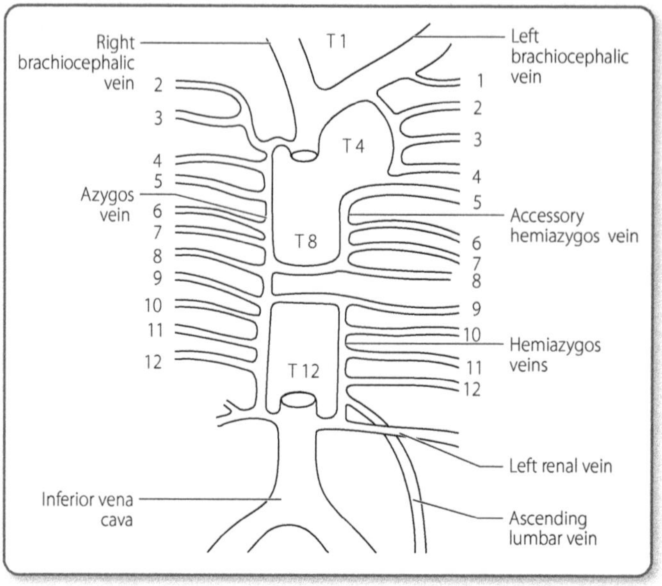

Figure 2.1 The azygos system.

The azygos system of veins lies on either side of the vertebral column in the posterior mediastinum and drains the mediastinal organs, thoracic and abdominal walls, and the back. Its course and anatomy are variable.

The azygos begins at the level of L2 as a branch of the IVC, or as a confluence of lumbar and subcostal veins. It enters the thorax behind the right crus of the diaphragm, and lies to the right of the aorta and thoracic duct. The azygos enters the SVC by arching over the right hilum from the posterior mediastinum.

The azygos receives blood from most of the intercostal veins on the right, as displayed in the diagram above. The hemiazygos and accessory hemiazygos receive blood from most of the intercostal veins on the left, and drain into the azygos at the midthoracic level.

The hemiazygos often begins at the left renal vein, and ascends into the thorax on the left side of the aorta. These structures are shown in **Figure 2.1**.

Moore KL, Dalley AF, Agur AMR. Clinically Oriented Anatomy, 6th edition. Philadelphia: Lippincott Williams & Wilkins, 2009:135–165.

Weir J, Abrahams P. Imaging Atlas of Human Anatomy, 4th edition. Edinburgh: Mosby, 2010:99.

Ryan S, McNicholas M, Eustace SJ. Anatomy for Diagnostic Imaging, 3rd edition. Edinburgh: Saunders, 2010:132–135.

Case 2.12

A Left main stem coronary artery

B Circumflex

C First obtuse marginal branch

D Septal branch

E Left anterior descending

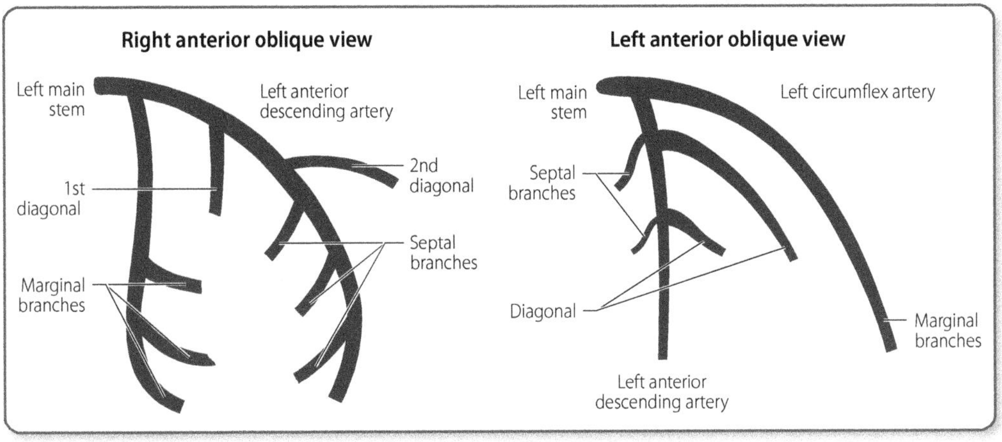

Figure 2.2 The left coronary artery.

Conventional coronary angiogram, right anterior oblique. Selective catheterisation of left main stem.

The left coronary artery (LCA) arises as the left main stem from the posterior sinus of Valsalva/left coronary sinus, and travels between the left atrial appendage and the pulmonary trunk in the left atrioventricular groove. It bifurcates early into the left anterior descending artery (LAD), which continues in the interventricular groove, and the left circumflex which continues laterally in the atrioventricular groove.

The LAD travels over the anterior aspect of the heart in the interventricular groove, it turns around the inferior border to anastomose with the posterior descending branch of the right coronary artery. The LAD gives off septal and diagonal branches.

The left circumflex travels down the posterior aspect of the heart and gives off obtuse marginal and atrial branches **(Figure 2.2)**.

The LCA supplies:

- The left atrium
- Most of the left ventricle
- Part of the right ventricle
- Most of the interventricular septum, including the bundle of His
- The sinoatrial node (in 40% of people)

Moore KL, Dalley AF, Agur AMR. Clinically Oriented Anatomy, 6th edition. Philadelphia: Lippincott Williams & Wilkins, 2009:135–165.

Weir J, Abrahams P. Imaging Atlas of Human Anatomy, 4th edition. Edinburgh: Mosby, 2010:113.

Ryan S, McNicholas M, Eustace SJ. Anatomy for Diagnostic Imaging, 3rd edition. Edinburgh: Saunders, 2010:135.

Case 2.13

A Right coronary artery

B Posterolateral branch

C Right ventricular branch

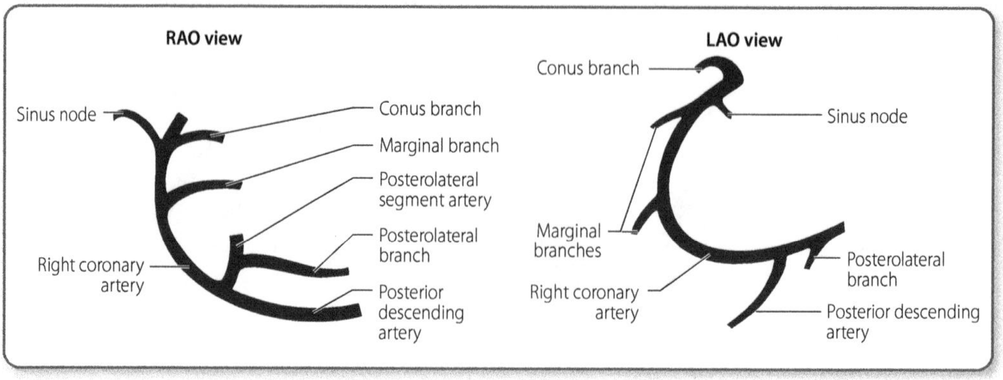

Figure 2.3 The right coronary artery.

D Atrioventricular nodal artery

E Posterior descending artery

Conventional coronary angiogram, left anterior oblique. Selective catheterisation of right coronary artery.

The right coronary artery (RCA) arises from the anterior sinus of Valsalva/right coronary sinus and travels between the right atrium and pulmonary trunk in the right atrioventricular groove. The sinoatrial nodal branch, given off near the origin of the RCA, supplies the sinoatrial node. The marginal branch supplies the right border of the heart. The RCA continues to the posterior aspect of the heart where it gives off the posterior descending artery (PDA). The dominance of the coronary system is defined by which coronary supplies the PDA **(Figure 2.3)**.

The RCA supplies:

- The right atrium
- Most of the right ventricle
- The diaphragmatic surface of the left ventricle
- Part of the atrioventricular septum
- The sinoatrial node (in 60% of people)
- The atrioventricular node (in 80% of people)

Moore KL, Dalley AF, Agur AMR. Clinically Oriented Anatomy, 6th edition. Philadelphia: Lippincott Williams & Wilkins, 2009:135–165.

Weir J, Abrahams P. Imaging Atlas of Human Anatomy, 4th edition. Edinburgh: Mosby, 2010:113.

Ryan S, McNicholas M, Eustace SJ. Anatomy for Diagnostic Imaging, 3rd edition. Edinburgh: Saunders, 2010:135.

Case 2.14

A Right subclavian artery

B Brachiocephalic artery

C Right vertebral artery

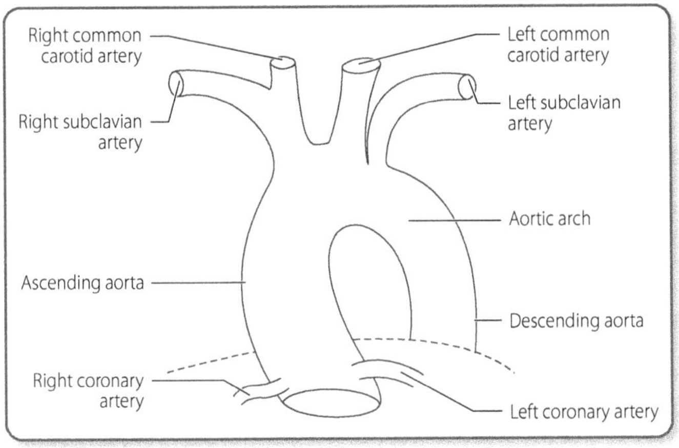

Figure 2.4 Branches of the arch of the aorta.

D Left common carotid artery

E Left subclavian artery

Digital subtraction arch aortogram.

The common pattern for the branches of the arch of the aorta (**Figure 2.4**) is:

- Brachiocephalic trunk, which gives off the right subclavian and right common carotid arteries
- Left common carotid artery
- Left subclavian artery

Moore KL, Dalley AF, Agur AMR. Clinically Oriented Anatomy, 6th edition. Philadelphia: Lippincott Williams & Wilkins, 2009:94.

Weir J, Abrahams P. Imaging Atlas of Human Anatomy, 4th edition. Edinburgh: Mosby, 2010:117.

Case 2.15

A Right internal mammary/thoracic artery

B Thymus

C Ascending aorta

D Main pulmonary artery

E Left main bronchus

Axial arterial phase CT chest in a paediatric patient.

The internal mammary/thoracic arteries originate from the subclavian arteries, and enter the thorax behind the clavicle and first costal cartilage. They run along the inside of the thoracic wall just lateral to the sternum, to the sixth intercostal space where they divide into the superior epigastric and musculophrenic arteries.

The thymus is a soft structure of the lymphatic system which sits in the anterior mediastinum. It has left and right lobes, and on CT it is a homogenous soft-tissue density.

The thymus normally involutes by around age 8, but may be seen as a small remnant of anterior mediastinal soft tissue on CT in adults.

Moore KL, Dalley AF, Agur AMR. Clinically Oriented Anatomy, 6th edition. Philadelphia: Lippincott Williams & Wilkins, 2009:135–165.

Weir J, Abrahams P. Imaging Atlas of Human Anatomy, 4th edition. Edinburgh: Mosby, 2010:99.

Case 2.16

A Left atrium

B Posterior leaflet of the mitral vale

C Fundus of the stomach

D Aortic valve

E Left ventricle

Three-chamber view gated cardiac CT.

This view includes the left atrium, left ventricle and the proximal aorta as its 'three chambers'. It is also known as the left ventricular outflow tract view, as is reformatted into a plane which includes the left ventricle apex and both the mitral and aortic valves.

The mitral valve is also known at the bicuspid valve, as it has two leaflets–anterior and posterior. In this image, although off axis for the usual axial plane, the vertebral body and sternum can still be seen, helping to orientate which is the anterior leaflet and which is posterior.

Case 2.17

A Thyrocervical trunk

B Catheter in left subclavian artery

C Ascending cervical artery

D Left vertebral artery

E Left internal thoracic artery

Selective catheterisation and angiogram of the left subclavian artery.

The branches of the subclavian artery (shown in **Figure 2.5**) can be recalled with the mnemonic VITamin C and D.

The first part (from origin to medial border of scalenus anterior):

- *Vertebral artery:* Runs in the foramen transversarium of the vertebra to supply the posterior circulation of the brain
- *Internal thoracic artery:* Runs along the inside of the thoracic cage
- *Thyrocervical trunk:* It is short in length and quickly divides into inferior thyroid, suprascapular and transverse cervical arteries

The second part (posterior to scalenus anterior):

- *Costocervical trunk:* Divides into superior intercostal and deep cervical arteries

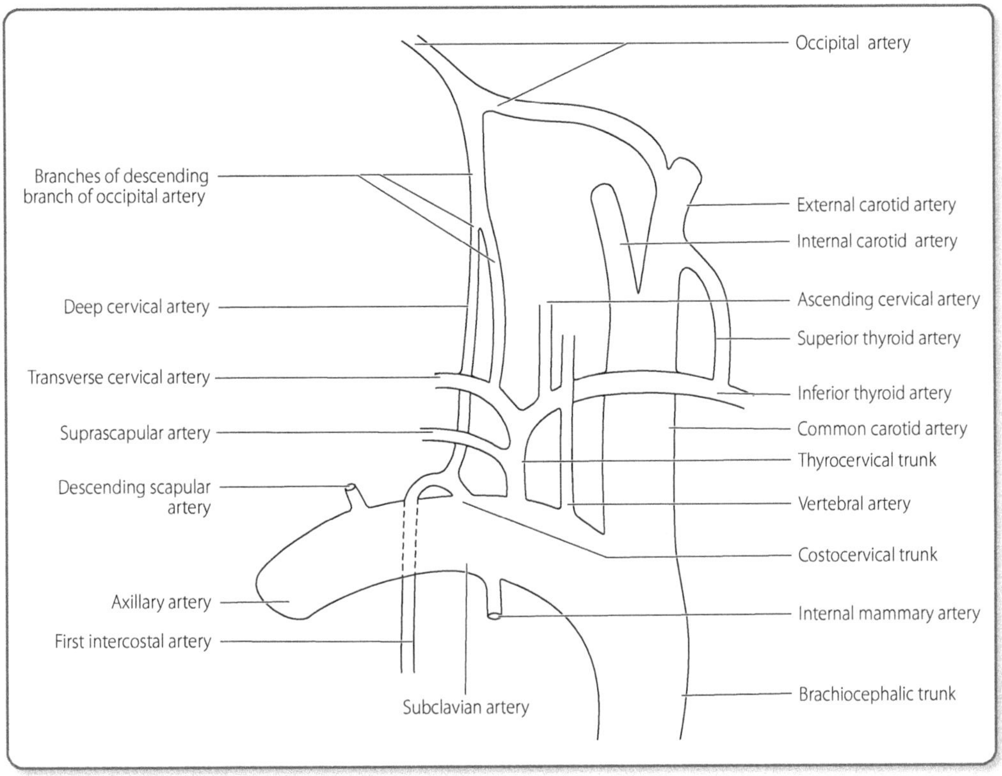

Figure 2.5 Branches of the subclavian artery.

The third part (between scalenus anterior and first rib):

- Dorsal scapular artery, which may also originate from the second part of subclavian. This supplies the levator scapulae and rhomboid muscles

Moore KL, Dalley AF, Agur AMR. Clinically Oriented Anatomy, 6th edition. Philadelphia: Lippincott Williams & Wilkins, 2009:1003.

Weir J, Abrahams P. Imaging Atlas of Human Anatomy, 4th edition. Edinburgh: Mosby, 2010:33.

Case 2.18

A Brachiocephalic artery

B Left common carotid artery

C Left subclavian artery

D Coeliac axis

E Superior mesenteric artery

MR angiogram.

An MR angiogram showing the great vessels of the aorta. The first two unpaired abdominal aortic branches are the coeliac axis and the superior mesenteric artery.

Ryan S, McNicholas M, Eustace SJ. Anatomy for Diagnostic Imaging, 3rd edition. Edinburgh: Saunders, 2010:142.

Case 2.19

A Sternum

B Right coronary artery

C Anterior sinus of Valsalva/right aortic sinus

D Left atrium

E Left inferior pulmonary artery

Axial CT of the chest.

The sternum consists of three fused bones: manubrium, body of sternum and xiphoid process. Superiorly, the junction of the manubrium with the body of sternum is called the 'Angle of Louis'. This is at the level of T4/T5, where the second rib articulates. This is the same level as the aortic arch and the carina.

The right coronary artery (RCA) arises from the anterior sinus of Valsalva/right aortic sinus and travels between the right atrium and pulmonary trunk in the right atrioventricular groove. The RCA supplies:

- The right atrium
- Most of the right ventricle
- The diaphragmatic surface of the left ventricle
- Part of the atrioventricular septum
- The sinoatrial node (in 60% of people)
- The atrioventricular node (in 80% of people)

The left main pulmonary artery runs superoposteriorly, and arches over the left main bronchus before entering the hilum. At this point, it branches into its lobar branches.

Moore KL, Dalley AF, Agur AMR. Clinically Oriented Anatomy, 6th edition. Philadelphia: Lippincott Williams & Wilkins, 2009:135–165.

Weir J, Abrahams P. Imaging Atlas of Human Anatomy, 4th edition. Edinburgh: Mosby, 2010:99.

Ryan S, McNicholas M, Eustace SJ. Anatomy for Diagnostic Imaging, 3rd edition. Edinburgh: Saunders, 2010:139.

Case 2.20

A Trachea

B Right upper lobe bronchus

C Bronchus intermedius

D Left clavicle

E Carina

Coronal reformatted CT of the thorax.

The trachea begins at C6 level at the lower border of the cricoid cartilage. The trachea is approximately 15 cm long, 2 cm in diameter, and made of 15–20 incomplete rings of cartilage which are completed posteriorly by the trachealis muscle. The lower trachea is supplied by branches of the bronchial artery. The upper trachea is supplied by the inferior thyroid artery. The arch of the aorta may indent the left side of the trachea just above the carina.

Weir J, Abrahams P. Imaging Atlas of Human Anatomy, 4th edition. Edinburgh: Mosby, 2010:102.

Ryan S, McNicholas M, Eustace SJ. Anatomy for Diagnostic Imaging, 3rd edition. Edinburgh: Saunders, 2010:122–125.

Case 2.21

A Horizontal fissure

B Middle lobe bronchus

C Oblique fissure

D Right lower lobe bronchus

E Left lower lobe bronchus

High-resolution CT (HRCT).

The fissures are well demonstrated on HRCT. The oblique fissures appear as:

- Thin curvilinear lines which are concaved anteriorly in the upper thorax
- Flat lines in the midthorax
- Convex anterior lines in the lower chest

The horizontal fissure is seen as an avascular zone in the midthorax (**Figure 2.6**).

Ryan S, McNicholas M, Eustace SJ. Anatomy for Diagnostic Imaging, 3rd edition. Edinburgh: Saunders, 2010:122.

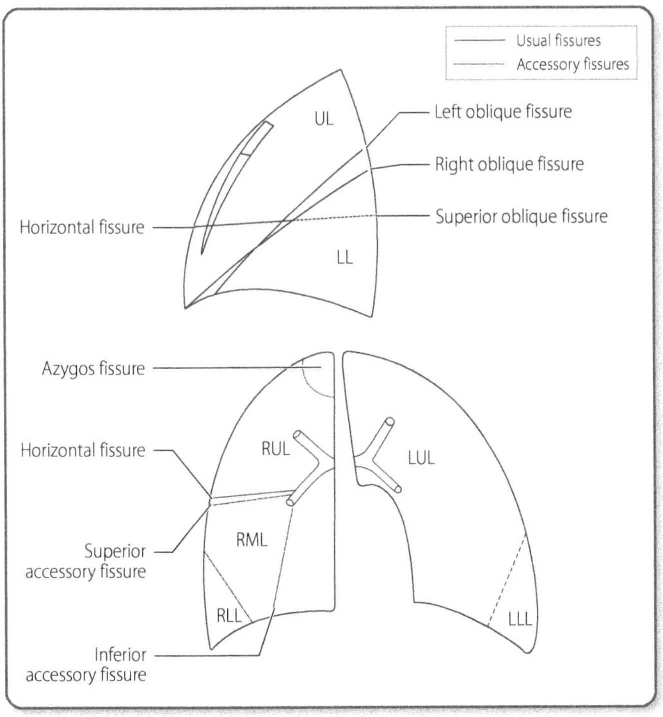

Figure 2.6 The pulmonary lobes and fissures. UL, upper lobe; ML, middle lobe; LL, lower lobe; RUL, right upper lobe; RML, right middle lobe; RLL, right lower lobe; LUL, left upper lobe; LLL, left lower lobe.

Case 2.22

A Paratracheal stripe

B Right hilar point

C Right costophrenic angle

D Left coracoid process

E Descending thoracic aorta

Chest radiograph.

The paratracheal stripe is normally <3–4 mm wide and formed by the pleura in contact with the right lateral wall of the trachea. The pleura is in contact with the trachea from the clavicles down to the azygous vein at the right tracheobronchial angle. The left lateral wall of the trachea is not normally distinguishable from the mediastinum.

The left coracoid process projects anteriorly from the upper border of the neck of the scapula.

Most lung markings are due to vessels. The hilar point is where the superior pulmonary vein crosses the descending pulmonary artery. The right is 1 cm lower than the left, and is projected over the sixth posterior interspace. The angle between the vessels at the hilar point (hilar angle) is normally 120°.

Weir J, Abrahams P. Imaging Atlas of Human Anatomy, 4th edition. Edinburgh: Mosby, 2010:90.

Ryan S, McNicholas M, Eustace SJ. Anatomy for Diagnostic Imaging, 3rd edition. Edinburgh: Saunders, 2010:120.

Weber E, Netter FH, Vilensky JA, Carmichael SW. Netter's Concise Radiologic Anatomy. Philadelphia: Saunders/Elsevier, 2009:183.

Case 2.23

A Left upper lobe

B Left lower lobe

C Left oblique fissure

D Left anterior hemidiaphragm

E Stomach with gastric contents

Sagittal reformatted high-resolution CT.

The left upper lobe is anterior and superior to the left lower lobe. The left oblique fissure separates the two lobes, and travels from T4/T5 posteriorly to the diaphragm anteroinferiorly.

The stomach is situated just inferior to the left hemidiaphragm, which is demonstrated well here.

Ryan S, McNicholas M, Eustace SJ. Anatomy for Diagnostic Imaging, 3rd edition. Edinburgh: Saunders, 2010:125–126.

Case 2.24

A Right upper lobe

B Horizontal fissure

C Middle lobe

D Right oblique fissure

E Right lower lobe

Sagittal reformatted high-resolution CT.

The right upper lobe is superior and anterior. The middle lobe sits anterior and inferior, and the right lower lobe sites posterior and inferior. The right oblique fissure follows a similar course to the left oblique fissure.

The horizontal fissure travels from the hilum laterally at the level of the 4th costal cartilage. It meets the oblique fissure posteriorly in the midaxillary line at the level of the sixth rib. It is absent in 10% of people and complete in only 30%.

Ryan S, McNicholas M, Eustace SJ. Anatomy for Diagnostic Imaging, 3rd edition. Edinburgh: Saunders, 2010:125–126.

Case 2.25

A Medial segment of middle lobe bronchus

B Middle lobe bronchus

C Right lower lobe bronchus

D Sternum

E Left scapula

Axial contrast enhanced CT chest.

Bronchus intermedius bifurcates to give rise to the middle and lower lobar bronchi (**m**iddle **l**obe = **me**dial and **l**ateral segments). The middle lobe bronchus has two branches the medial and lateral segmental bronchi. The right lower lobe branches into five segmental bronchi, the superior, medial basal, anterior, lateral basal and posterior basal.

Case 2.26

A Right atrial border

B Azygos fissure

C Anatomical neck of right humerus

D Superior vena cava

E Acromion of right scapula

Shoulder radiograph.

The azygos fissure is a normal variant. The azygos vein travels through the right apical lobe, where it has four pleural layers: two parietal and two visceral.

The anatomical neck of the humerus separates the greater and lesser tuberosities. The surgical neck is the narrow area of shaft just inferior to the tuberosities and anatomical neck. The surgical neck is fractured more frequently than the anatomical neck, and the axillary nerve is at risk here.

The acromion articulates with the clavicle at the acromioclavicular joint to help to provide stability to the shoulder joint.

Ryan S, McNicholas M, Eustace SJ. Anatomy for Diagnostic Imaging, 3rd edition. Edinburgh: Saunders, 2010:125–126.

Moore KL, Dalley AF, Agur AMR. Clinically Oriented Anatomy, 6th edition. Philadelphia: Lippincott Williams & Wilkins, 2009:114.

Case 2.27

A Right fourth rib

B T9 vertebral body

C Sternum (ossification centre)

D Left humerus diaphysis

E Left hemidiaphragm

Left lateral oblique paediatric chest radiograph.

These views are most commonly performed as part of skeletal surveys and sometimes for suspected rib abnormalities. Prior to complete fusion between 6 and 12 years of age, the sternum exists as multiple rounded ossification centres. This is important to recognise, because sometimes these rounded ossification centres can each line up and project over ribs on oblique projections and mimic a row of healing rib fractures.

Weir J, Abrahams P. Imaging Atlas of Human Anatomy, 4th edition. Edinburgh: Mosby, 2010:90.

Ryan S, McNicholas M, Eustace SJ. Anatomy for Diagnostic Imaging, 3rd edition. Edinburgh: Saunders, 2010:120.

Case 2.28

A Right main pulmonary artery

B Right hemidiaphragm

C Stomach bubble

D Left hemidiaphragm

E Right ventricle

Plain lateral chest radiograph.

The right diaphragm is usually higher than the left, and you can see the heart through it, i.e. the heart therefore cannot be in contact with it. The inferior vena cava may be seen to pass through the right diaphragm.

Aerated lung is adjacent to the right hemidiaphragm and therefore its contour is visible from its posterior to anterior aspects.

The left diaphragm is usually lower than the right and the heart is in contact with it, i.e. the heart is sitting on the left diaphragm and the gastric bubble can be seen to lie below it.

The right ventricle is the most anterior chamber of the heart. It is crescent shaped, and has a thinner wall than the larger, more muscular left ventricle. The left ventricle is so large that it bulges into the right ventricle, giving it its crescent shape. Inflow is from the right atrium via the tricuspid valve (three leaflets). Outflow is into the pulmonary artery via the pulmonary valve.

Weir J, Abrahams P. Imaging Atlas of Human Anatomy, 4th edition. Edinburgh: Mosby, 2010:91.

Ryan S, McNicholas M, Eustace SJ. Anatomy for Diagnostic Imaging, 3rd edition. Edinburgh: Saunders, 2010:121.

Weber E, Netter FH, Vilensky JA, Carmichael SW. Netter's Concise Radiologic Anatomy. Philadelphia: Saunders/Elsevier, 2009:203.

Case 2.29

A Left atrial border

B Left scapula

C Trachea

D Right eighth rib

E Body of sternum

Plain lateral chest radiograph.

The left atrium forms the left posterior heart border. The left ventricle can be identified as the most posterior and inferior of the cardiac chambers.

The lower trachea is supplied by branches of the bronchial artery. The upper trachea is supplied by the inferior thyroid artery. The arch of the aorta may be seen to indent the left side of the trachea just above the carina.

The sternum consists of three fused bones: manubrium, body of sternum and xiphoid process. Superiorly, the junction of the manubrium with the body of sternum is called the 'Angle of Louis'. This is at the level of T4/T5, where the 2nd rib articulates. This is the same level as the aortic arch and the carina.

In order to ascertain which rib is labelled, one can use the 'big rib sign'. On a well-positioned left lateral chest radiograph, the left ribs are in contact with the film. The right ribs are farther from the film than the left, and are therefore magnified and look bigger.

Weir J, Abrahams P. Imaging Atlas of Human Anatomy, 4th edition. Edinburgh: Mosby, 2010:91.

Ryan S, McNicholas M, Eustace SJ. Anatomy for Diagnostic Imaging, 3rd edition. Edinburgh: Saunders, 2010:121.

Kurihara Y, Yakushiji YK, Matsumoto J, et al. The ribs: anatomic and radiologic considerations. Radiographics 1999; 19:105–119.

Case 2.30

A T4 vertebral body

B Right 5th rib

C Left lower lobe pulmonary artery

D Left lower lobe pulmonary vein

E Left crus of the diaphragm

Coronal CT pulmonary angiogram of the thorax.

This is a posterior section as the vertebral bodies and the aorta can be seen. There is contrast in the pulmonary arteries and thus they are of higher attenuation than the aorta.

Bony structures A and B are easily recognised as a vertebral body and a rib. It is of paramount importance not to rush into writing these answers down; the number and laterality of the ribs must be given. Forgetting to include these details will cost precious points. In this case, the first rib can be seen and the numbers of the labelled structures can be determined by counting down. If you cannot find anything that helps to determine the number of a labelled vertebral body, simply indicate whether it is cervical, thoracic or lumbar.

The branching of the pulmonary arteries closely follows the branching of the airways; this is not the case with the branching of the pulmonary veins. Remembering this fact will prevent mistaking pulmonary arteries for veins.

The main divisions of the pulmonary trunk are the right and left pulmonary arteries. At the left hilum, the left pulmonary artery divides into the upper and lower lobe branches.

Weir J, Abrahams P. Imaging Atlas of Human Anatomy, 4th edition. Edinburgh: Mosby, 2010:110–111.

Ryan S, McNicholas M, Eustace SJ. Anatomy for Diagnostic Imaging, 3rd edition. Edinburgh: Saunders, 2010:126–127.

Weber E, Netter FH, Vilensky JA, Carmichael SW. Netter's Concise Radiologic Anatomy. Philadelphia: Saunders/Elsevier, 2009:205.

Case 2.31

A Right internal thoracic artery/mammary artery

B Right main bronchus

C Pulmonary trunk/main pulmonary artery

D Costotransverse joint on the right

E Left erector spinae

Axial CT of the chest.

This is an axial section through the thorax at the level of the pulmonary trunk division. The pulmonary trunk begins at the pulmonary valve inferior to the level seen here. At first, it lies anterior to the aorta and then passes to its left to lie in the concavity of the arch where it divides.

The internal thoracic/internal mammary artery arises from the subclavian artery near its origin. It is a paired artery that supplies the anterior chest wall and the breast. It divides into the superior epigastric and musculophrenic arteries.

The facet of the tubercle of the rib forms an articulation with the transverse process of the vertebra. This is called the costotransverse joint. It is not possible to assign a number to the costotransverse joint in this image as there are no solid landmarks to count from. Therefore, only laterality can be indicated.

The erector spinae is a large muscular and tendinous mass which acts as an extensor of the spine. Its superior part attaches to the transverse processes of the lumbar vertebra and the 11th and 12th rib.

Weir J, Abrahams P. Imaging Atlas of Human Anatomy, 4th edition. Edinburgh: Mosby, 2010:93.

Ryan S, McNicholas M, Eustace SJ. Anatomy for Diagnostic Imaging, 3rd edition. Edinburgh: Saunders, 2010:133.

Case 2.32

A Right pectoralis minor

B Oesophagus

C Left brachiocephalic vein/innominate vein

D Right brachiocephalic trunk/artery

E Left subclavian artery

Axial CT of the thorax.

The pectoralis minor lies beneath the larger pectoralis major. Its attachments are the anterior third to fifth ribs and the coracoid process of the scapula. It lies in the anterior wall of the axilla, and nerves and vessels travel under it to enter the arm. Its functions are to draw the scapula anteriorly and inferiorly to stabilise it against the chest wall, and to elevate the ribs in deep inspiration. It is innervated by the medial pectoral nerve.

The left brachiocephalic trunk, or innominate vein is the common drainage vessel of the left arm and the left of the neck, formed by the left internal jugular vein and left subclavian vein. It courses anterior to the arch vessels to join the right brachiocephalic vein to become the superior vena cava. This is why the IV contrast injection should be in the right arm for a CT angiogram aorta, as high-density contrast draining centrally via the left brachiocephalic vein may cause streak artefact that obscures the arch and its branch vessels.

Moore KL, Dalley AF, Agur AMR. Clinically Oriented Anatomy, 6th edition. Philadelphia: Lippincott Williams & Wilkins, 2009:709.

Weir J, Abrahams P. Imaging Atlas of Human Anatomy, 4th edition. Edinburgh: Mosby, 2010:96.

Ryan S, McNicholas M, Eustace SJ. Anatomy for Diagnostic Imaging, 3rd edition. Edinburgh: Saunders, 2010:153.

Case 2.33

A Pericardium

B Right lobe of liver

C Inferior vena cava

D Left ventricle

E Left latissimus dorsi

Axial CT of the thorax.

The pericardium is a double-walled sac which is draped over the heart and great vessels and has a visceral and parietal layer. The visceral layer is attached to the myocardium. The parietal layer is loose except superiorly where it is attached to the great vessels, and inferiorly where it is attached to the central tendon of the diaphragm by the pericardiophrenic ligament.

Ryan S, McNicholas M, Eustace SJ. Anatomy for Diagnostic Imaging, 3rd edition. Edinburgh: Saunders, 2010:132.

Moore KL, Dalley AF, Agur AMR. Clinically Oriented Anatomy, 6th edition. Philadelphia: Lippincott Williams & Wilkins, 2009:107.

Case 2.34

A Thymus

B Left cardiophrenic angle

C Ossification centre of left humeral proximal femoral epiphysis.

D Right clavicle

E Left posterior 5th rib

Frontal chest radiograph.

The thymus is hugely variable in size and shape, and because of its soft density, the lateral edges may appear 'wavy' as they conform to the overlying ribs and intercostal spaces. Lung markings may be seen through it, and a normal thymus should never deviate other structures.

Ryan S, McNicholas M, Eustace SJ. Anatomy for Diagnostic Imaging, 3rd edition. Edinburgh: Saunders, 2010:147–148.

Case 2.35

A Pectoral muscle

B Skin line

C Glandular tissue

D Nipple

E Inframammary fold

Mammogram.

The breast lies on the second to sixth ribs. It consists of fatty and glandular tissue, which is held in place by Cooper's ligaments that attach to skin and underlying pectoralis muscle fascia. It is supplied by the internal mammary artery and the lateral thoracic branch of the axillary artery. Venous drainage follows the arterial supply.

Most of the lymph drainage is to the axillary chain, with 5% draining to the internal mammary chain.

Weir J, Abrahams P. Imaging Atlas of Human Anatomy, 4th edition. Edinburgh: Mosby, 2010:120–122.

Ryan S, McNicholas M, Eustace SJ. Anatomy for Diagnostic Imaging. Edinburgh: Saunders, 2004:313–325.

Chapter 3

Abdomen and pelvis

Bowel

Case 3.1

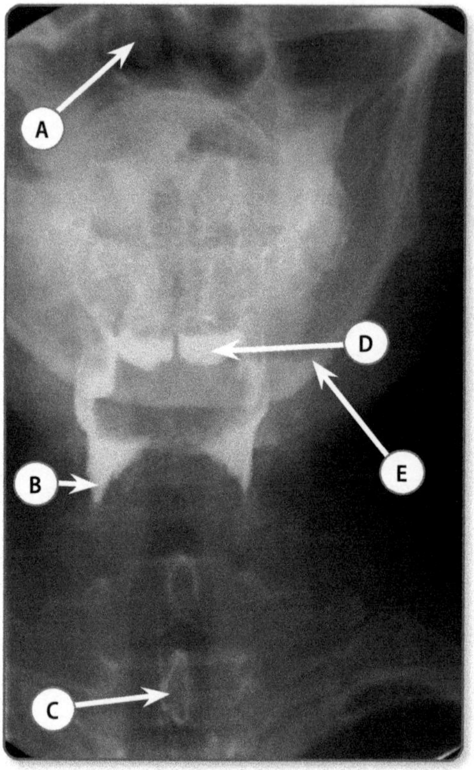

Case 3.1

QUESTION		WRITE YOUR ANSWER HERE
A	Name the structure labelled A.	
B	Name the structure labelled B.	
C	Name the structure labelled C.	
D	Name the structure labelled D.	
E	Name the structure labelled E.	

Case 3.2

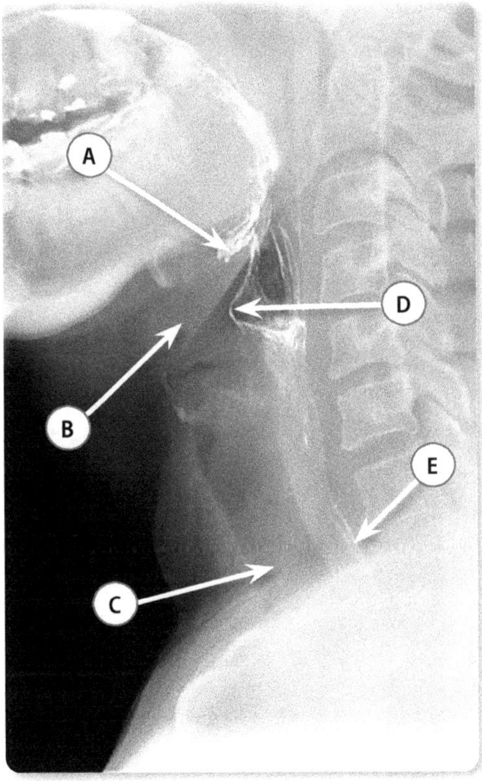

Case 3.2

QUESTION		WRITE YOUR ANSWER HERE
A	Name the structure labelled A.	
B	Name the structure labelled B.	
C	Name the structure labelled C.	
D	Name the structure labelled D.	
E	Name the structure labelled E.	

Case 3.3

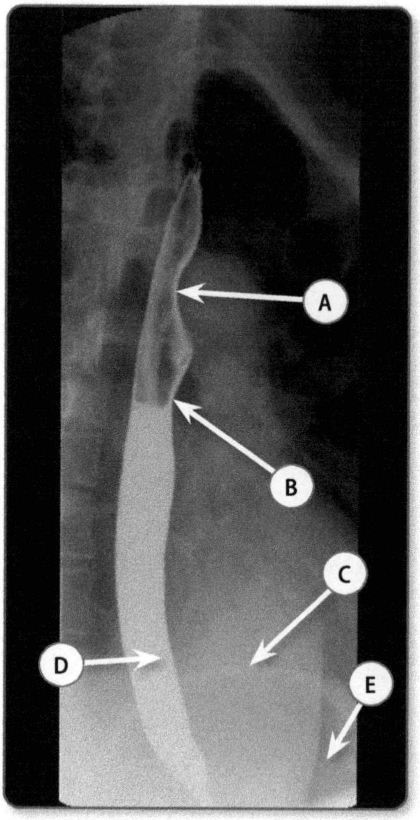

Case 3.3

QUESTION		WRITE YOUR ANSWER HERE
A	Name the structure labelled A.	
B	Name the structure labelled B.	
C	Name the structure labelled C.	
D	Name the structure labelled D.	
E	Name the structure labelled E.	

Case 3.4

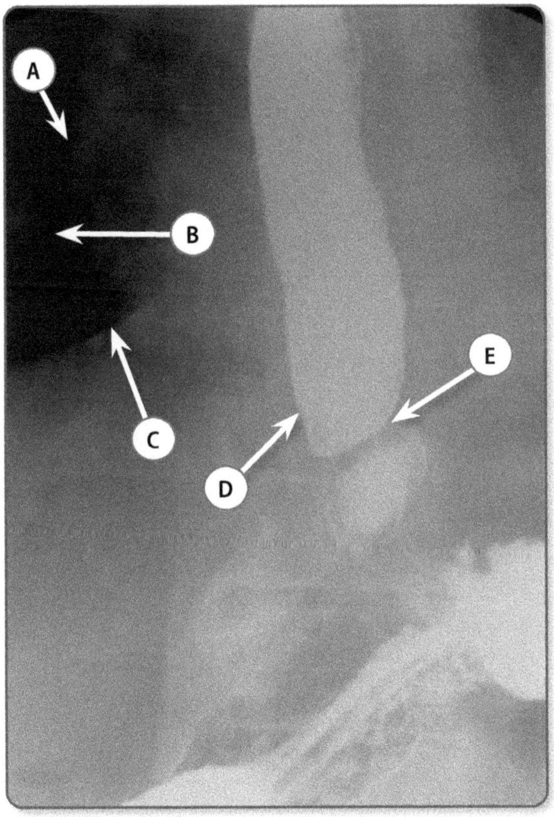

Case 3.4

QUESTION		WRITE YOUR ANSWER HERE
A	Name the structure labelled A.	
B	Name the structure labelled B.	
C	Name the structure labelled C.	
D	Name the structure labelled D.	
E	Name the structure labelled E.	

Case 3.5

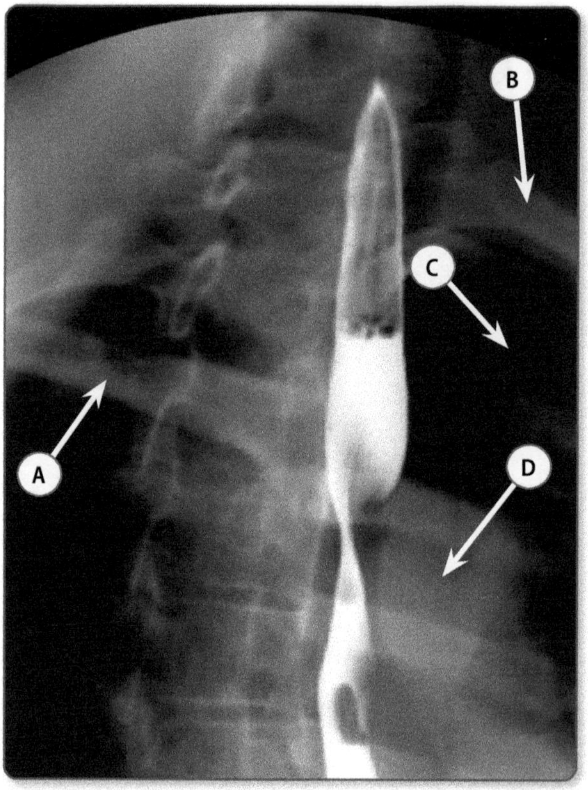

Case 3.5

QUESTION		WRITE YOUR ANSWER HERE
A	Name the structure labelled A.	
B	Name the structure labelled B.	
C	Name the structure labelled C.	
D	Name the structure labelled D.	
E	Which normal variant is demonstrated?	

Case 3.6

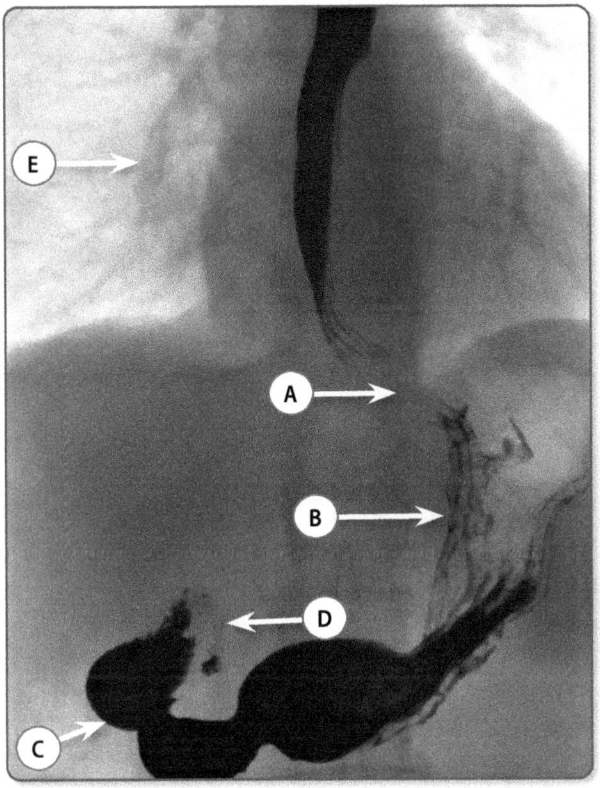

Case 3.6

QUESTION		WRITE YOUR ANSWER HERE
A	Name the structure labelled A.	
B	Name the structure labelled B.	
C	Name the structure labelled C.	
D	Name the structure labelled D.	
E	Name the structure labelled E.	

Case 3.7

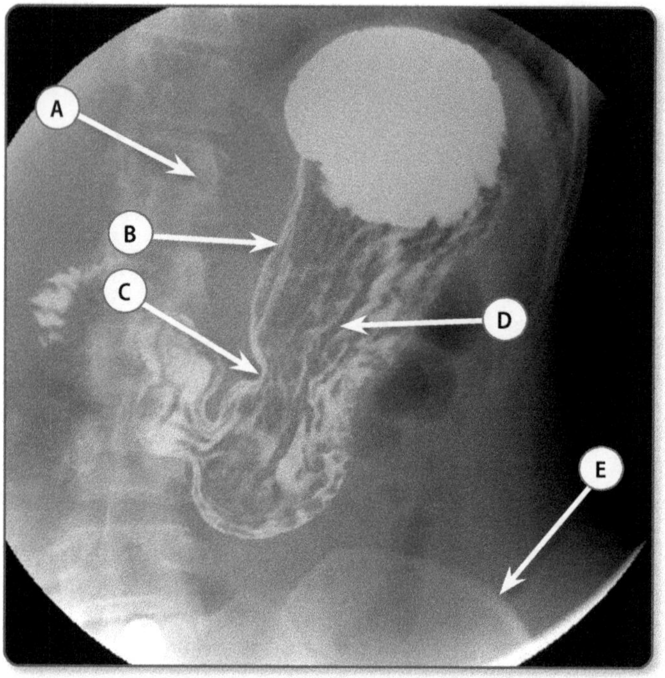

Case 3.7

QUESTION		WRITE YOUR ANSWER HERE
A	Name the structure labelled A.	
B	Name the structure labelled B.	
C	Name the structure labelled C.	
D	Name the structure labelled D.	
E	Name the structure labelled E.	

Case 3.8

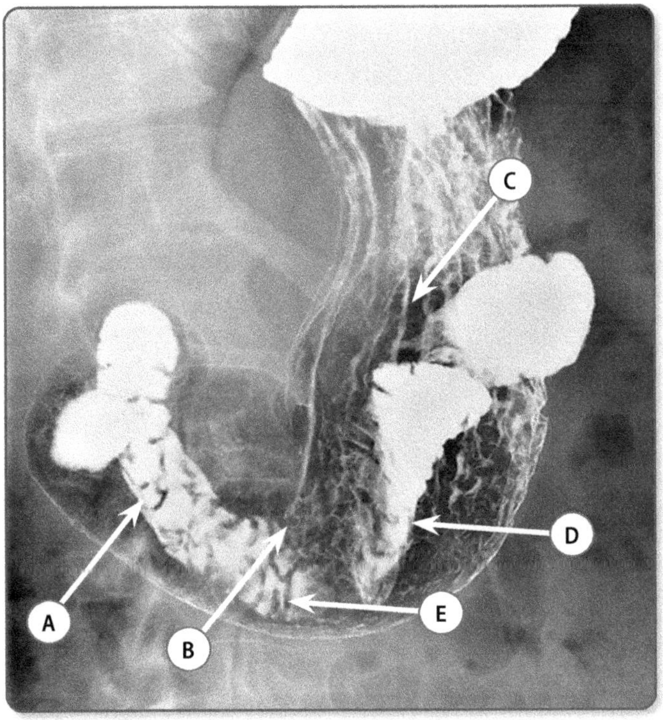

Case 3.8

QUESTION		WRITE YOUR ANSWER HERE
A	Name the structure labelled A.	
B	Name the structure labelled B.	
C	Name the structure labelled C.	
D	Name the structure labelled D.	
E	Name the structure labelled E.	

Case 3.9

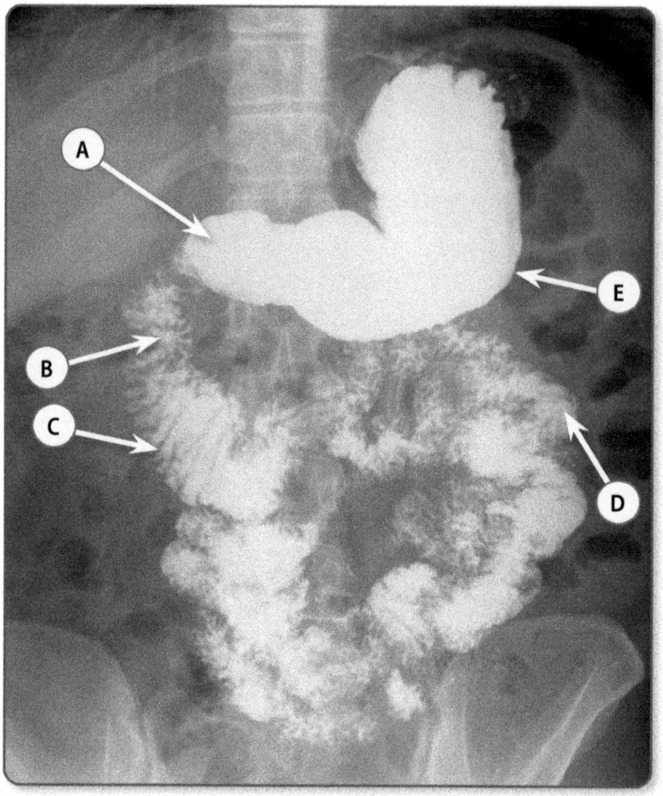

Case 3.9		
QUESTION		WRITE YOUR ANSWER HERE
A	Name the structure labelled A.	
B	Name the structure labelled B.	
C	Name the structure labelled C.	
D	Name the structure labelled D.	
E	Name the structure labelled E.	

Case 3.10

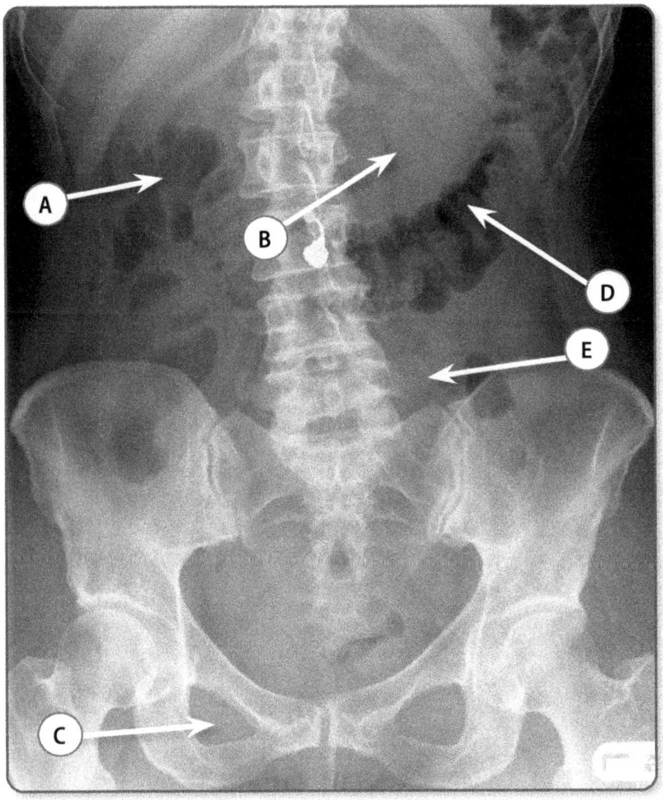

Case 3.10

QUESTION		WRITE YOUR ANSWER HERE
A	Name the structure labelled A.	
B	Name the structure labelled B.	
C	Name the structure labelled C.	
D	Name the structure labelled D.	
E	Name the structure labelled E.	

Case 3.11

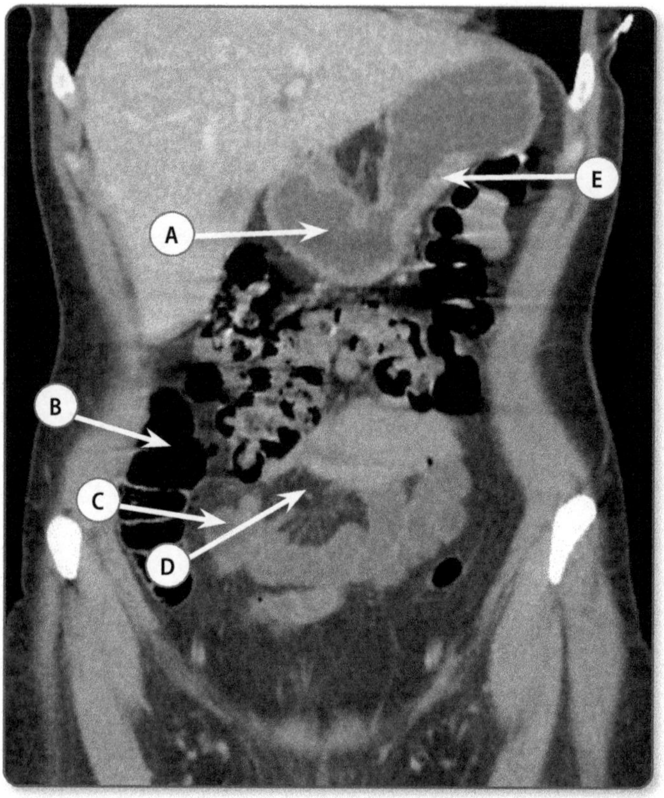

Case 3.11

QUESTION		WRITE YOUR ANSWER HERE
A	Name the structure labelled A.	
B	Name the structure labelled B.	
C	Name the structure labelled C.	
D	Name the structure labelled D.	
E	Name the structure labelled E.	

Case 3.12

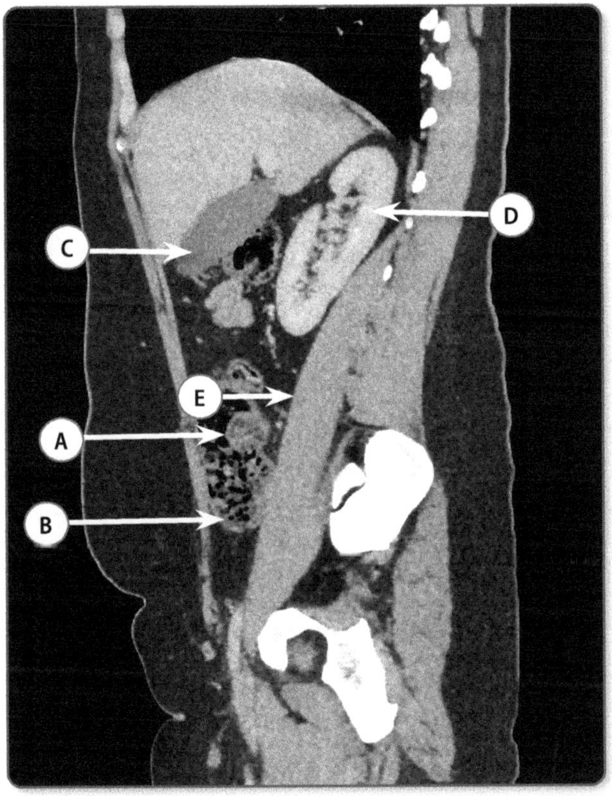

Case 3.12

QUESTION		WRITE YOUR ANSWER HERE
A	Name the structure labelled A.	
B	Name the structure labelled B.	
C	Name the structure labelled C.	
D	Name the structure labelled D.	
E	Name the structure labelled E.	

Case 3.13

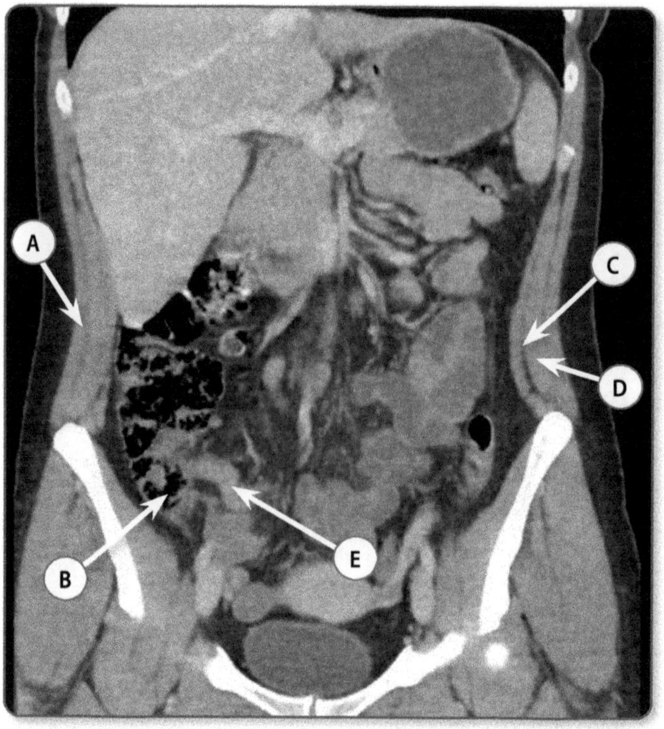

Case 3.13

QUESTION		WRITE YOUR ANSWER HERE
A	Name the structure labelled A.	
B	Name the structure labelled B.	
C	Name the structure labelled C.	
D	Name the structure labelled D.	
E	Name the structure labelled E.	

Case 3.14

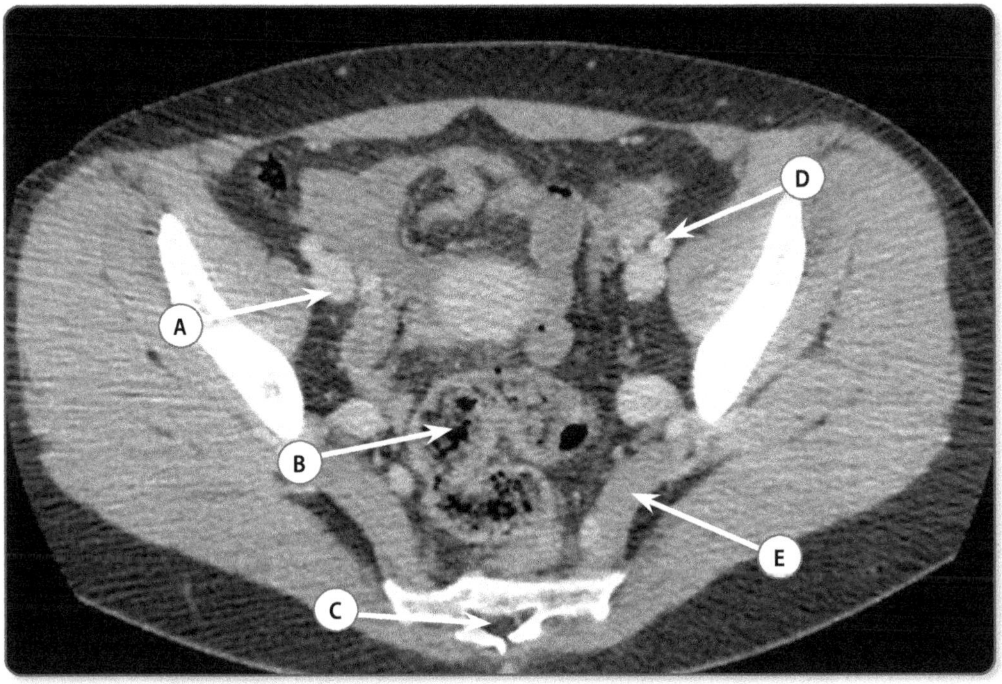

Case 3.14		
QUESTION		WRITE YOUR ANSWER HERE
A	Name the structure labelled A.	
B	Name the structure labelled B.	
C	Name the structure labelled C.	
D	Name the structure labelled D.	
E	Name the structure labelled E.	

Upper abdominal viscera

Case 3.15

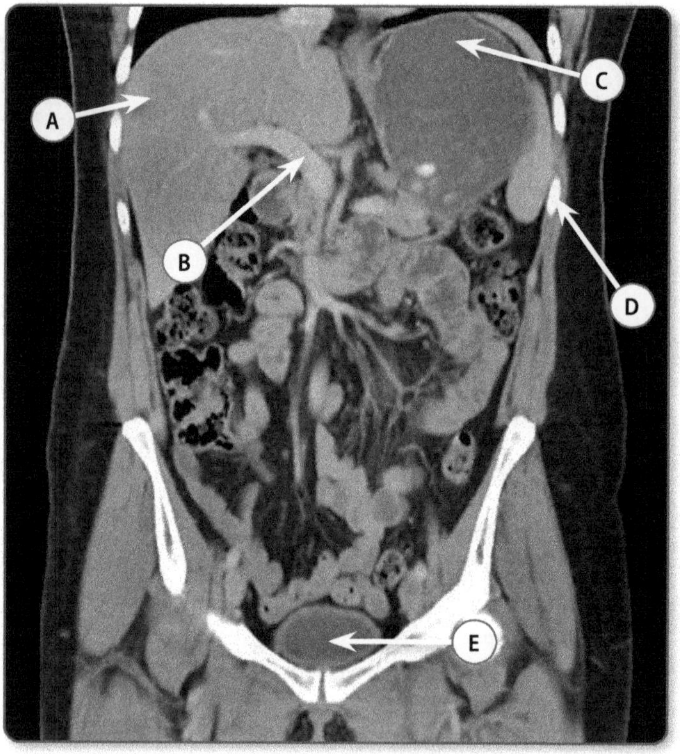

Case 3.15

QUESTION		WRITE YOUR ANSWER HERE
A	Name the structure labelled A.	
B	Name the structure labelled B.	
C	Name the structure labelled C.	
D	Name the structure labelled D.	
E	Name the structure labelled E.	

Case 3.16

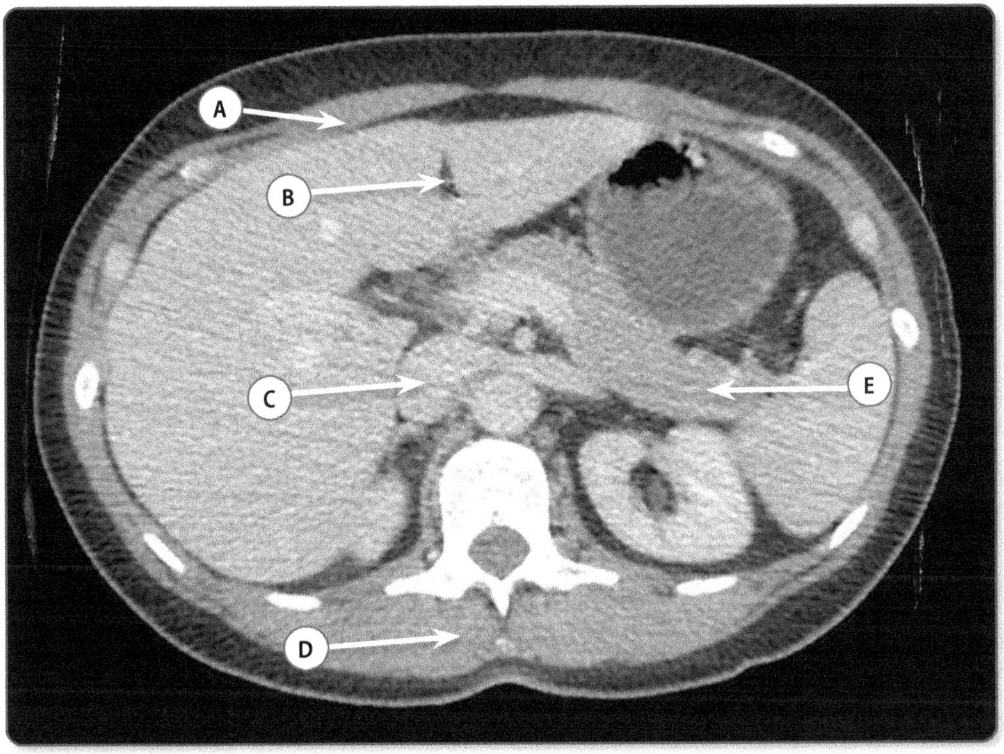

Case 3.16

	QUESTION	WRITE YOUR ANSWER HERE
A	Name the structure labelled A.	
B	Name the structure labelled B.	
C	Name the structure labelled C.	
D	Name the structure labelled D.	
E	Name the structure labelled E.	

Case 3.17

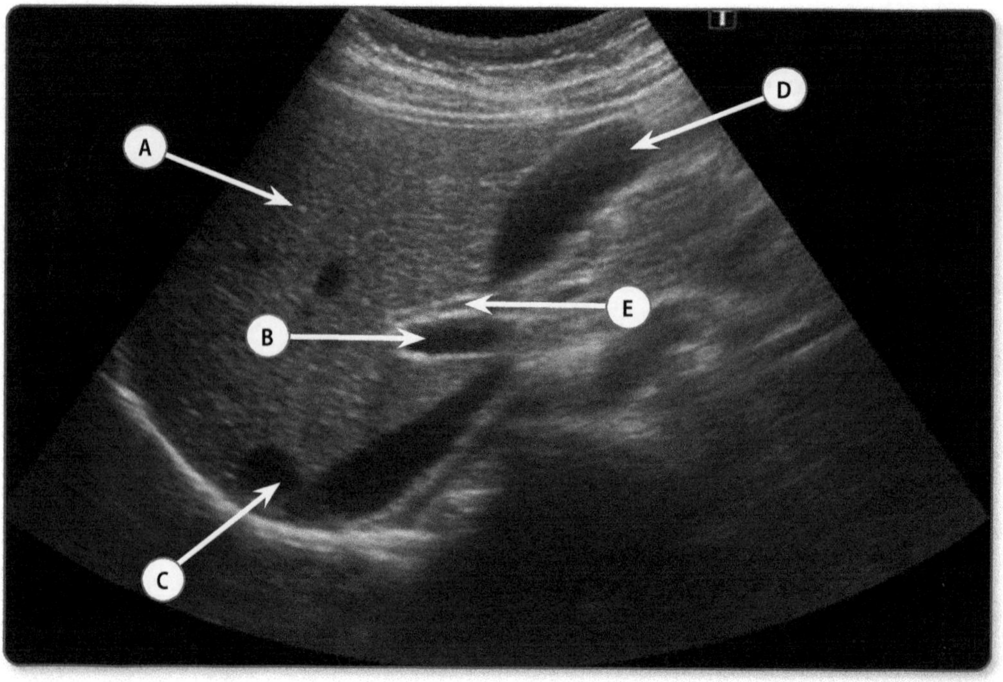

Case 3.17		
QUESTION		**WRITE YOUR ANSWER HERE**
A	Name the structure labelled A.	
B	Name the structure labelled B.	
C	Name the structure labelled C.	
D	Name the structure labelled D.	
E	Name the structure labelled E.	

Case 3.18

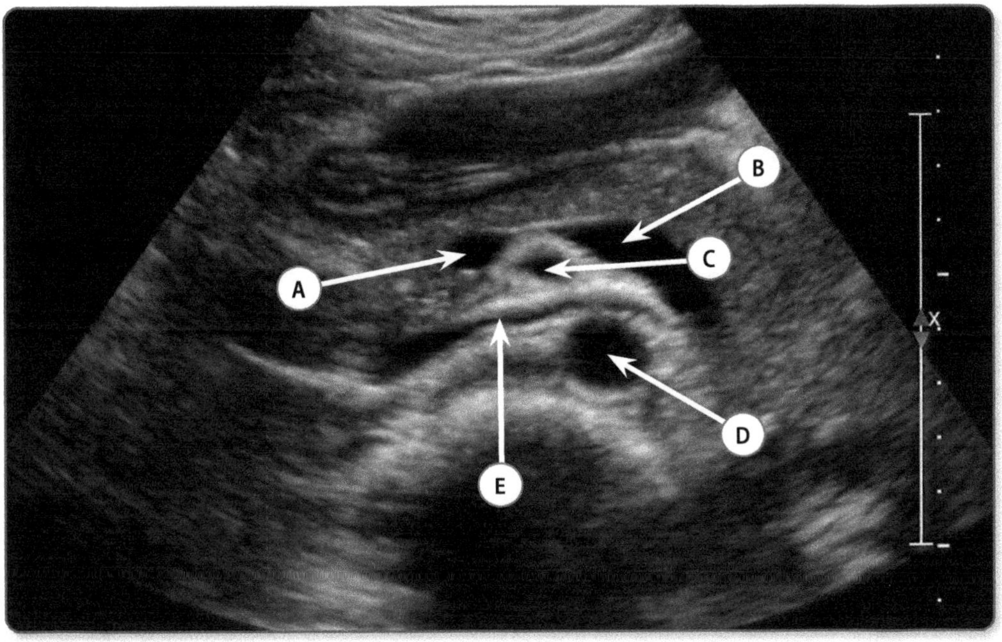

Case 3.18

QUESTION		WRITE YOUR ANSWER HERE
A	Name the structure labelled A.	
B	Name the structure labelled B.	
C	Name the structure labelled C.	
D	Name the structure labelled D.	
E	Name the structure labelled E.	

Case 3.19

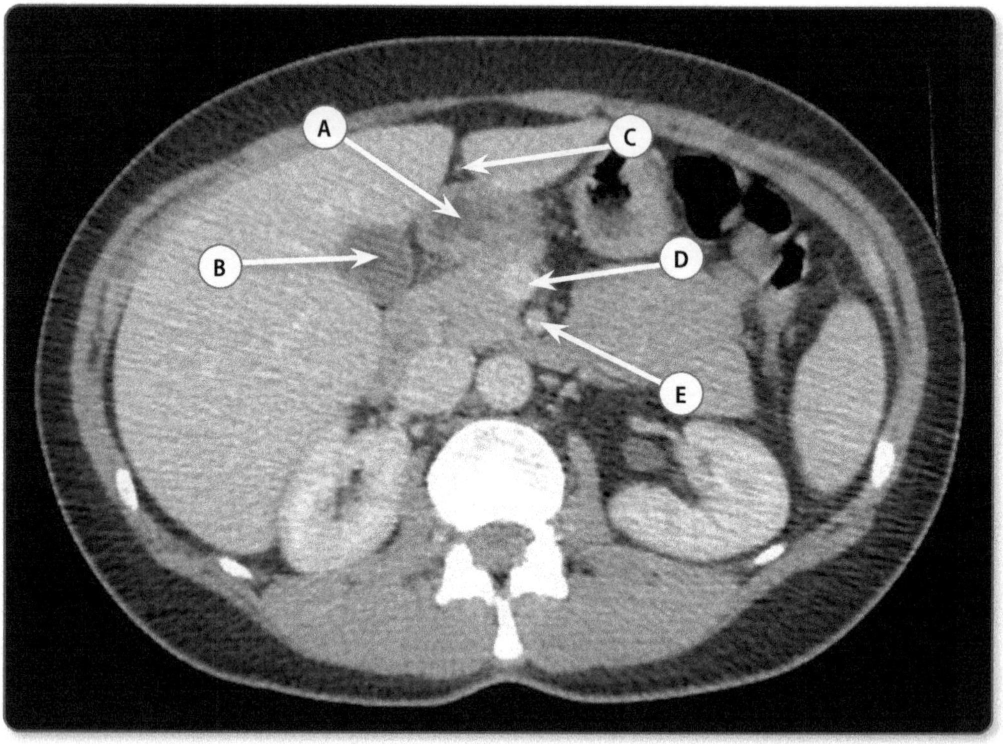

Case 3.19		
QUESTION		WRITE YOUR ANSWER HERE
A	Name the structure labelled A.	
B	Name the structure labelled B.	
C	Name the structure labelled C.	
D	Name the structure labelled D.	
E	Name the structure labelled E.	

Case 3.20

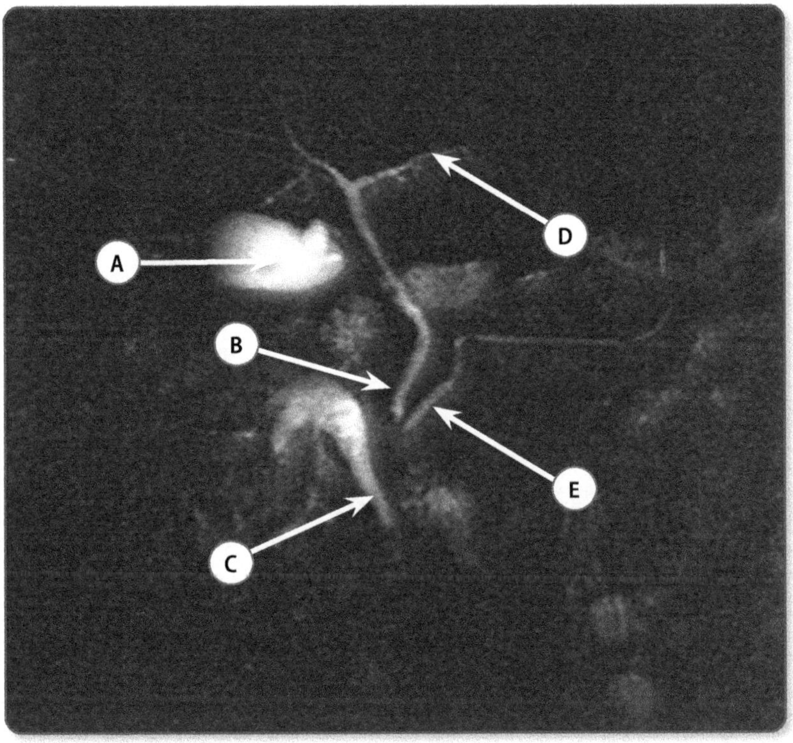

Case 3.20

QUESTION		WRITE YOUR ANSWER HERE
A	Name the structure labelled A.	
B	Name the structure labelled B.	
C	Name the structure labelled C.	
D	Name the structure labelled D.	
E	Name the structure labelled E.	

Case 3.21

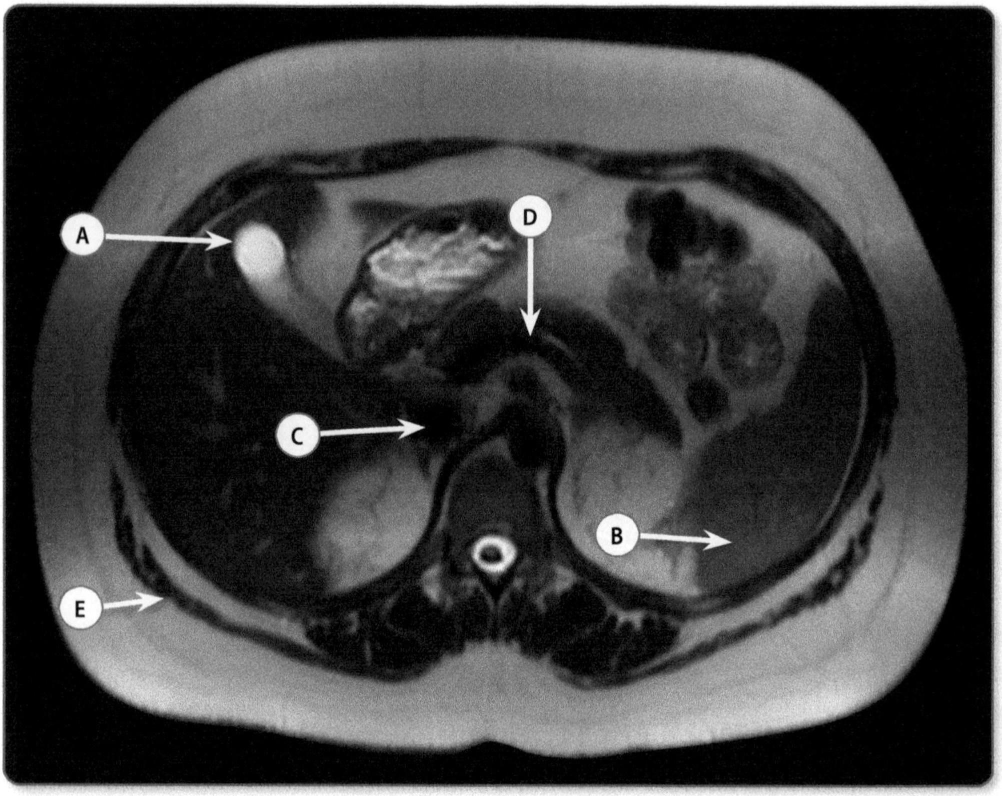

Case 3.21

QUESTION		WRITE YOUR ANSWER HERE
A	Name the structure labelled A.	
B	Name the structure labelled B.	
C	Name the structure labelled C.	
D	Name the structure labelled D.	
E	Name the structure labelled E.	

Abdominal wall

Case 3.22

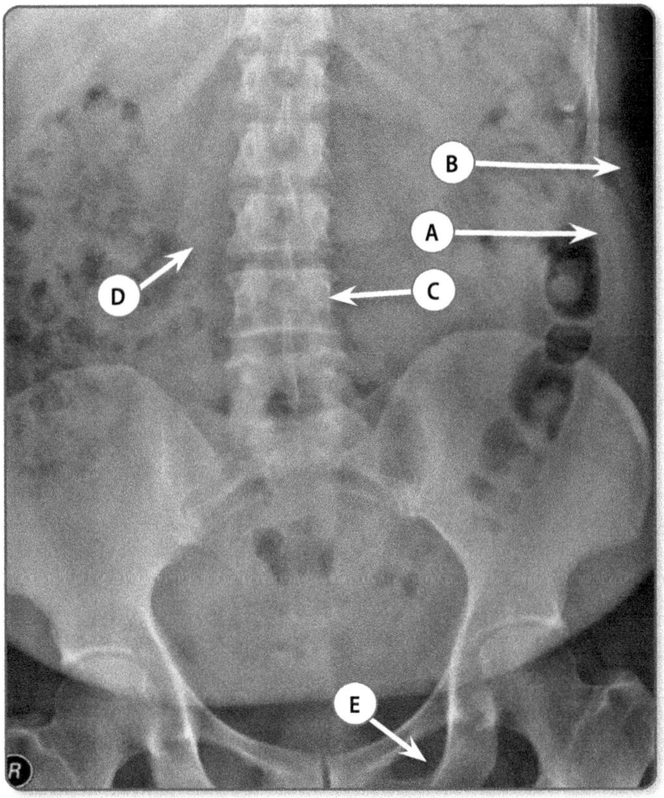

Case 3.22

QUESTION		WRITE YOUR ANSWER HERE
A	Name the structure labelled A.	
B	Name the structure labelled B.	
C	Name the structure labelled C.	
D	Name the structure labelled D.	
E	Name the structure labelled E.	

Case 3.23

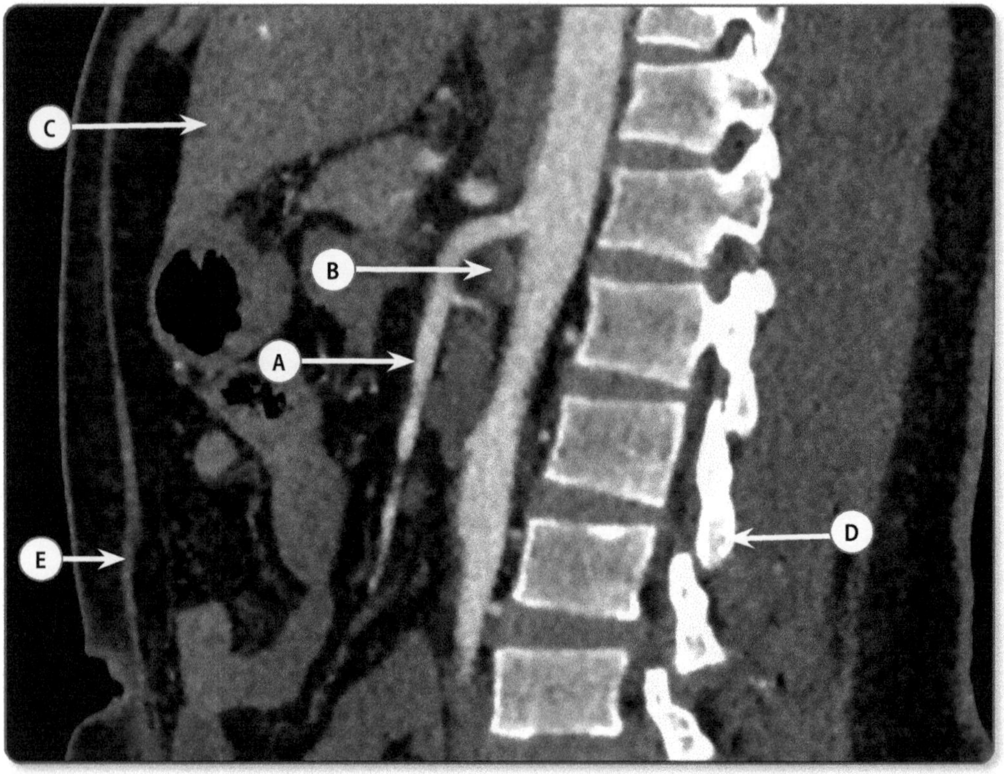

Case 3.23

QUESTION		WRITE YOUR ANSWER HERE
A	Name the structure labelled A.	
B	Name the structure labelled B.	
C	Name the structure labelled C.	
D	Name the structure labelled D.	
E	Name the structure labelled E.	

Case 3.24

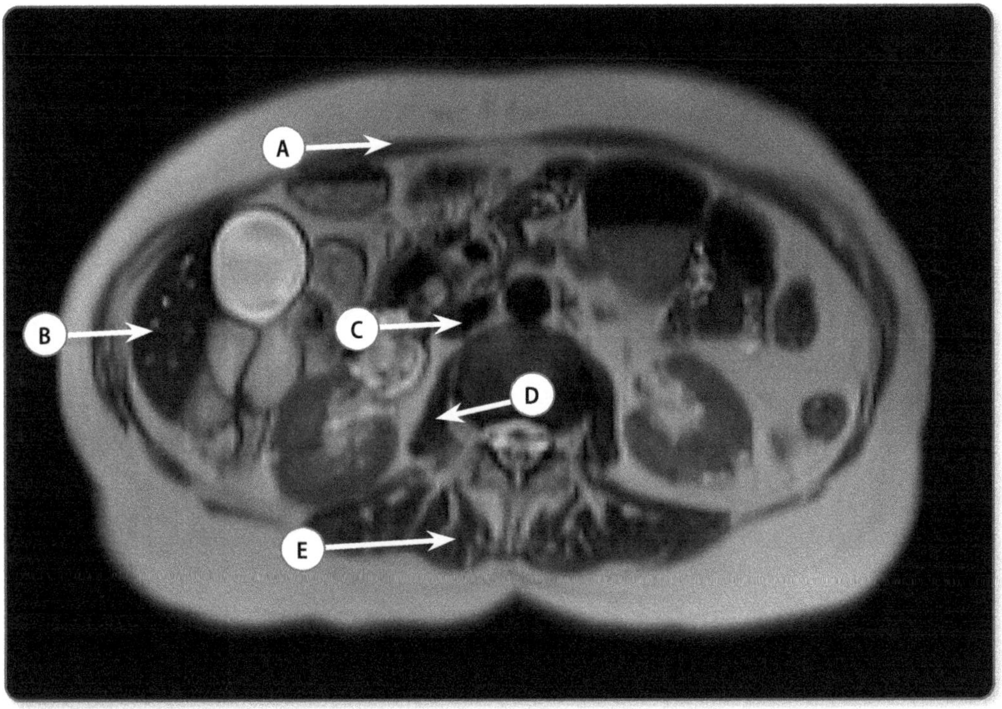

Case 3.24

QUESTION		WRITE YOUR ANSWER HERE
A	Name the structure labelled A.	
B	Name the structure labelled B.	
C	Name the structure labelled C.	
D	Name the structure labelled D.	
E	Name the structure labelled E.	

Case 3.25

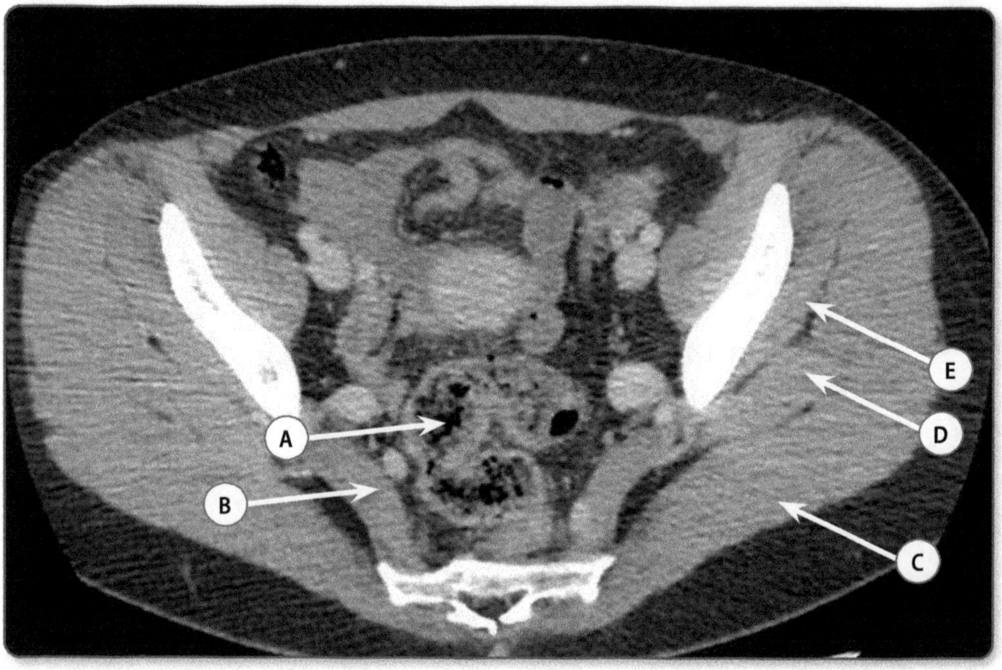

Case 3.25

QUESTION		WRITE YOUR ANSWER HERE
A	Name the structure labelled A.	
B	Name the structure labelled B.	
C	Name the structure labelled C.	
D	Name the structure labelled D.	
E	Name the structure labelled E.	

Case 3.26

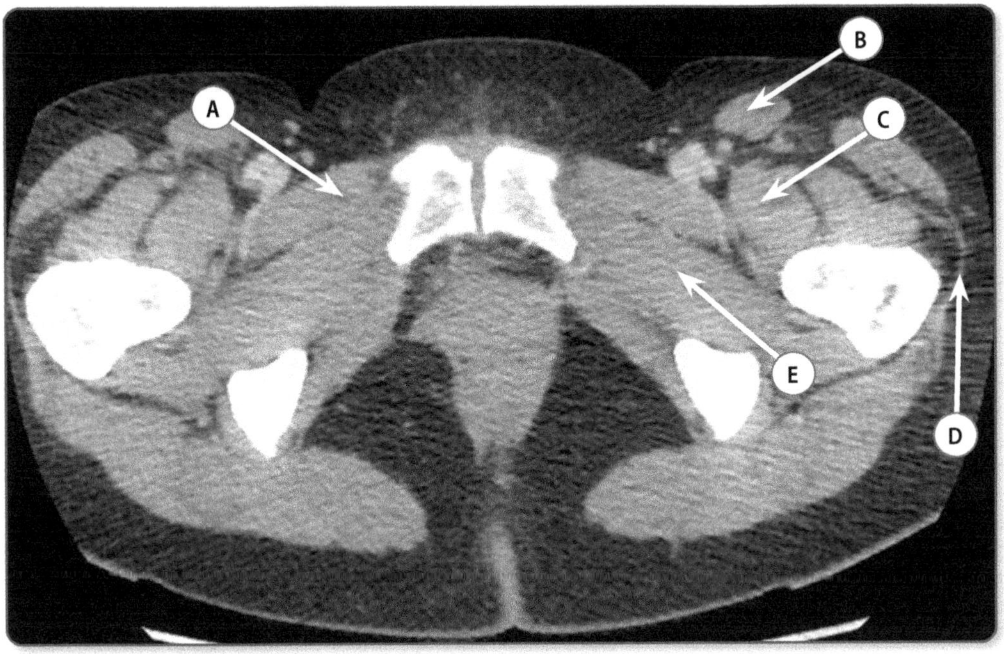

Case 3.26		
QUESTION		WRITE YOUR ANSWER HERE
A	Name the structure labelled A.	
B	Name the structure labelled B.	
C	Name the structure labelled C.	
D	Name the structure labelled D.	
E	Name the structure labelled E.	

Case 3.27

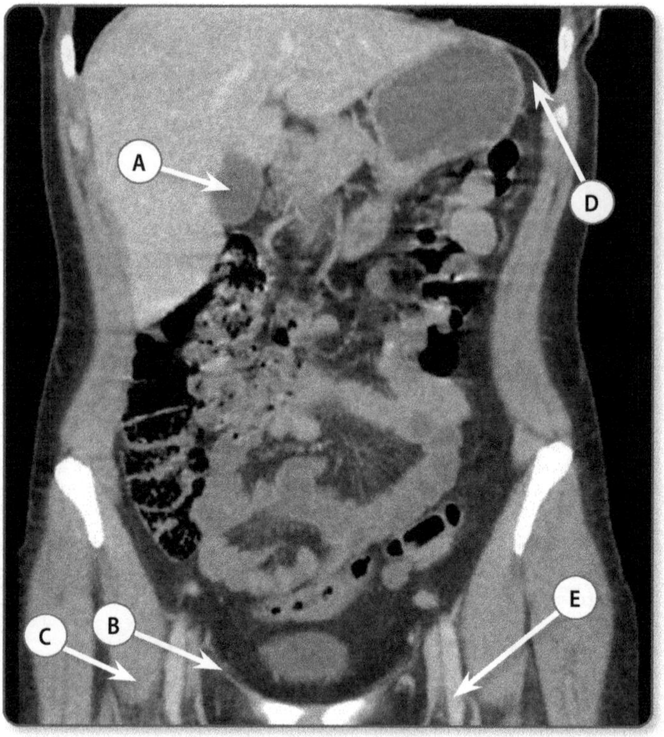

Case 3.27

	QUESTION	WRITE YOUR ANSWER HERE
A	Name the structure labelled A.	
B	Name the structure labelled B.	
C	Name the structure labelled C.	
D	Name the structure labelled D.	
E	Name the structure labelled E.	

Spaces and planes

Case 3.28

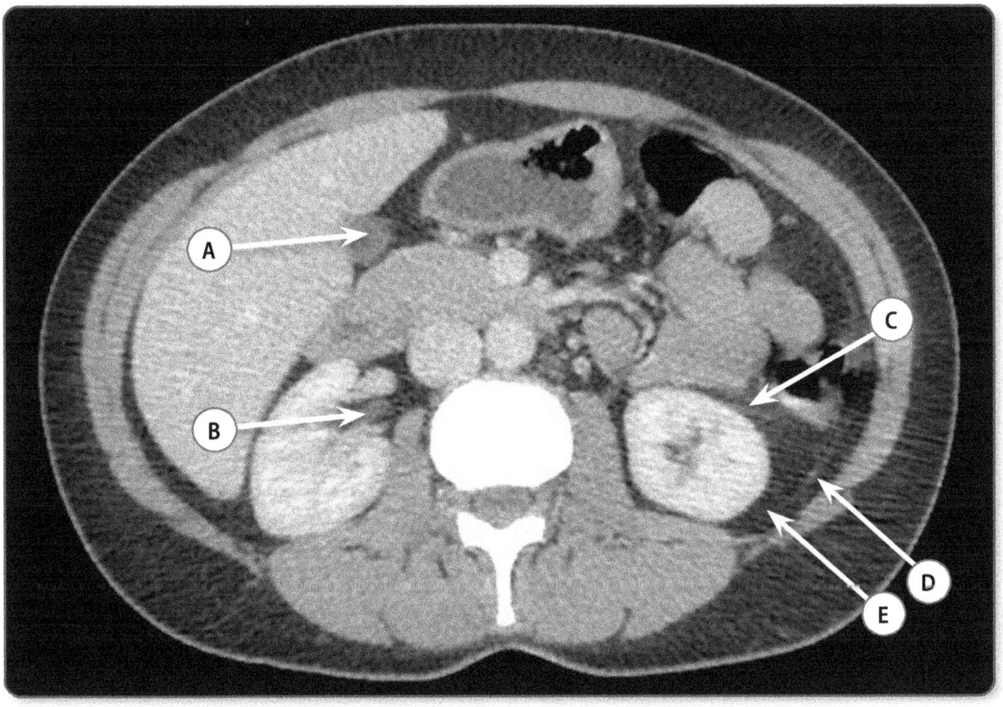

Case 3.28		
QUESTION		WRITE YOUR ANSWER HERE
A	Name the structure labelled A.	
B	Name the structure labelled B.	
C	Name the structure labelled C.	
D	Name the structure labelled D.	
E	Name the structure labelled E.	

Case 3.29

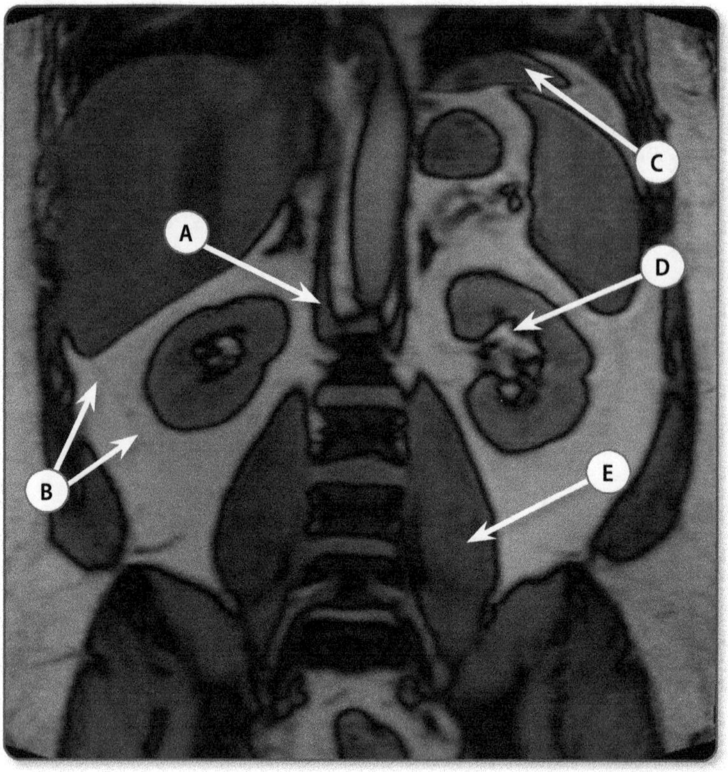

Case 3.29

QUESTION		WRITE YOUR ANSWER HERE
A	Name the structure labelled A.	
B	Name the structure labelled B.	
C	Name the structure labelled C.	
D	Name the structure labelled D.	
E	Name the structure labelled E.	

Case 3.30

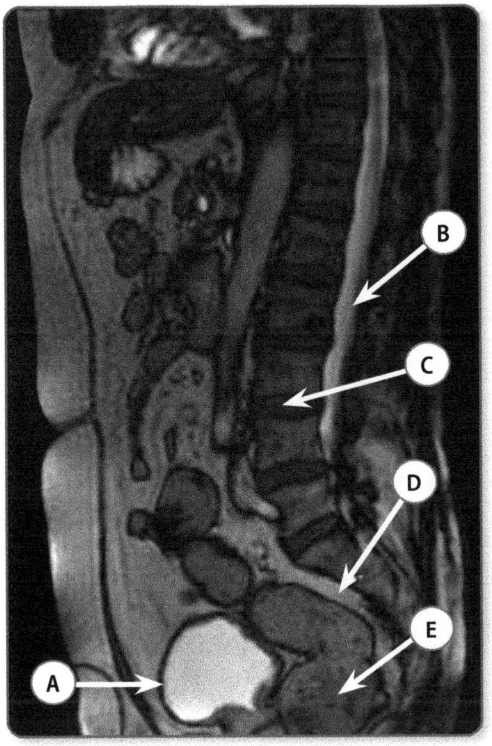

Case 3.30

QUESTION		WRITE YOUR ANSWER HERE
A	Name the structure labelled A.	
B	Name the structure labelled B.	
C	Name the structure labelled C.	
D	Name the structure labelled D.	
E	Name the structure labelled E.	

Case 3.31

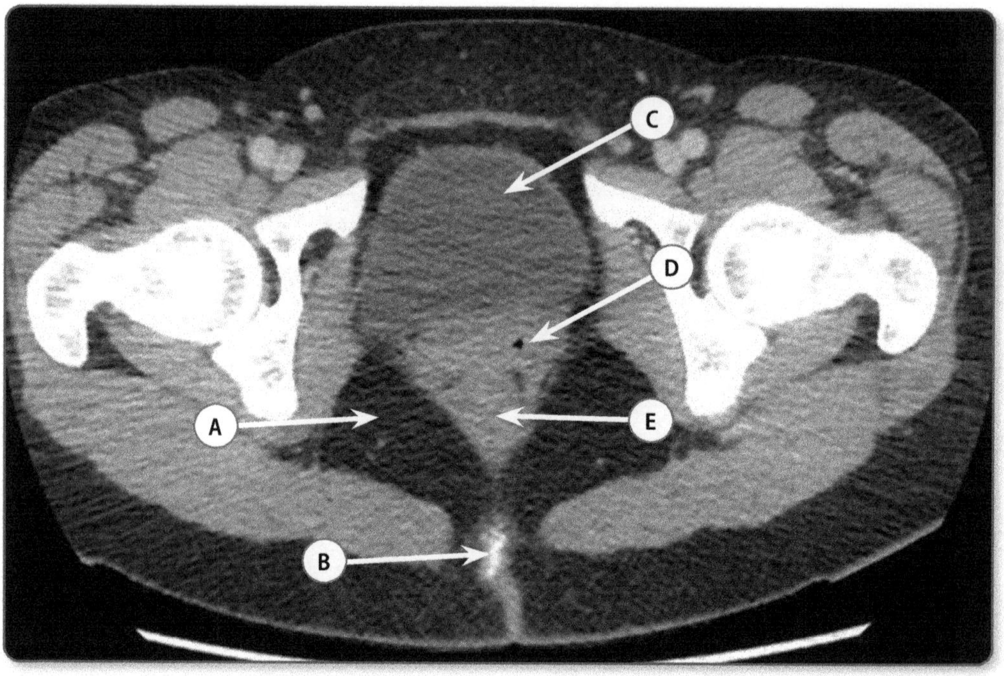

Case 3.31

QUESTION		WRITE YOUR ANSWER HERE
A	Name the structure labelled A.	
B	Name the structure labelled B.	
C	Name the structure labelled C.	
D	Name the structure labelled D.	
E	Name the structure labelled E.	

Case 3.32

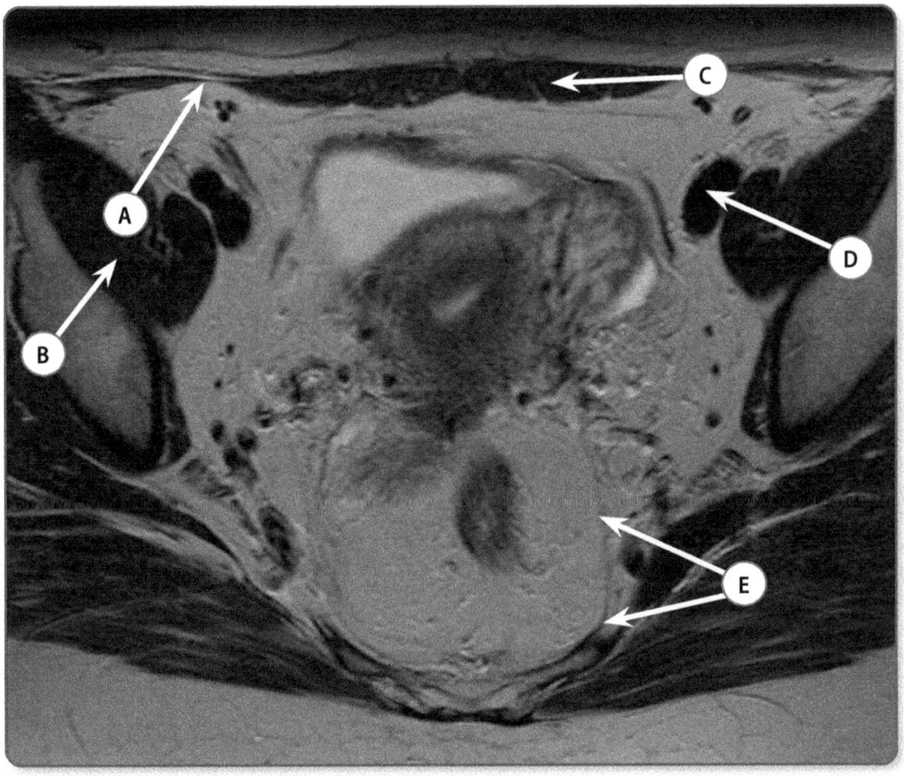

Case 3.32		
QUESTION		WRITE YOUR ANSWER HERE
A	Name the structure labelled A.	
B	Name the structure labelled B.	
C	Name the structure labelled C.	
D	Name the structure labelled D.	
E	Name the structure labelled E.	

Genitourinary

Case 3.33

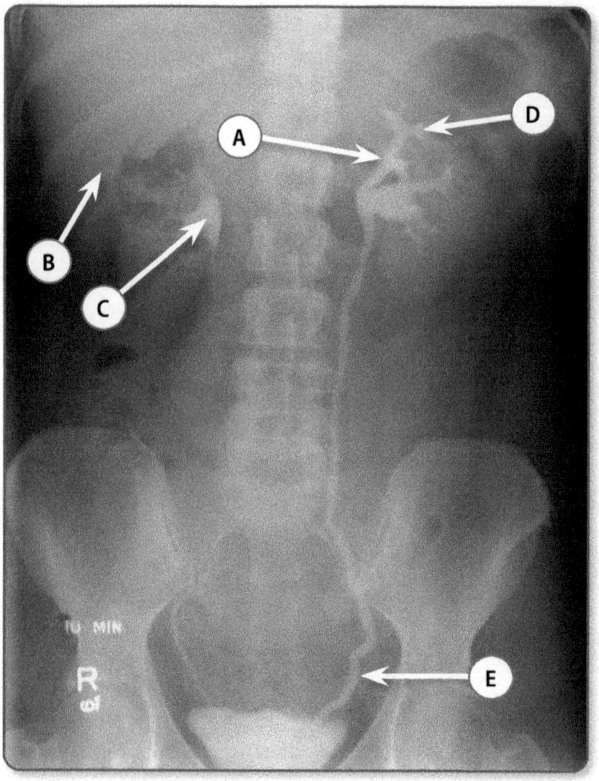

Case 3.33

QUESTION		WRITE YOUR ANSWER HERE
A	Name the structure labelled A.	
B	Name the structure labelled B.	
C	Name the structure labelled C.	
D	Name the structure labelled D.	
E	Name the structure labelled E.	

Case 3.34

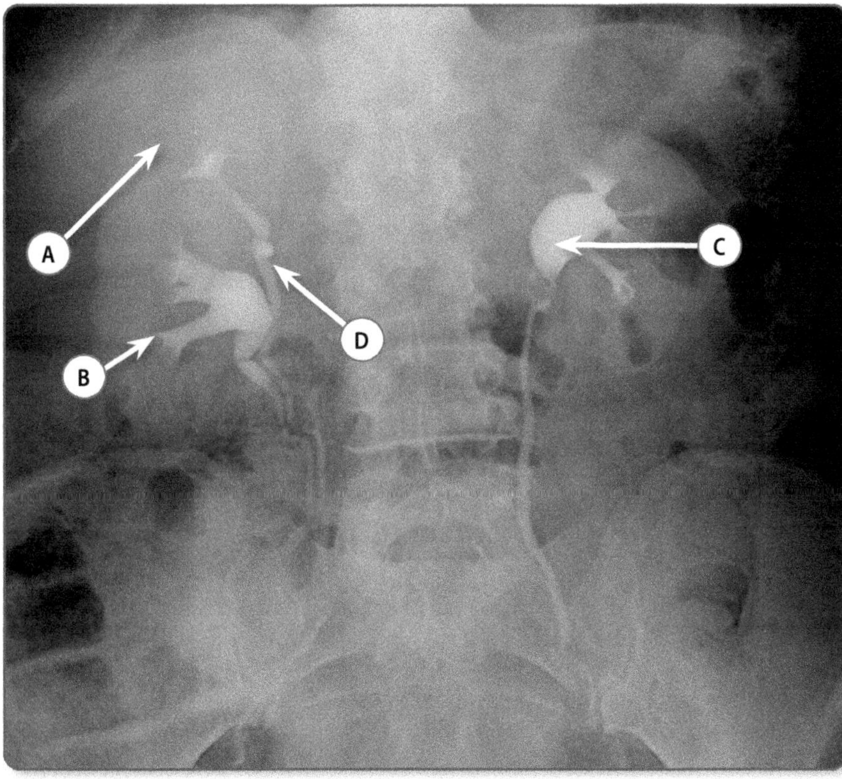

Case 3.34

QUESTION		WRITE YOUR ANSWER HERE
A	Name the structure labelled A.	
B	Name the structure labelled B.	
C	Name the structure labelled C.	
D	Name the structure labelled D.	
E	What congenital abnormality is shown here?	

Case 3.35

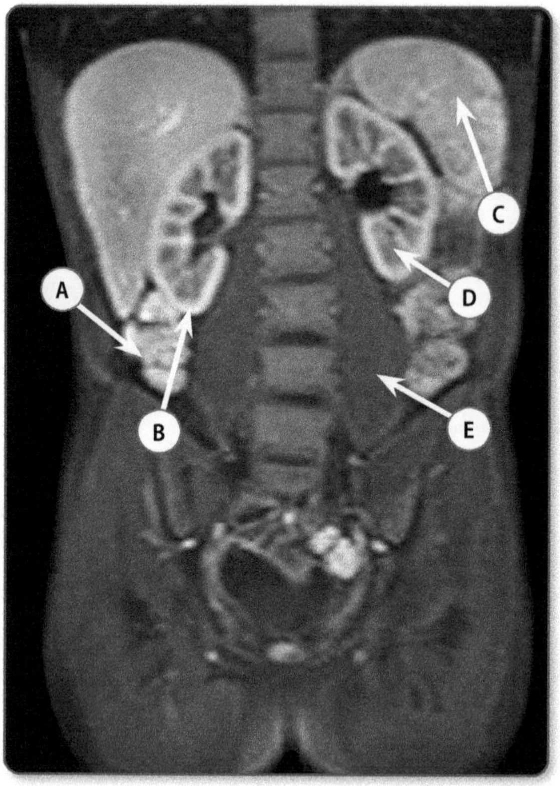

Case 3.35

QUESTION		WRITE YOUR ANSWER HERE
A	Name the structure labelled A.	
B	Name the structure labelled B.	
C	Name the structure labelled C.	
D	Name the structure labelled D.	
E	Name the structure labelled E.	

Case 3.36

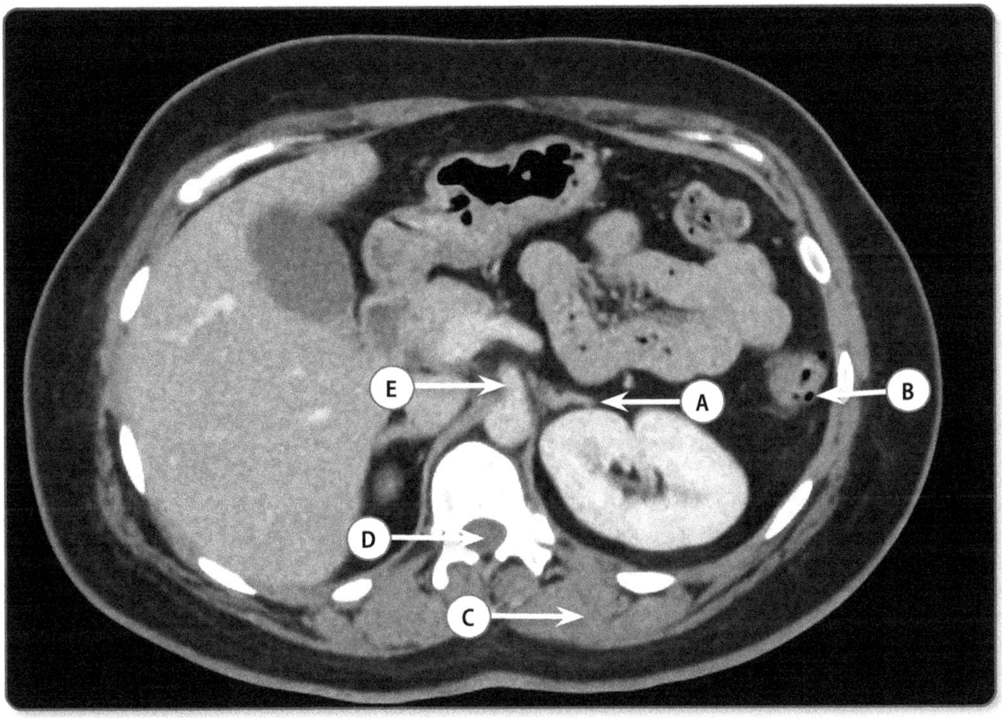

Case 3.36		
QUESTION		WRITE YOUR ANSWER HERE
A	Name the structure labelled A.	
B	Name the structure labelled B.	
C	Name the structure labelled C.	
D	Name the structure labelled D.	
E	Name the structure labelled E.	

Case 3.37

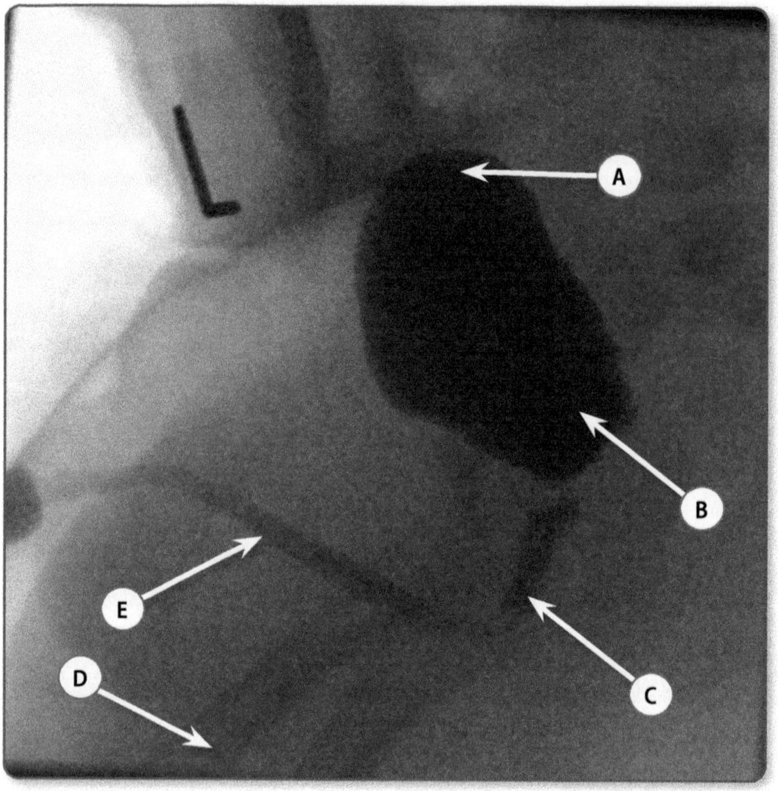

Case 3.37

QUESTION		WRITE YOUR ANSWER HERE
A	Name the structure labelled A.	
B	Name the structure labelled B.	
C	Name the structure labelled C.	
D	Name the structure labelled D.	
E	Name the structure labelled E.	

Case 3.38

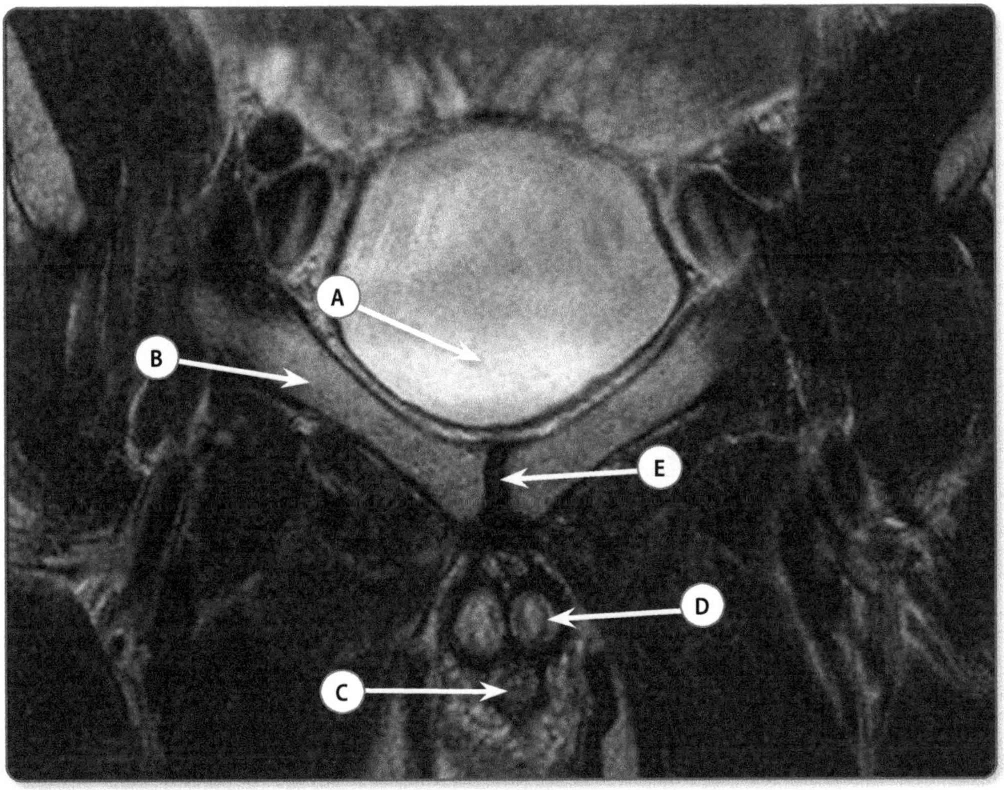

Case 3.38

QUESTION		WRITE YOUR ANSWER HERE
A	Name the structure labelled A.	
B	Name the structure labelled B.	
C	Name the structure labelled C.	
D	Name the structure labelled D.	
E	Name the structure labelled E.	

Case 3.39

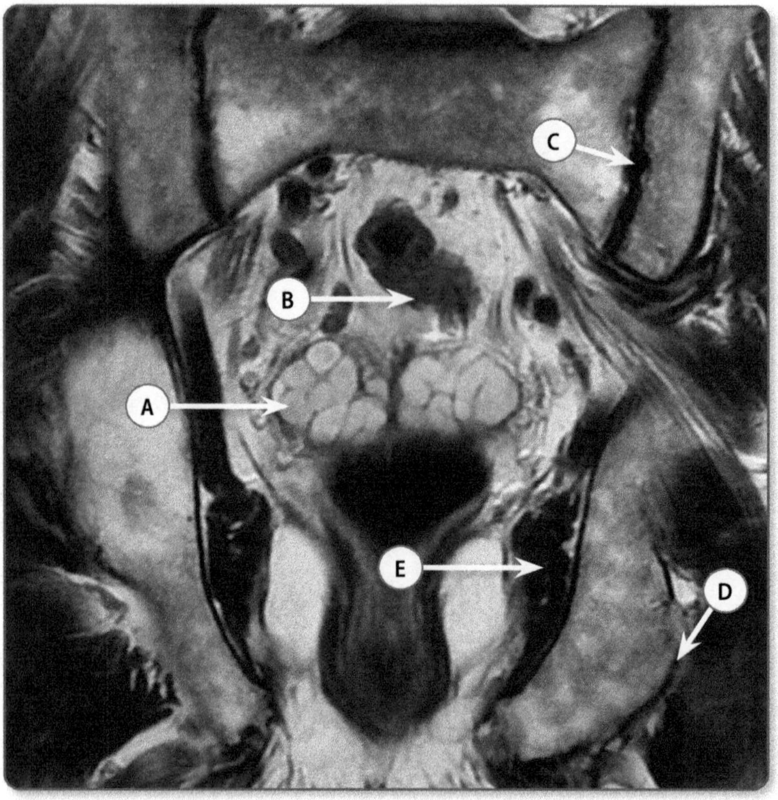

Case 3.39

QUESTION		WRITE YOUR ANSWER HERE
A	Name the structure labelled A.	
B	Name the structure labelled B.	
C	Name the structure labelled C.	
D	Name the structure labelled D.	
E	Name the structure labelled E.	

Case 3.40

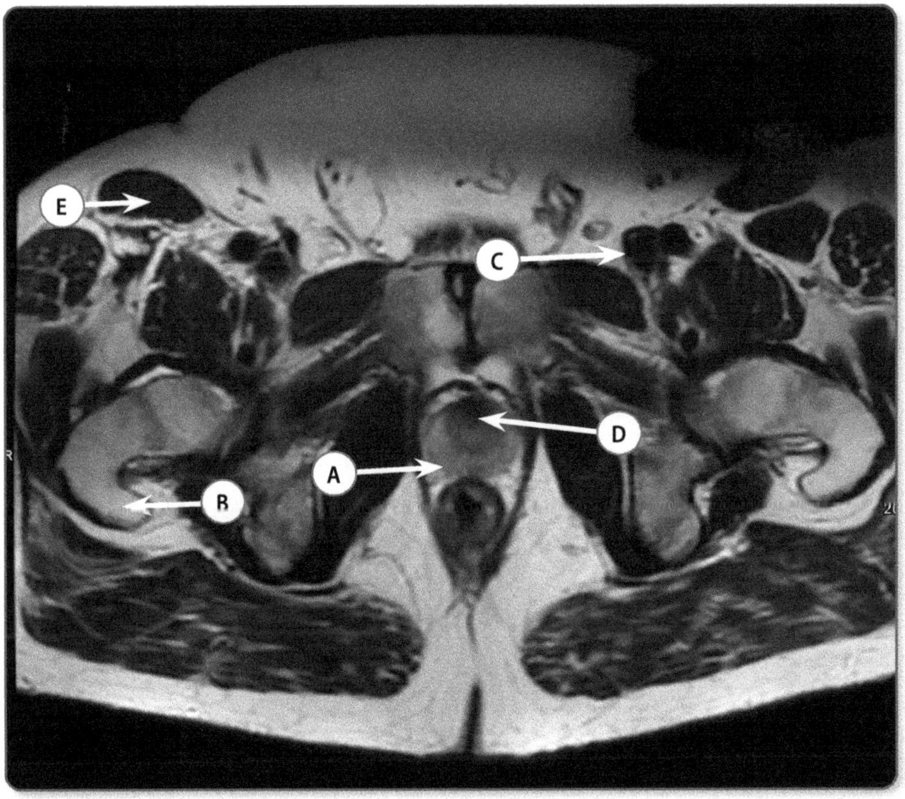

Case 3.40

QUESTION		WRITE YOUR ANSWER HERE
A	Name the structure labelled A.	
B	Name the structure labelled B.	
C	Name the structure labelled C.	
D	Name the structure labelled D.	
E	Name the structure labelled E.	

Case 3.41

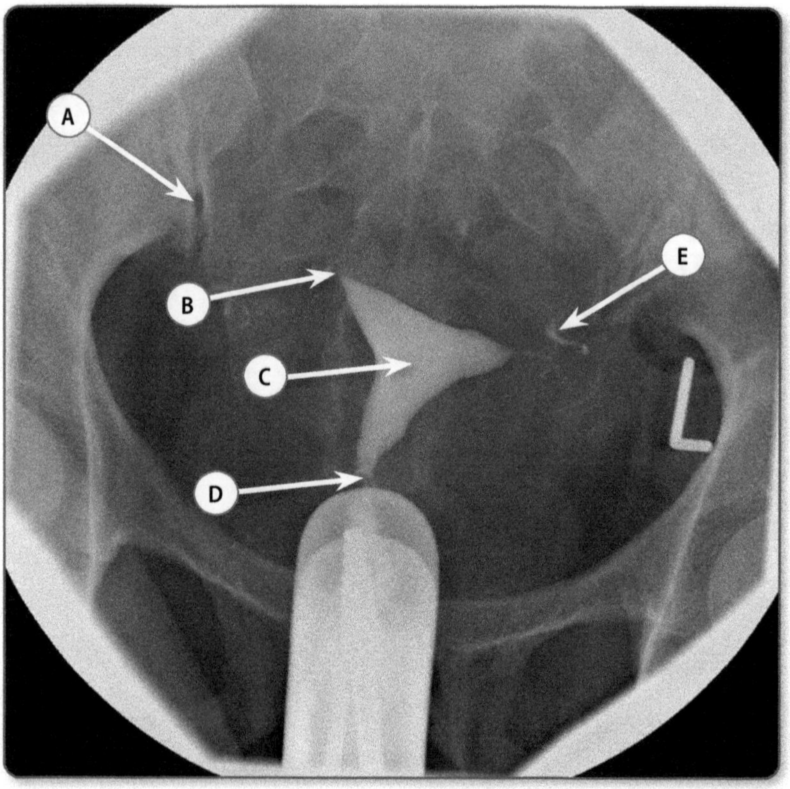

Case 3.41

QUESTION		WRITE YOUR ANSWER HERE
A	Name the structure labelled A.	
B	Name the structure labelled B.	
C	Name the structure labelled C.	
D	Name the structure labelled D.	
E	Name the structure labelled E.	

Case 3.42

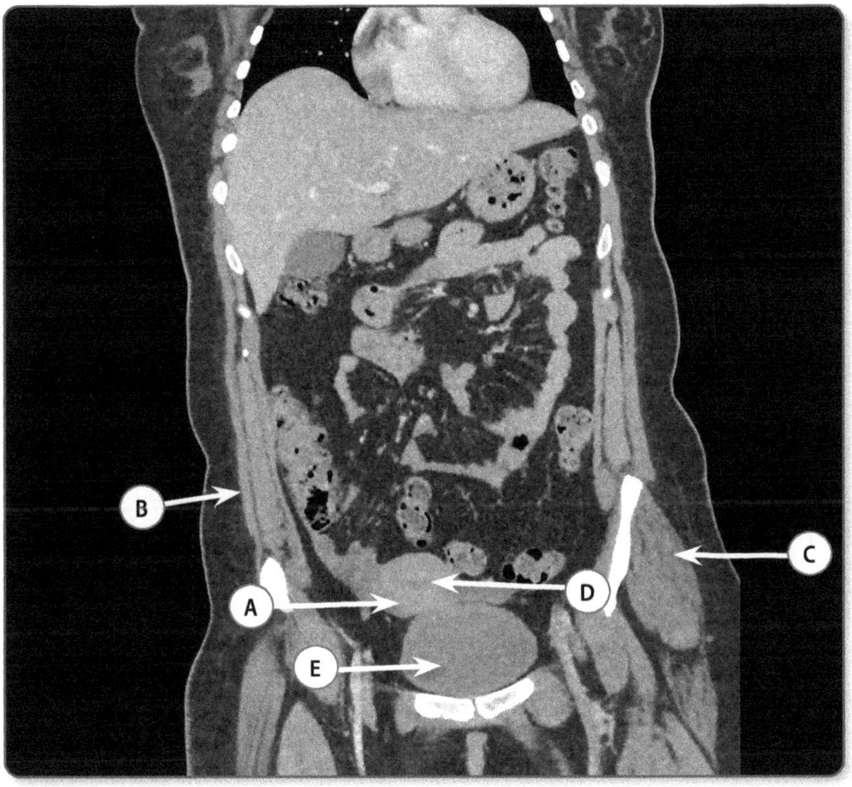

Case 3.42

QUESTION		WRITE YOUR ANSWER HERE
A	Name the structure labelled A.	
B	Name the structure labelled B.	
C	Name the structure labelled C.	
D	Name the structure labelled D.	
E	Name the structure labelled E.	

Case 3.43

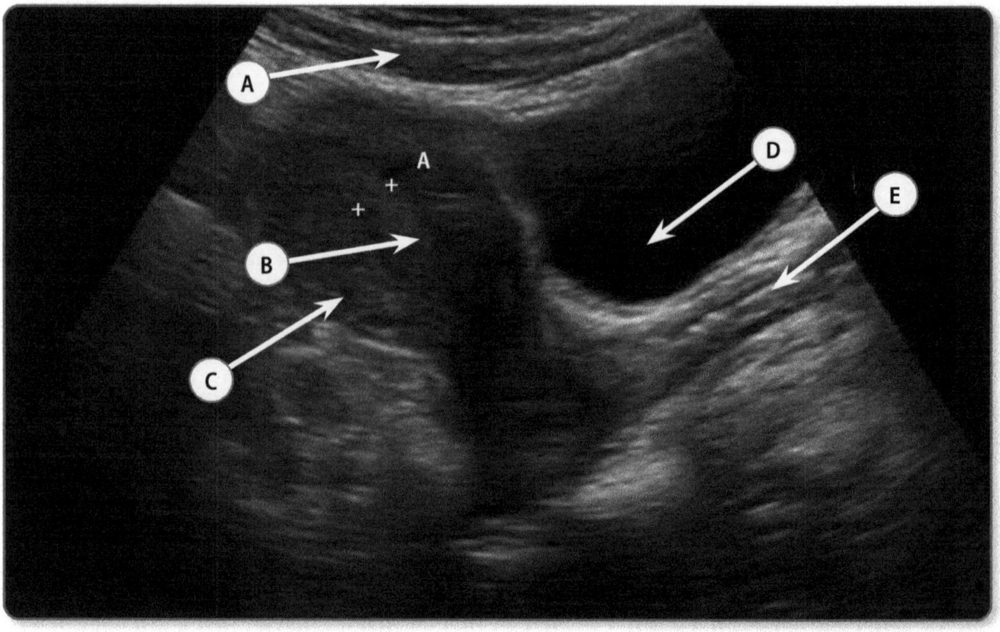

Case 3.43

QUESTION		WRITE YOUR ANSWER HERE
A	Name the structure labelled A.	
B	Name the structure labelled B.	
C	Name the structure labelled C.	
D	Name the structure labelled D.	
E	Name the structure labelled E.	

Case 3.44

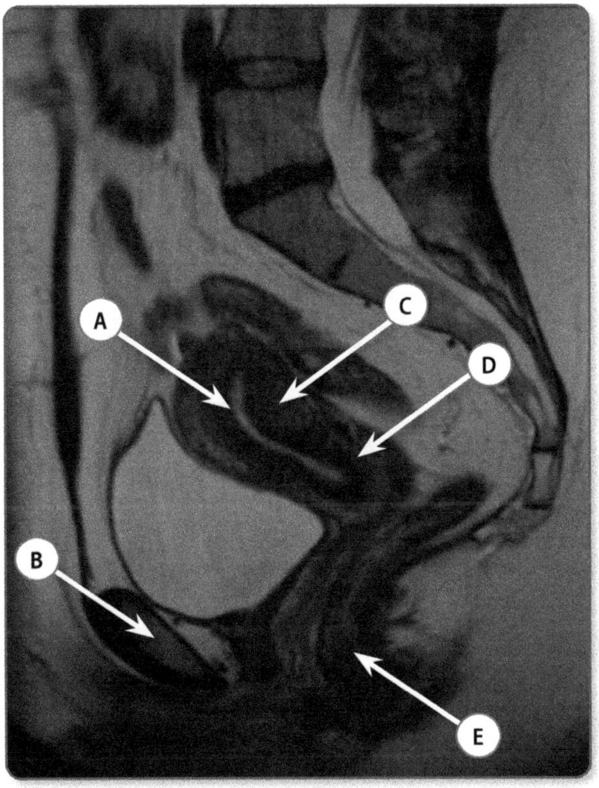

Case 3.44

QUESTION		WRITE YOUR ANSWER HERE
A	Name the structure labelled A.	
B	Name the structure labelled B.	
C	Name the structure labelled C.	
D	Name the structure labelled D.	
E	Name the structure labelled E.	

Case 3.45

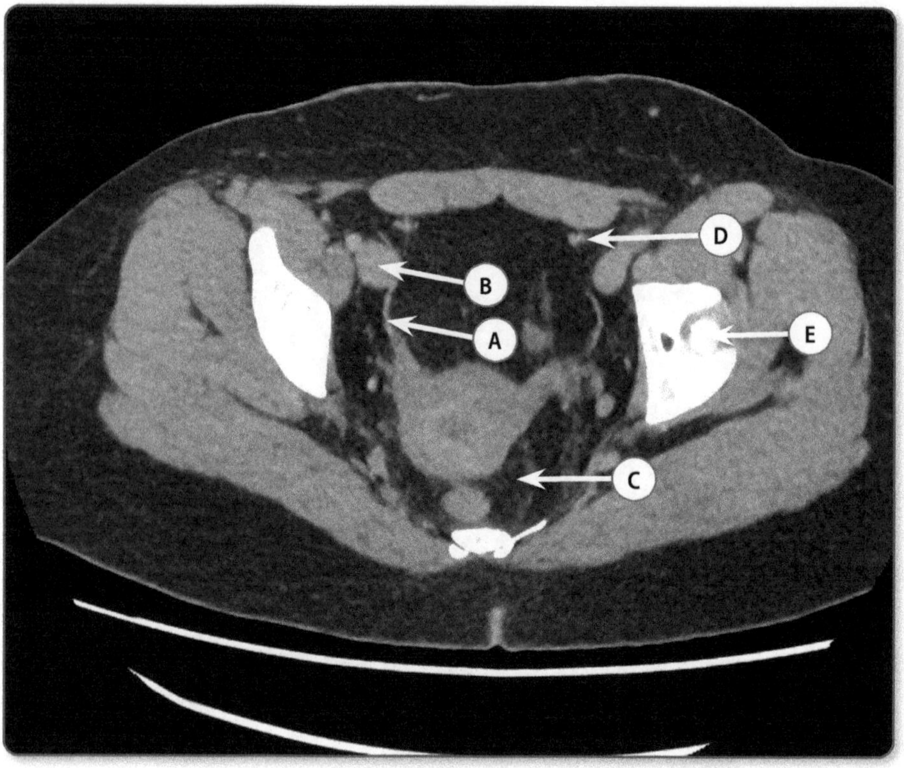

Case 3.45

QUESTION		WRITE YOUR ANSWER HERE
A	Name the structure labelled A.	
B	Name the structure labelled B.	
C	Name the structure labelled C.	
D	Name the structure labelled D.	
E	Name the structure labelled E.	

Case 3.46

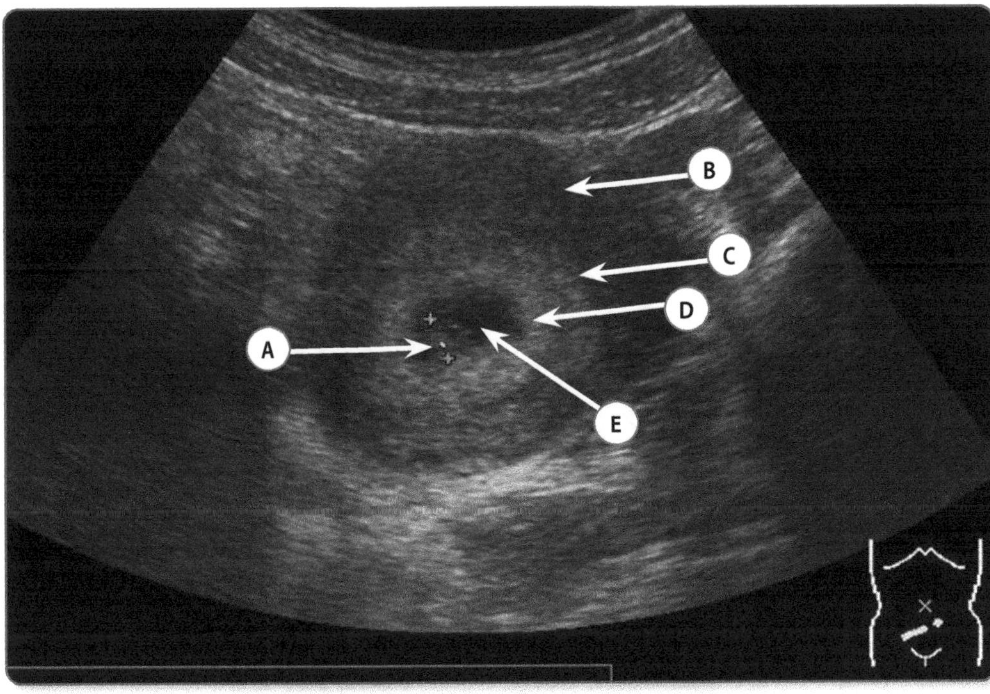

Case 3.46		
QUESTION		WRITE YOUR ANSWER HERE
A	Name the structure labelled A.	
B	Name the structure labelled B.	
C	Name the structure labelled C.	
D	Name the structure labelled D.	
E	Name the structure labelled E.	

Case 3.49

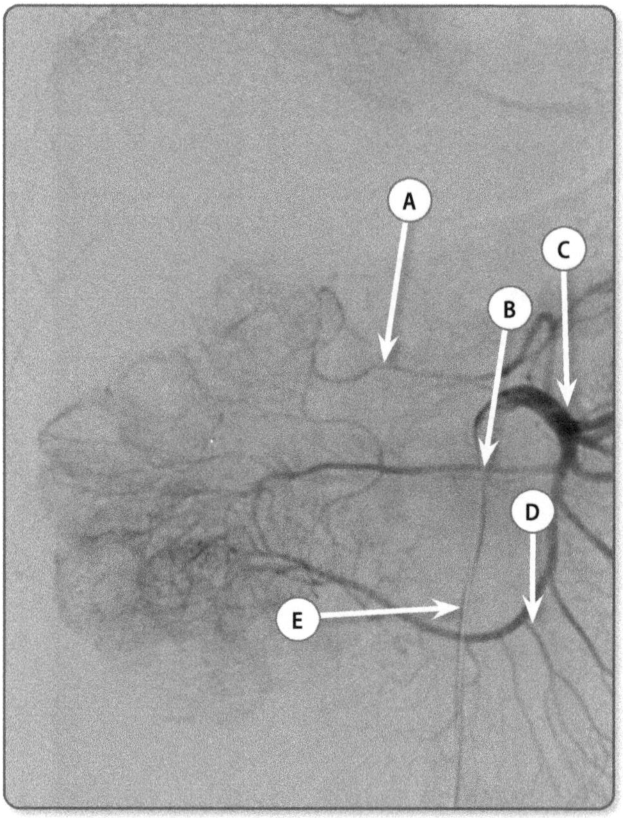

Case 3.49

QUESTION		WRITE YOUR ANSWER HERE
A	Name the structure labelled A.	
B	Name the structure labelled B.	
C	Name the structure labelled C.	
D	Name the structure labelled D.	
E	Name the structure labelled E.	

Case 3.50

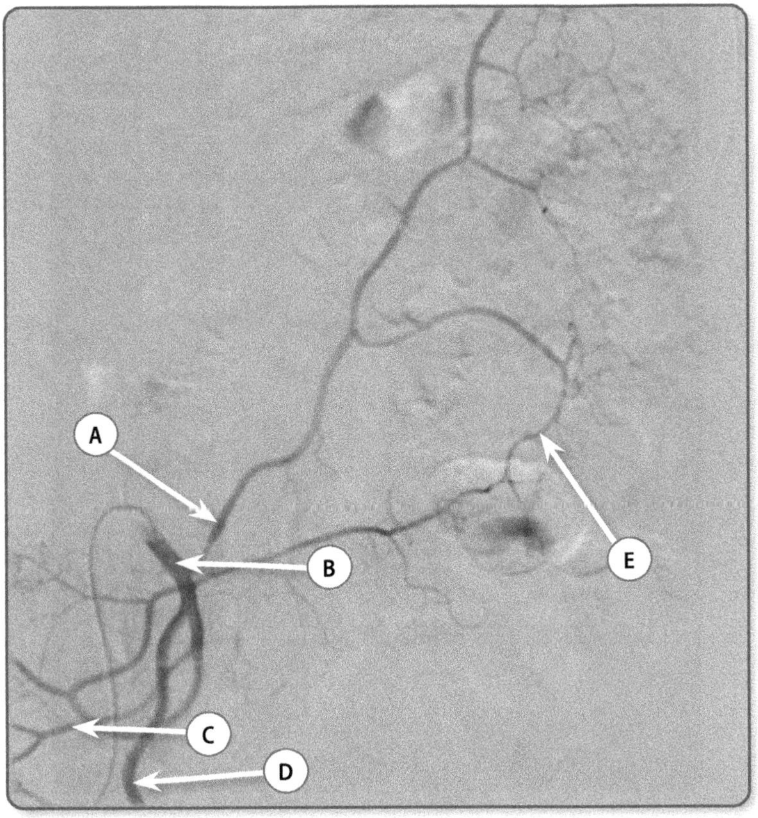

Case 3.50

QUESTION		WRITE YOUR ANSWER HERE
A	Name the structure labelled A.	
B	Name the structure labelled B.	
C	Name the structure labelled C.	
D	Name the structure labelled D.	
E	Name the structure labelled E.	

Case 3.51

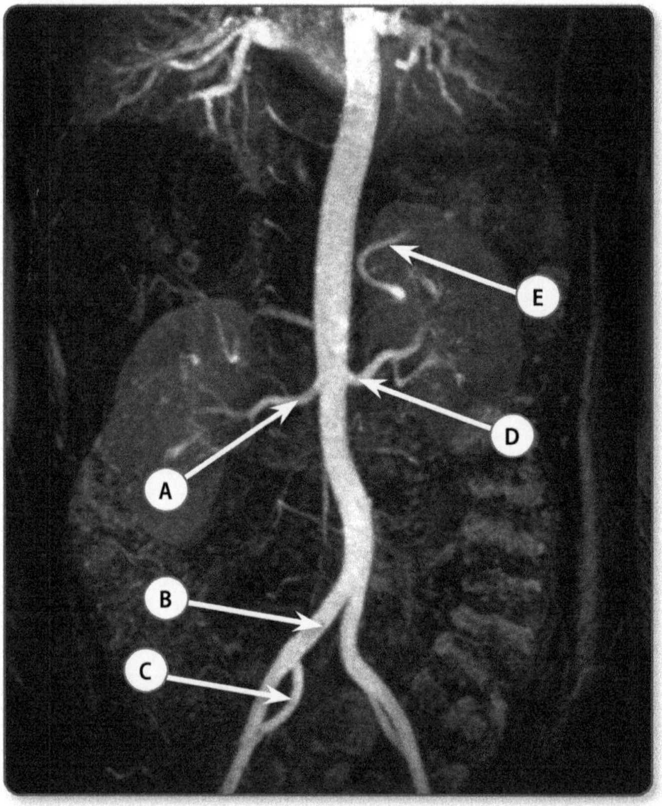

Case 3.51

QUESTION		WRITE YOUR ANSWER HERE
A	Name the structure labelled A.	
B	Name the structure labelled B.	
C	Name the structure labelled C.	
D	Name the structure labelled D.	
E	Name the structure labelled E.	

Case 3.52

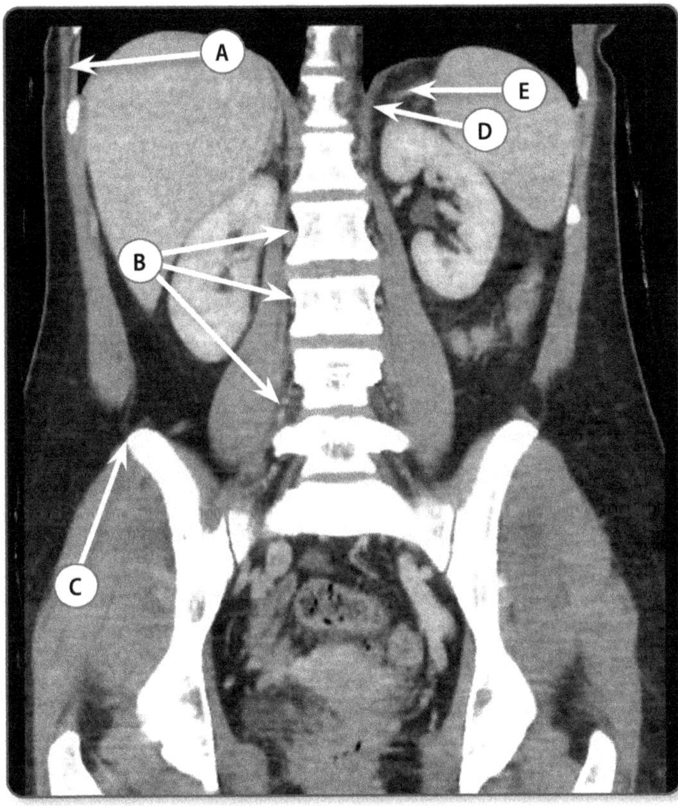

Case 3.52

QUESTION		WRITE YOUR ANSWER HERE
A	Name the structure labelled A.	
B	Name the structure labelled B.	
C	Name the structure labelled C.	
D	Name the structure labelled D.	
E	Name the structure labelled E.	

Case 3.53

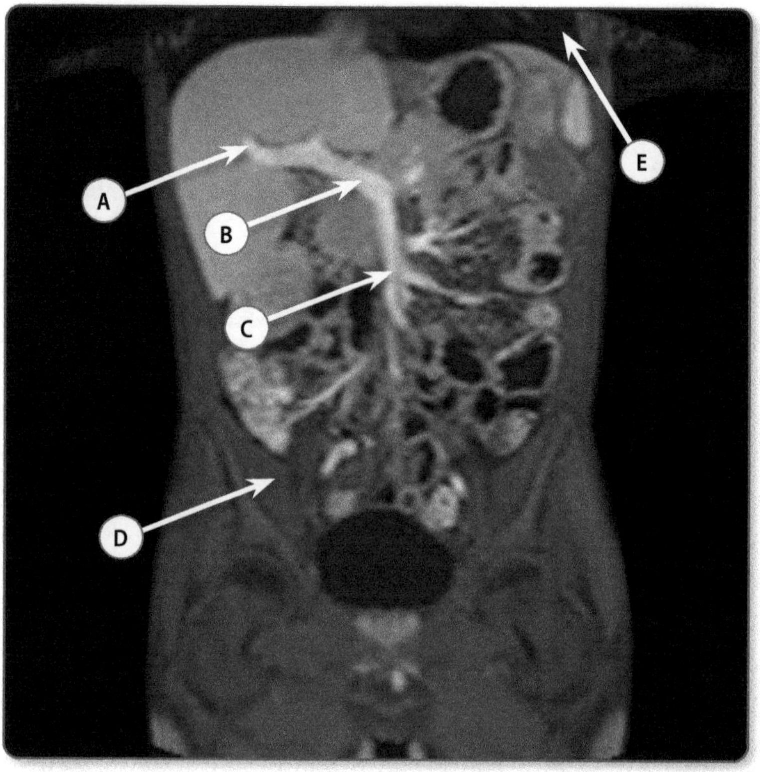

Case 3.53

QUESTION		WRITE YOUR ANSWER HERE
A	Name the structure labelled A.	
B	Name the structure labelled B.	
C	Name the structure labelled C.	
D	Name the structure labelled D.	
E	Name the structure labelled E.	

Case 3.54

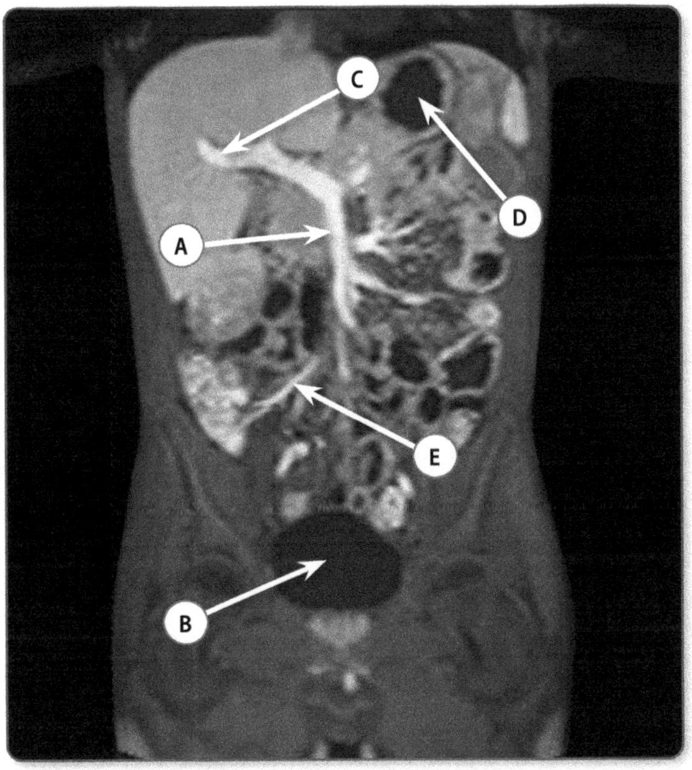

Case 3.54

QUESTION		WRITE YOUR ANSWER HERE
A	Name the structure labelled A.	
B	Name the structure labelled B.	
C	Name the structure labelled C.	
D	Name the structure labelled D.	
E	Name the structure labelled E.	

Case 3.55

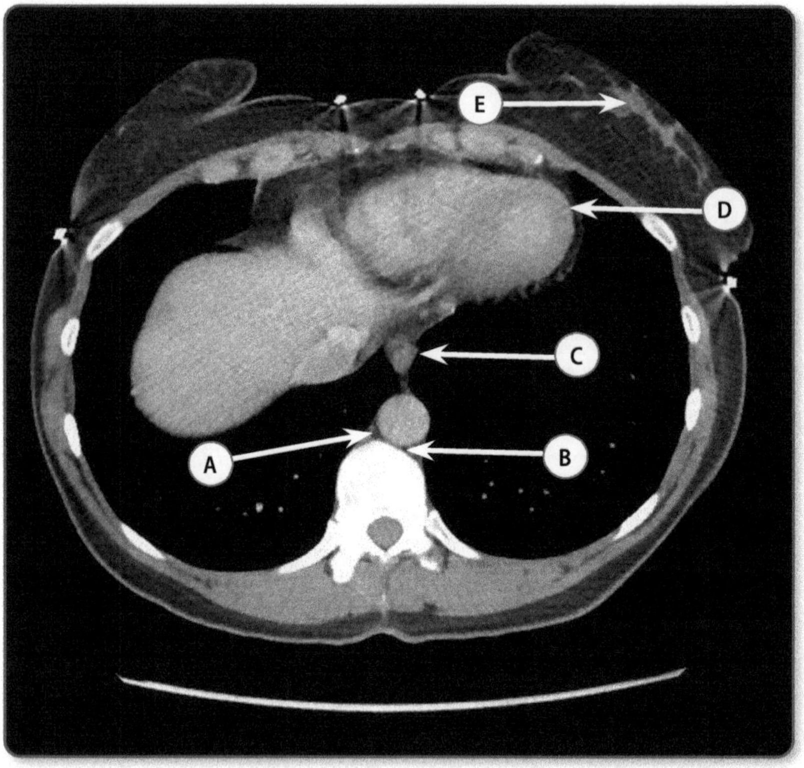

Case 3.55

QUESTION		WRITE YOUR ANSWER HERE
A	Name the structure labelled A.	
B	Name the structure labelled B.	
C	Name the structure labelled C.	
D	Name the structure labelled D.	
E	Name the structure labelled E.	

Case 3.56

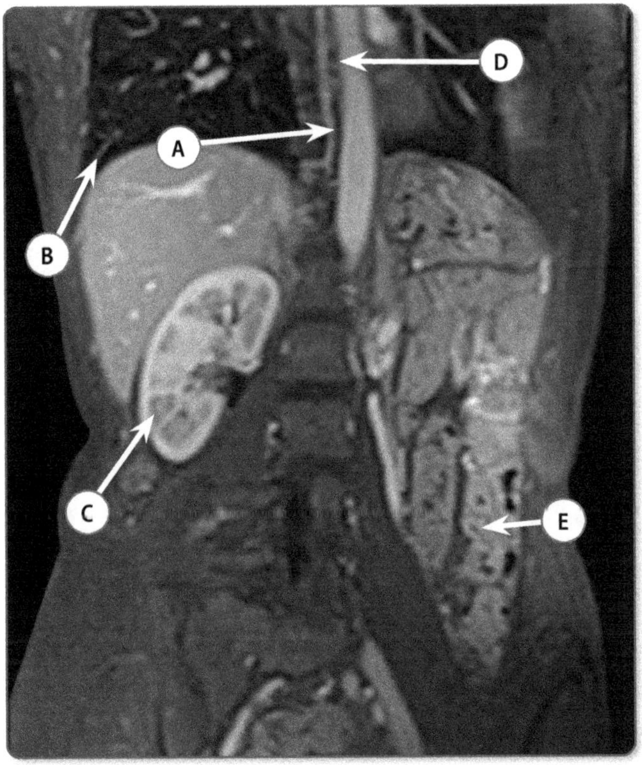

Case 3.56

QUESTION		WRITE YOUR ANSWER HERE
A	Name the structure labelled A.	
B	Name the structure labelled B.	
C	Name the structure labelled C.	
D	Name the structure labelled D.	
E	Name the structure labelled E.	

Case 3.57

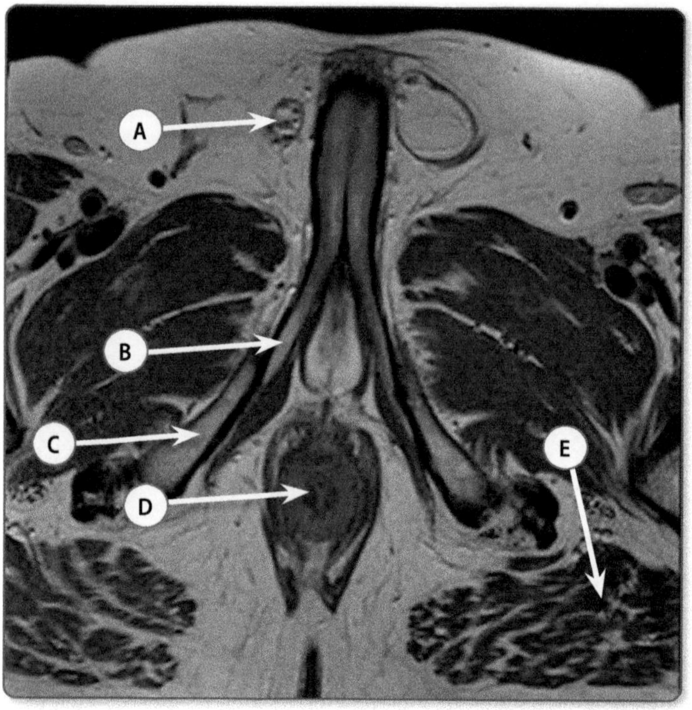

Case 3.57

	QUESTION	WRITE YOUR ANSWER HERE
A	Name the structure labelled A.	
B	Name the structure labelled B.	
C	Name the structure labelled C.	
D	Name the structure labelled D.	
E	Name the structure labelled E.	

Case 3.58

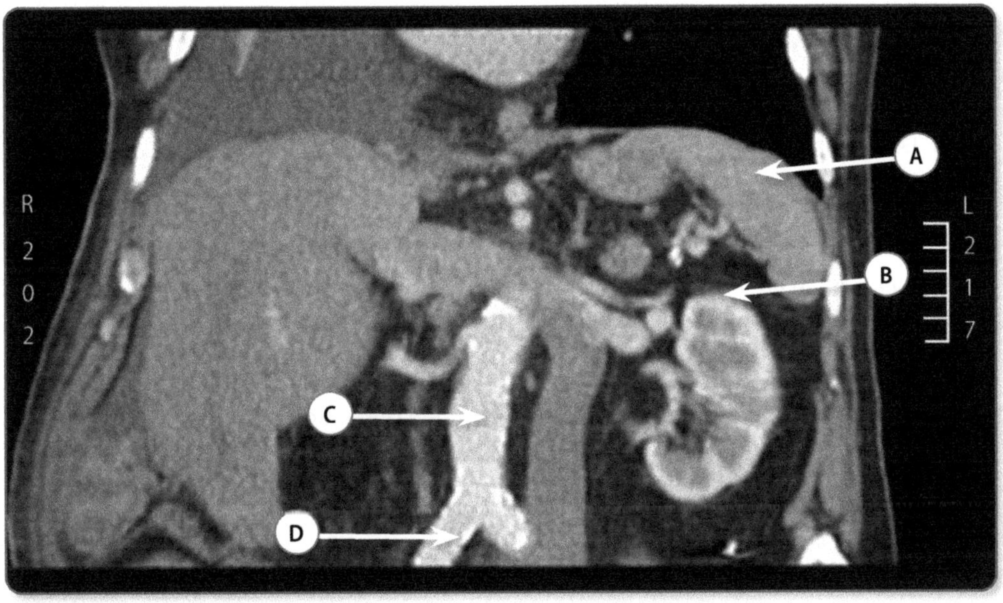

Case 3.58

QUESTION		WRITE YOUR ANSWER HERE
A	Name the structure labelled A.	
B	Name the structure labelled B.	
C	Name the structure labelled C.	
D	Name the structure labelled D.	
E	What normal variant is shown here?	

Answers

Case 3.1

A Right inferior nasal turbinate

B Right piriform fossa

C Spinous process T1

D Left vallecula

E Left body of mandible

Fluoroscopic image from a barium swallow taken in a frontal projection.

The valleculae are two shallow depressions formed by mucosal folds between the base of the tongue and the epiglottis. They are separated by the median glosso-epiglottic fold, and are bounded laterally by the lateral glosso-epiglottic folds. The piriform, fossae are located between the aryepiglottic folds and the thyroid cartilage on either side. These structures can be examined dynamically during a barium swallow.

Sinnatamby C. Last's Anatomy: Regional and Applied. London: Churchill Livingstone, 2011: 402.

Butler P, Mitchell AM, Ellis H. Applied Radiological Anatomy. Cambridge: Cambridge University Press, 1999: 112.

Case 3.2

A Vallecula

B Epiglottis

C Trachea

D Piriform fossa

E Cervical oesophagus

Lateral view of a barium swallow.

The epiglottis is attached at its base to the thyroid cartilage, along with the anterior aspect of the vocal cords. From here, it projects upwards behind the base of the tongue. Its function is to direct boluses of food into the piriform fossae at either side, thus protecting the airway during swallowing. The valleculae are two paired recesses found within the glossoepiglottic folds, which extend from the base of the tongue to the anterior surface of the epiglottis. These structures are made up of three mucosal folds – two lateral glossoepiglottic folds and a central one.

The larynx is separated from the piriform fossae by the aryepiglottic folds, which run from the lateral margin of the epiglottis to the arytenoid cartilages posteriorly.

Ryan S, McNicholas M, Eustace SJ. Anatomy for Diagnostic Imaging, 3rd edition. Edinburgh: Saunders, 2011: 38–39.

Case 3.3

A Oesophageal impression from aortic knuckle

B Oesophageal impression from left main bronchus

C Left hemi-diaphragm

D Lower third of the oesophagus, distended with barium

E Gas within the gastric fundus

Fluoroscopic image from a barium swallow in a right anterior oblique position.

There are three normal anatomical structures which cause an impression on the anterior aspect of the oesophagus:

1. Most cranially, there is an impression from the aortic knuckle – this is seen as a soft tissue density on the image – causing a smooth indentation of the upper oesophagus
2. Below this is a second impression from the left main bronchus. This is identifiable as an ovoid lucency to the left of the oesophagus
3. Lastly, the left-sided cardiac chambers can cause an impression on the anterior aspect of the oesophagus in its distal portion. The most posterior cardiac chamber is the left atrium, which lies just anterior to the oesophagus. Enlargement of this chamber can cause dysphagia

Ryan S, McNicholas M, Eustace SJ. Anatomy for Diagnostic Imaging, 3rd edition. Edinburgh: Saunders, 2011: 144.

Case 3.4

A Right heart border/right atrium

B Right lung base

C Right cardio-phrenic angle

D Oesophageal vestibule

E B ring/Schatzki ring/transverse mucosal fold

Fluoroscopic image taken from a barium swallow in a right anterior oblique position.

At the distal oesophagus, there is a focal dilatation just proximal to the gastro-oesophageal junction – this is known as the oesophageal vestibule or phrenic ampulla. The upper border of the vestibule is known as the 'A' ring, and the lower border the 'B' ring, Schatzki ring, or transverse mucosal fold. The 'B' ring marks the junction between the squamous epithelium of the oesophagus and columnar epithelium of the stomach. This mucosal change can sometimes be appreciated as a faint line on barium swallow, which is known as the 'Z' line.

B rings are composed of mucosa and submucosa, and are approximately 2–3 mm thick. They are usually located below the diaphragm, and therefore are typically only visualised in the presence of a small hiatal hernia, as demonstrated on this image.

Butler P, Mitchell AM, Ellis H. Applied Radiological Anatomy. Cambridge: Cambridge University Press, 1999: 211.

Case 3.5

A Right clavicle

B Left 1st rib

C Left lung apex

D Aortic knuckle

E Aberrant right subclavian artery

Fluoroscopic image from a barium swallow in a right anterior oblique position.

This study demonstrates the presence of an aberrant right subclavian artery. This is the most common congenital anomaly of the great vessels. With a left sided aortic arch, the right subclavian artery arises as the last branch from the arch. It then takes an oblique course, rising from left to right, crossing behind the oesophagus as it does so. It, therefore, causes a posterior impression on the oesophagus at barium swallow. The displacement of the oesophagus by the aberrant vessel is said to produce a 'bayonet deformity'.

There are three normal anatomical impressions on the oesophagus that can be seen at barium swallow. These are seen anteriorly and to the left and are caused by the aortic arch, the left main bronchus, and the heart (left atrium). An aberrant right subclavian artery should therefore be differentiated from these normal impressions. On this image, the subclavian artery is seen to cause an oblique impression just above the aortic knuckle, passing from left to right.

Freed K, Low VH. The aberrant subclavian artery. Am J Roentgenol 1997; 168: 481–484.

Butler P, Mitchell AM, Ellis H. Applied Radiological Anatomy. Cambridge: Cambridge University Press, 1999: 210.

Case 3.6

A Distal oesophagus

B Gastric cardia

C Duodenal bulb

D Second part of duodenum

E Right lower lobe pulmonary artery

Fluoroscopic image from a barium meal taken in a frontal projection.

The oesophagus crosses the diaphragm at the level of T10, where it is surrounded by fibres from the right diaphragmatic crus. The oesophageal mucosa forms longitudinal folds, which measure approximately 3 mm in thickness. They are outlined by barium in a non-distended oesophagus. The rugal folds in the stomach are much thicker, and can help to define the location of the gastro-oesophageal junction. The cardia describes the area of the stomach into which the oesophagus opens – the cardiac orifice. Above the cardia is the fundus, and below the cardia up to the level of the incisura is the gastric body. Beyond the incisura is the antrum.

Ryan S, McNicholas M, Eustace SJ. Anatomy for Diagnostic Imaging, 3rd edition. Edinburgh: Saunders, 2011: 144, 161–167.

Case 3.7

A Left pedicle of L1

B Lesser curve of the stomach

C Incisura angularis

D Rugal fold

E Left iliac crest

Fluoroscopic image from a double contrast barium meal in a frontal projection in the supine position.

The stomach is made up of the fundus, body, antrum and pylorus (from proximal to distal). The incisura angularis describes a notch at the distal end of the lesser curve of the stomach, which is located between the gastric body and antrum.

The way the barium collects can help to work out the patient's position – on an erect film the fundus would be gas-filled. The mucosal folds of the stomach are called rugae, and can easily be appreciated on barium studies. In the region of the lesser curve, they are arranged longitudinally. On this barium meal, they can be seen as parallel lucent lines, as the barium collects in between them. The mucosal surface is covered in a nodular texture caused by 'areae gastricae'; these are best appreciated in the antrum.

Butler P, Mitchell AM, Ellis H. Applied Radiological Anatomy. Cambridge: Cambridge University Press, 1999: 211.

Case 3.8

A Barium within the third part of duodenum

B Areae gastricae within antrum

C Rugal fold

D Barium within the fourth part of duodenum

E Valvulae conniventes

Fluoroscopic image taken from a barium meal in an oblique position.

This image demonstrates the mucosal relief in the body and antrum of stomach, with both the rugal folds and area gastricae being shown. The area gastricae are small nodules, or undulations in the gastric mucosa, which give a 'cobblestone' effect. They are approximately 2–3 mm in diameter, and have grooves in between them that collect barium. This results in a 'mosaic' type pattern on barium meal. This pattern is stable, and remains unaltered by the degree of stretch or the contraction of muscularis mucosae. The rugal fold pattern, however, does change with the peristaltic activity of the stomach. Along the lesser curve, the rugae are arranged longitudinally, in parallel rows known as *Magenstrasse* (main street). In other areas of the stomach, the rugae have a more random pattern.

The duodenum forms a 'C' shape around the head of pancreas, and then continues across the aorta and inferior vena cava before turning superiorly towards its junction with the jejunum. The path taken by the duodenum is demonstrated in this image, with its distinctive mucosal fold pattern projected over the stomach.

Mackintosh CE. Anatomy and radiology of the area gastricae. Gut 1977; 18: 855–864.

Ryan S, McNicholas M, Eustace SJ. Anatomy for Diagnostic Imaging, 3rd edition. Edinburgh: Saunders, 2011: 161–163.

Case 3.9

A Pylorus

B Second part of duodenum

C Valvulae conniventes

D Barium within proximal jejunum

E Greater curve of stomach

Fluoroscopic image from a barium meal in a frontal projection.

The duodenum has four parts; it begins with the duodenal bulb, and forms a 'C' shape as it runs around the head of the pancreas, and crosses the midline, over the aorta and inferior vena cava to its junction with the jejunum at the ligament of Treitz. The first part of the duodenum (D1) is intraperitoneal, and makes up the duodenal bulb or cap. The remainder of the duodenum is retroperitoneal. The pancreatic and biliary ducts drain into the second (descending) part of the duodenum, and the duodenal papilla may be seen as a filling defect on barium studies. The third part of the duodenum has a horizontal course, which follows the lower margin of the pancreatic head. Finally, the fourth part has a course which runs superolaterally, over the left psoas, and it finishes by turning forwards, to join the jejunum at the level of L2.

The small bowel mucosa has numerous folds called valvulae conniventes or plicae circulares, which encircle two-thirds of the inner surface. These are absent from D1, but become more numerous towards the distal duodenum. The jejunum can be differentiated from the ilium on barium studies not only by its position, but also by its mucosal fold pattern. The jejunum is located more towards the left upper quadrant, and has more prominent valvulae conniventes than the ilium, which is located more towards the right lower quadrant.

Butler P, Mitchell AM, Ellis H. Applied Radiological Anatomy. Cambridge: Cambridge University Press, 1999: 213.

Case 3.10

A Gas within the colon; hepatic flexure

B Left renal outline, lower pole

C Right obturator foramen

D Gas within the transverse colon

E Left transverse process of the L5 vertebra

Plain supine abdominal radiograph.

Structures on plain film are differentiated from one another based on their differing densities. Some abdominal organs are clearly outlined by the fat which surrounds them. On this film, the left kidney can be clearly identified, with its upper pole projected over the lower ribs, and its lower pole adjacent to the left psoas.

Gas within bowel can outline valvulae conniventes and haustral markings, which helps to identify small and large bowel respectively. Haustrae are fixed structures in the proximal colon, but are formed by muscular contraction more distally, and so are variable. Haustral markings may be absent from the mid transverse colon onwards. Small and large bowel can be further differentiated by their position within the abdomen. The large bowel is located around the periphery, and can be said to 'frame the abdomen'. **Table 3.1** outlines the anatomical features which differentiate large from small bowel on plain film.

Table 3.1 Anatomical features of small bowel and large bowel on plain radiograph

	Small bowel	Large bowel
Position	Central	Peripheral
Septations	Complete (valvulae conniventes)	Incomplete (haustrae)
Diameter	<3 cm	<5.5 cm
Contents	• Air • Fluid	Solid faeces may be present

Ryan S, McNicholas M, Eustace SJ. Anatomy for Diagnostic Imaging, 3rd edition. Edinburgh: Saunders, 2011: 167–174.

Case 3.11

A Gastric antrum

B Gas within ascending colon

C Small bowel loop; ileum

D Small bowel mesentery

E Stomach wall, greater curve

Coronal contrast-enhanced CT in the portal venous phase.

The small bowel mesentery is made up of two folds of peritoneum, which connect the small bowel to the posterior abdominal wall. The mesentery is fan-shaped and within it run the blood vessels, nerves and lymphatics which supply the small bowel. The blood vessels can be easily appreciated on this image as fine linear branching structures, containing contrast, and outlined by fat. The root of the small bowel mesentery runs from the duodenojejunal flexure in the left upper quadrant, to the superior aspect of the right sacroiliac joint in the right lower quadrant.

The ileum makes up approximately 60% of the length of the small bowel. It forms the distal small bowel, running from the jejunum to the caecum via the ileocaecal valve. The ileum tends to lie in the right lower quadrant, whereas the jejunum tends to be located in the left upper quadrant. Other differences between jejunum and ileum include the diameter of the loops and the number of valvulae conniventes they contain; both being greater in the jejunal loops. **Table 3.2** summarises the differences in the appearance of jejunal and ilial loops.

Table 3.2 Anatomical features to differentiate jejunal from ilial loops

	Jejunum	Ileum
Location	Left upper quadrant	Right lower quadrant
Diameter	Wider (~ 3.5 cm)	Narrower (~ 2.5 cm)
Thickness of wall	Thicker	Thinner (1 mm)
Valvulae conniventes	• More numerous • Thicker (2mm)	• Less numerous • Thinner (1 mm)

Butler P, Mitchell AM, Ellis H. Applied Radiological Anatomy. Cambridge: Cambridge University Press, 1999: 196.

Ryan S, McNicholas M, Eustace SJ. Anatomy for Diagnostic Imaging, 3rd edition. Edinburgh: Saunders, 2011: 167–169.

Case 3.12

A Ileocaecal valve

B Caecal pole

C Gallbladder

D Left kidney

E Left psoas

Sagittal contrast-enhanced CT.

The ileocaecal valve is found in the right iliac fossa, and is the point at which the small bowel joins the large bowel. The ileocaecal valve opens into the postero-medial aspect of the large bowel, at the level of the first complete transverse haustral fold. This fold thickens posteriorly to become the frenula of the valve – these are typically up to 3 mm in thickness. Below this level is found the caecum, and above, the ascending colon. The appendix joins the caecum approximately 2 cm below the ileocaecal valve. The valve has an upper and a lower fold, and helps to prevent reflux of bowel contents from the large bowel into the terminal ileum due to thickening of the circular muscle at this point. It projects slightly into the lumen of the large bowel, and may be seen as a filling defect on barium enema. There is often some fat around the valve, which makes it easily identifiable on CT studies.

Butler P, Mitchell AM, Ellis H. Applied Radiological Anatomy. Cambridge: Cambridge University Press, 1999: 216.

Ryan S, McNicholas M, Eustace SJ. Anatomy for Diagnostic Imaging, 3rd edition. Edinburgh: Saunders, 2011: 169.

Case 3.13

A Right external oblique muscle

B Caecum

C Left transversus abdominis

D Left internal oblique

E Terminal ileum

Coronal contrast-enhanced CT of the abdomen.

The terminal ileum is the most distal part of the small bowel, and joins the large bowel at the junction of the caecum and the ascending colon via the ileocaecal valve. There are few valvulae conniventes in this part of the small bowel, and it tends to have a thinner and smaller calibre wall than the more proximal jejunum.

The ileocaecal valve opens into the posteromedial aspect of the large bowel, where it projects into the lumen somewhat. There is usually some fat around the ileocaecal valve, which makes it easily identifiable on CTs.

The muscles of the anterolateral abdominal wall are external oblique, most superficially, with internal oblique deep to this, and transversus abdominis as the third, and deepest muscle layer. All three form an aponeurosis that becomes the rectus sheath, surrounding the rectus abdominis muscles before inserting into the linea alba in the midline.

Ryan S, McNicholas M, Eustace SJ. Anatomy for Diagnostic Imaging, 3rd edition. Edinburgh: Saunders, 2011: 157, 167–169.

Case 3.14

A Right external iliac vein

B Sigmoid colon

C Sacral canal

D Left external iliac artery

E Left piriformis

Axial contrast-enhanced CT of the pelvis.

The sacrum is made up of five sacral vertebrae which are fused together. It has a triangular shape, with its base lying superiorly, articulating with L5. Anteriorly, it has a concave surface, which forms the posterior wall of the pelvis. In the central part of the sacrum runs the sacral canal, which is continuous with the spinal canal above. There are four pairs of anterior sacral foramina and four pairs of dorsal sacral foramina, which transmit the anterior and dorsal rami of S1–S4 respectively. On the dorsal surface, running longitudinally, between the dorsal foramina is the median sacral crest. The four sacral tubercles project from this crest in the midline. There are also two lateral sacral crests, which are found laterally to the dorsal foramina. Occasionally, there are transverse tubercles which arise from these crests – these represent vestigial transverse processes.

The sigmoid colon is found in the pelvis, and is quite variable in length. It begins at the pelvic brim, and extends to its junction with the rectum. It is surrounded by peritoneum, which also ends at the rectosigmoid junction. The sigmoid colon is attached to the posterior pelvic wall by the sigmoid mesocolon, the root of which is shaped like an inverted 'V'. The sigmoid vessels, arising from the inferior mesenteric vessels, are transmitted in the sigmoid mesocolon.

Butler P, Mitchell AM, Ellis H. Applied Radiological Anatomy. Cambridge: Cambridge University Press, 1999: 218, 354.

Case 3.15

A Right lobe of liver

B Portal vein

C Gastric fundus

D Left 12th rib

E Urinary bladder

Coronal contrast-enhanced CT of the abdomen in the portal venous phase.

The liver is divided into right and left lobes, and further subdivided into eight segments by the portal and hepatic veins. **Figure 3.1** illustrates the segmental anatomy of the liver.

The portal vein is formed by the confluence of the superior mesenteric vein and the splenic vein, behind the pancreatic neck, just to the right of midline. It travels superiorly, within the hepatoduodenal ligament, towards the porta hepatis, where it divides into right and left branches. The right portal vein divides further into anterior

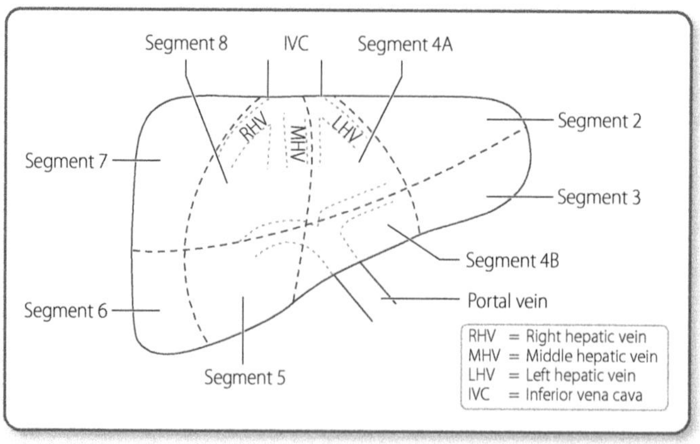

Figure 3.1 Segmental anatomy of the liver. RHV, right hepatic vein; MHV, middle hepatic vein; LHV, left hepatic vein; IVC, inferior vena cava.

and posterior branches. The left portal vein gives off branches to the caudate and quadrate lobes (segments I and IV), before going on to divide into superior and inferior branches more distally. The superior and inferior branches supply segments II, III and the inferior aspect of segment IV.

Butler P, Mitchell AM, Ellis H. Applied Radiological Anatomy. Cambridge: Cambridge University Press, 1999: 234–235.

Case 3.16

A Right rectus abdominis

B Ligamentum teres

C Inferior vena cava

D Right erector spinae

E Pancreatic tail

Coronal contrast-enhanced CT of the abdomen in the portal venous phase.

The ligamentum teres (also known as the round ligament) is formed by the obliterated left umbilical vein. It runs in the falciform ligament (a peritoneal fold) from the umbilicus to the liver. The falciform ligament divides the liver into right and left lobes. In this image, the ligamentum teres appears as a soft-tissue density structure surrounded by fat.

The extensors of the spine can be described by their location – deep, intermediate and superficial. Erector spinae is the most powerful of these groups, and is made up by the superficial extensors. These muscles lie in the groove either side of the spinal column and run the length of the spine.

Ryan S, McNicholas M, Eustace SJ. Anatomy for Diagnostic Imaging, 3rd edition. Edinburgh: Saunders, 2011: 175.

Butler P, Mitchell AM, Ellis H. Applied Radiological Anatomy. Cambridge: Cambridge University Press, 1999: 308.

Case 3.17

A Right lobe of liver

B Portal vein

C Intrahepatic IVC

D Gallbladder fundus

E Common bile duct

Longitudinal abdominal ultrasound at the porta hepatis.

The common bile duct (CBD), hepatic artery and portal vein are all very closely related to each other at the porta hepatis. Here the CBD is demonstrated running anterior and parallel to the portal vein.

Butler P, Mitchell AM, Ellis H. Applied Radiological Anatomy. Cambridge: Cambridge University Press, 1919: 252.

Ryan S, McNicholas M, Eustace SJ. Anatomy for Diagnostic Imaging, 3rd edition. Edinburgh: Saunders, 2010: 182–192

Case 3.21

A Gallbladder

B Spleen

C Hepatic IVC

D Splenic vein

E Right latissimus dorsi

Axial T2 MRI of the abdomen.

The spleen is found in the left upper quadrant of the abdomen, and measures up to 12 cm in length, 7 cm in width and 4 cm in breadth. It is attached from its hilum to the posterior abdominal wall via the splenorenal and phrenicosplenic ligaments. The gastrosplenic ligament attaches the spleen to the stomach, and separates the lesser sac from the greater sac anteriorly. The splenic surface which abuts the diaphragm is smooth and rounded, and it is protected in this position by the 9th–11th ribs which overly it. The 'visceral' surface is contoured where it abuts the adjacent organs. This surface has impressions from the left kidney posteriorly, the splenic flexure inferiorly, the pancreatic tail at the splenic hilum, and an anterior impression from the stomach. The splenic vessels enter at the hilum between the gastric and renal impressions. The red and white pulps of the spleen enhance at different rates, and can therefore cause a mottled appearance particularly in the arterial phase.

Ryan S, McNicholas M, Eustace SJ. Anatomy for Diagnostic Imaging, 3rd edition. Edinburgh: Saunders, 2011: 192–193.

Case 3.22

A Pro-peritoneal fat line

B Left anterolateral abdominal wall

C Left L4 pedicle

D Right psoas

E Left obturator foramen

Plain pelvic radiograph.

In this image, the soft tissues can be easily outlined due to the fat which is surrounding them. There is a layer of fat which separates the muscles of the anterior abdominal wall from the peritoneum, which is known as properitoneal fat. This can be seen as a hypodense line or stripe on abdominal plain radiographs: the properitoneal fat line.

The anterolateral abdominal wall has three muscle layers, which are interposed with fat. The largest and most superficial of these muscles is the external oblique. It arises as slips from the inferolateral borders of the eight inferior ribs, and its posterior fibres extend to insert into the anterior half of the iliac crests. The middle and uppermost fibres are continuous with the aponeurosis of the muscle, anteriorly. This aponeurosis continues medially and becomes part of the rectus sheath and linea alba. Inferiorly, the aponeurosis extends to the pubic symphysis. The free edge of the aponeurosis, between the anterior superior iliac spine and the pubic tubercle, forms the inguinal ligament.

Deep to external oblique, forming the other two muscle layers of the anterolateral abdominal wall are internal oblique and transversus abdominis.

There are four different densities which can be appreciated on plain radiograph: air, fat, fluid/soft tissue, and bone. Edges and borders can only be seen on plain film if there is an interface with a tissue of differing density (silhouette sign).

Ryan S, McNicholas M, Eustace SJ. Anatomy for Diagnostic Imaging, 3rd edition. Edinburgh: Saunders, 2011: 158.

Butler P, Mitchell AM, Ellis H. Applied Radiological Anatomy. Cambridge: Cambridge University Press, 2012.

Case 3.23

A Superior mesenteric artery

B D3 duodenum

C Left lobe of liver

D Spinous process of lumbar vertebrae

E Linea alba

Case 3.24

A Right rectus abdominis

B Right lobe of liver

C Inferior vena cava

D Right crus of diaphragm

E Right erector spinae

Axial T2 MRI.

The diaphragm is a strong muscular sheet which forms the floor of the thorax. It has origins arising from the sternum, ribs and vertebrae, as well as the central tendon. The central tendon is fused with the pericardium at its midportion, and posteriorly it extends towards the paraspinal gutters. The sternal attachment is via two small slips, which extend to the posterior aspect of the xiphisternum. There are further diaphragmatic slips which arise from the six lower costal cartilages to form the costal attachments.

From the lower thoracic and upper lumbar vertebrae arise the crura and arcuate ligaments. The right crus is attached to the bodies of L1–3, whereas the smaller left crus extends only from L1 to L2. The median arcuate ligament is formed by a fibrous thickening of the medial aspects of both crura. Lateral to this, are found the medial arcuate ligaments, which overlie the psoas muscles, and are formed from a thickening of the psoas fascia. Lastly, the lateral arcuate ligament is found overlying the quadratus lumborum muscles, and is formed by a thickening of its fascia.

Ryan S, McNicholas M, Eustace SJ. Anatomy for Diagnostic Imaging, 3rd edition. Edinburgh: Saunders, 2011: 117–119.

Butler P, Mitchell AM, Ellis H. Applied Radiological Anatomy. Cambridge: Cambridge University Press, 1999: 270.

Case 3.25

A Sigmoid colon

B Right piriformis

C Left gluteus maximus

D Left gluteus medius

E Left gluteus minimus

Axial contrast-enhanced CT scan.

The gluteal muscles arise from the iliac bones and pass around the outside of the pelvis, to insert into the proximal femur. Gluteus maximus is the largest and most superficial of the gluteal muscles. Of the three, gluteus maximus arises most posteriorly with its origin from the posterior surface of the ilium, including the sacrum, coccyx and sacrotuberous ligament. The muscle fibres from gluteus maximus converge to form a tough tendinous sheath which becomes part of the iliotibial tract. The deep fibres then attach to the gluteal tuberosity on the proximal femur. Gluteus medius arises anteriorly and deep to gluteus maximus, and inserts onto the greater trochanter. Gluteus minimus is the smallest and deepest of the gluteal muscles, arising below gluteus medius. It too inserts onto the greater trochanter.

Piriformis arises from the anterior surface of the sacrum and passes through the greater sciatic foramen to insert into the greater trochanter.

Ryan S, McNicholas M, Eustace SJ. Anatomy for Diagnostic Imaging, 3rd edition. Edinburgh: Saunders, 2011: 220.

Case 3.26

A Right pectineus

B Left sartorius

C Left iliopsoas

D Left iliotibial tract

E Obturator externus

Axial contrast-enhanced CT of the pelvis.

The iliotibial tract is a thickened band of connective tissue, that is part of the fascia lata (the deep fascia of the lateral thigh), and inserts into the lateral tibial condyle. The tensor fascia lata is one of the anterior thigh muscles, arising from the anterior superior iliac spine, and inserts into the iliotibial tract.

Sartorius is the longest muscle in the human body. It is a thin strap muscle which runs along the anterior thigh, from the anterior superior iliac spine to the medial tibial condyle, where it inserts as part of the pes anserinus. It acts to flex the hip and knee, as well as rotate the femur laterally.

Obturator externus is one of the muscles of the pelvic girdle. It arises from the outer aspect of the obturator membrane, and runs inferiorly to the hip joint to insert onto the posterior aspect of the greater trochanter. When flexed, it acts to externally rotate the femur.

Pectineus is one of the hip adductors. It is a flat muscle, which has its origin on the superior surface of the pubis. It then passes posterolaterally to insert into the femur, from the lesser trochanter to the linea aspera.

Butler P, Mitchell AM, Ellis H. Applied Radiological Anatomy. Cambridge: Cambridge University Press, 1999: 355, 362.

Wheeless, CR. Wheeless' Textbook of Orthopaedics, 2011. http://www.wheelessonline.com/ortho/sartorius (Last accessed April 2024).

Case 3.27

A Gallbladder

B Right inguinal ligament

C Right iliopsoas

D Fat in the left subphrenic space

E Left common femoral artery

Coronal contrast-enhanced CT of the abdomen and pelvis in the portal venous phase.

The aponeurosis of the external oblique muscle is thickened inferiorly at its free edge to form the inguinal ligament. This ligament runs from the pubic tubercle superolaterally to the anterior superior iliac spine. Its fibres continue inferiorly to merge with the fascia lata. The inguinal ligament forms the base of the inguinal canal, and forms the medial wall of the femoral ring.

The external iliac artery becomes the common femoral artery as it passes under the mid-point of the inguinal ligament (the midinguinal point). The common femoral artery enters the thigh below the inguinal ligament, and is found laterally to the common femoral vein at this point. As it enters the thigh it gives off four superficial branches:

1. Superficial epigastric artery passes superomedially through the rectus sheath to run in the anterior abdominal wall
2. Superficial circumflex iliac artery runs laterally on a course towards the anterior superior iliac spine

3. Superficial external pudendal artery passes medially and supplies the superficial portions of the external genitalia and skin
4. Deep external pudendal artery also passes medially and supplies the skin overlying the external genitalia

From here, the common femoral artery continues a course inferiorly through the femoral triangle, below sartorius to enter the adductor canal. The main branch of the common femoral is the profunda femoris artery, which arises approximately 5 cm distal to the inguinal ligament, and takes an inferoposterior course and comes to lie behind the femoral artery.

Butler P, Mitchell AM, Ellis H. Applied Radiological Anatomy. Cambridge: Cambridge University Press, 1999: 201, 387.

Case 3.28

A Gallbladder

B Right proximal ureter

C Left Gerota's fascia

D Left fascia of Zuckerkandl

E Left perirenal space/perirenal fat

Axial contrast-enhanced CT scan.

Each kidney is invested in fascia, which has an anterior and posterior leaf; these are referred to as Gerota's and Zuckerkandl's fascia, respectively. These fascial layers are approximately 1 mm thick, and are best seen on CT when they are at right angles to the beam. Laterally, Gerota's and Zuckerkandl's fascias merge to form the lateral conal fascia, which runs along the lateral abdominal wall and is continuous with the fascial covering of transversus abdominis.

The perirenal space is bounded by the renal fascia which contains the kidneys, their vessels, fat and the adrenal glands (the adrenal glands are found within the perirenal fascia, but are separate from the kidney as they are contained within their own compartment).

The anterior pararenal space lies between Gerota's fascia and the posterior peritoneum. It contains the duodenum, ascending and descending colon, and pancreas. The posterior pararenal space lies between Zuckerkandl's fascia and the muscles of the posterior abdominal wall. This space is bounded medially by the attachment of the renal fascia to the fascia of psoas muscle and laterally is continuous with the extraperitoneal fat, below transversus abdominis; it contains only fat.

The right ureter is nicely demonstrated on this image, with its water density helping to differentiate it from the surrounding vessels at the renal hilum.

Figure 3.2 demonstrates the relationships of the retroperitoneal fascial planes and spaces.

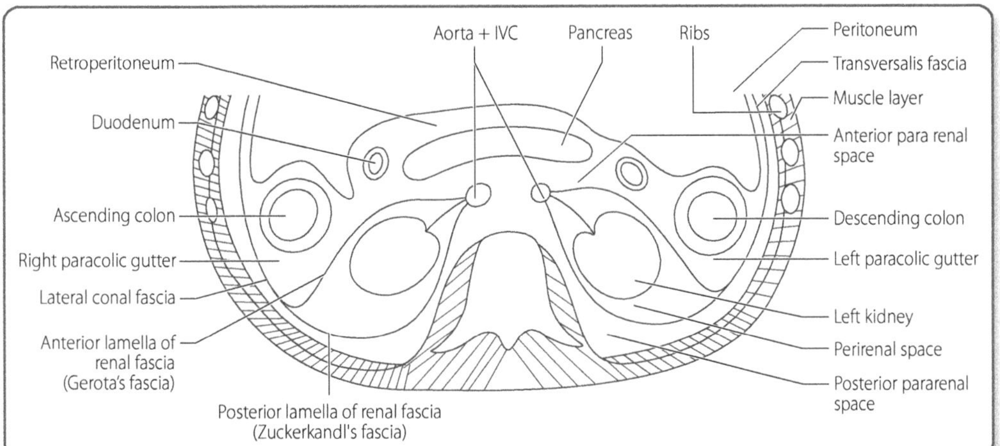

Figure 3.2 Fascial planes and anatomical spaces of the retroperitoneum.

Ryan S, McNicholas M, Eustace SJ. Anatomy for Diagnostic Imaging, 3rd edition. Edinburgh: Saunders, 2011: 196–199.

Case 3.29

A Right diaphragmatic crus

B Right Zuckerkandl's fascia

C Left lobe of liver

D Left renal sinus fat

E Left psoas

Coronal T1-weighted, out of phase MRI through the posterior abdomen.

Out of phase imaging gives this 'India ink' appearance. This is due to signal drop out from voxels which contain both fatty and non-fatty tissue. Therefore, it tends to occur at interfaces of fat with soft tissue. This sequence is often used to characterise adrenal lesions.

The kidney is surrounded by a fibrous capsule and the space immediately surrounding this is known as the perirenal space. This space is filled with perirenal fat and is bounded by the renal fascia. This fascia can be seen as a fine low signal line running around the kidney and is best visualised on images where the plane intersects it at right angles. On this image, it is outlined nicely on either side by the high signal fat surrounding it. The renal fascia has an anterior and a posterior leaf, which merge laterally to become the lateral conal fascia. The posterior pararenal space is found behind the posterior leaf of the renal fascia, which is also known as Zuckerkandl's fascia. The anterior pararenal space is found posterior to the peritoneum, in front of the anterior renal fascia, which is also known as Gerota's fascia. The retroperitoneum is therefore divided into three compartments by the renal fascias.

Ryan S, McNicholas M, Eustace SJ. Anatomy for Diagnostic Imaging, 3rd edition. Edinburgh: Saunders, 2011: 198–199.

Case 3.30

A Anterior bladder wall

B Cerebrospinal fluid (CSF) within spinal canal

C L3/4 intervertebral disc

D Fat within the presacral space

E Rectum

Sagittal T2-weighted abdominal MRI.

T2-weighting can help to identify structures, e.g. the urine within the bladder returns a high signal but the adjacent muscular bladder wall appears dark and the CSF within the spinal canal appears bright.

The presacral space is located between the rectum and sacrum/coccyx. It typically measures up to 15 mm in the anteroposterior dimension, although this figure may be higher in older or obese patients. Superiorly, this space is bounded by reflections of the peritoneum. Its inferior border is made up of the levator ani and coccygeus muscles, and the ureter and iliac vessels are found laterally.

The rectum begins at the level of S3, and is approximately 13 cm long. The rectum does not have haustrations, but it does have three lateral folds, which are known as the valves of Houston. These are formed by the curved shape that the rectum adopts, due to the convexity of the rectal ampulla (a focal dilation) as it sits on the pelvic diaphragm. There are two left-sided valves and one on the right. The rectum is extraperitoneal, with the pelvic peritoneum draped over the superior and lateral aspects of the upper and middle thirds, leaving the lower third uncovered.

Butler P, Mitchell AM, Ellis H. Applied Radiological Anatomy. Cambridge: Cambridge University Press, 1999: 219.

Kocaoglu M, Frush DP. Paediatric pre-sacral masses. Radiographics 2006; 26: 833–857.

Case 3.31

A Fat within the right ischiorectal fossa

B Coccyx

C Bladder

D Vagina

E Rectum

Axial contrast-enhanced CT of the pelvis.

The ischiorectal fossa is found below the posterior fibres of levator ani and anterior to the sacrotuberous ligaments and gluteus maximus. The urogenital perineum forms its anterior border and the lateral border reaches to the fascia overlying obturator internus. This space is important due to its propensity for sepsis, via the rectum or anal canal, and the subsequent development of ischiorectal abscesses.

The vagina is found between the bladder and urethra anteriorly, and the rectum posteriorly. There is a small bubble of air visible on this section within the vaginal vault, which may help to identify it. Between the upper third of the vagina and the rectum is found the pouch of Douglas, or recto-uterine pouch. This is the most dependent part of the peritoneal cavity when a person is in an erect position.

The urethra, vagina and rectum are all parallel to the pelvic brim, and to each other. The vagina is a muscular tube which extends from the vulva superiorly and posteriorly, piercing the urogenital diaphragm to surround the cervix. Anterior to the cervix is a shallow anterior vaginal fornix. The lateral and posterior fornices of the vagina are deeper in comparison.

Butler P, Mitchell AM, Ellis H. Applied Radiological Anatomy. Cambridge: Cambridge University Press, 1999: 281, 295.

Case 3.32

A Spigelian fascia/linea semilunaris

B Right iliopsoas

C Left rectus abdominis

D Left external iliac artery

E Mesorectal fascia

Axial T2-weighted pelvic MRI.

The spigelian fascia is formed from the aponeuroses of the internal and external obliques and transversus abdominis. It extends from the medial edge of these muscles to the lateral edge of the rectus muscles. These fibres then surround the rectus abdominis muscles, forming the rectus sheath and attaching them to the linea alba in the midline.

The mesorectal fascia is an important structure in the evaluation of rectal cancer as total mesorectal excision – removal of the rectum and mesorectum en-bloc within their enveloping fascia – has been shown to reduce local recurrence rates. The mesorectal fascia is seen as a thin, low signal intensity line surrounding the mesorectal tissue. It is best visualised on axial section. The mesorectal tissue is seen as high signal intensity, similar to fat, and contains blood vessels and lymphatics.

Brown G. High Resolution MRI of the Anatomy Important in Total Mesorectal Excision of the Rectum. Am J Roentgenol 2004; 182: 431–439.

Skandalakis LJ, Skandalakis JE, Skandalakis PN. Surgical Anatomy and Technique: a Pocket Manual, 3rd edition. New York: Springer, 2009: 174.

Case 3.33

A Infundibulum draining left upper pole calyx

B Right lobe of liver

C Right renal pelvis

D Left upper pole calyx

E Left distal ureter

Intravenous urogram.

There are approximately 12 collecting ducts which open onto the surface of each renal papilla. Each duct drains into a minor calyx, which drain via infundibula towards the renal pelvis. The angle at which the collecting ducts meet the convex surface of the renal pyramids is designed to prevent reflux of urine into the renal parenchyma. However, compound calyces (with multiple papillae projecting into them) are more prone to reflux, as the crowding of the papillae results in a suboptimal angle for a higher proportion of the ducts. Compound calyces are therefore often thought to be involved in reflux nephropathy.

From the renal pelvis drains the ureter, a fibromuscular tube which extends from the kidney to the posterolateral corner of the bladder. The ureter descends inferiorly and anteriorly within the retroperitoneum, from the kidneys towards the pelvis. Once it crosses the iliac vessels the ureter stays in close proximity to the internal iliac artery, along the pelvic side wall; when the ureter reaches the level of the anterior ischial spines its course changes to run anteromedially towards the bladder.

The narrowest parts of the ureter are found at the pelviureteric junction, the pelvic brim (where the ureter crosses the iliac vessels) and the vesicoureteric junction. These are the most likely sites for a kidney stone to become impacted. A normal calibre ureter on an intravenous urogram will measure up to 7 mm within the pelvis and 5 mm above the pelvic brim.

Butler P, Mitchell AM, Ellis H. Applied Radiological Anatomy. Cambridge: Cambridge University Press, 1999: 267.

Case 3.34

A Nephrogram of right kidney, upper pole

B Fornix of right lower pole calyx

C Left renal pelvis

D Ureter draining the right upper moiety

E Partial duplex collecting system, right kidney

Intravenous urogram.

A partial duplex collecting system is seen on the right of this image. This variant is relatively common, and is seen in approximately 1/70 people. The ureters can fuse before they reach the bladder or they may remain separate throughout their course. In the latter case, the ureter which drains the lower moiety enters the bladder in a normal anatomical position but is prone to vesicoureteric reflux. The upper moiety drains via a ureter which inserts in a more distal position and is prone to obstruction due to the increased incidence of ureterocele formation. **Figure 3.3** demonstrates renal anatomy.

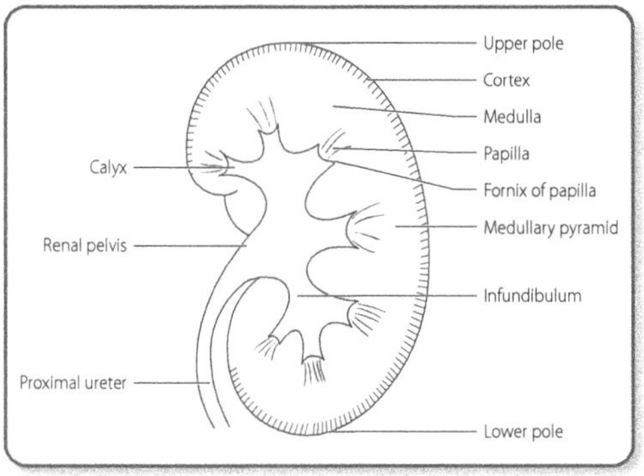

Figure 3.3 Renal anatomy.

Butler P, Mitchell AM, Ellis H. Applied Radiological Anatomy. Cambridge: Cambridge University Press, 1999: 426.
Babyn, PS. Teaching Atlas of Paediatric Imaging. New York: Thieme Medical Publishers, 2006: 363.

Case 3.35

A Ascending colon

B Right kidney, lower pole cortex

C Spleen

D Left kidney, lower pole medullary pyramid

E Left psoas

Coronal contrast-enhanced, fluid attenuated abdominal MRI.

The kidney is made up of an outer cortex, and an inner medulla. In contrast-enhanced imaging the cortex enhances first, followed by the medulla. Excretion of contrast then results in enhancement of the pelvicalyceal system. The renal medulla is made up of multiple pyramids, separated by columns of cortex (columns of Bertin). The apices of the pyramids form the renal papillae – these have a convex contour, cupped by the adjacent draining calyx. There are typically seven pairs of minor calyces (anterior and posterior). These join into two or three major calyces, which drain via their infundibula to the renal pelvis.

The psoas muscles are retroperitoneal structures, medial to the lower poles of the kidneys. They lie to either side of the lumbar spine and act as flexors and stabilisers. They originate from the transverse processes of L1–5 and, more superficially, from the bodies of T12–L5. As they descend they fuse with iliacus to form iliopsoas, which runs under the inguinal ligament and attaches to the lesser trochanter of the femur.

Ryan S, McNicholas M, Eustace SJ. Anatomy for Diagnostic Imaging, 3rd edition. Edinburgh: Saunders, 2011: 196–201, 220.

Butler P, Mitchell AM, Ellis H. Applied Radiological Anatomy. Cambridge: Cambridge University Press, 1999: 308.

Case 3.36

A Lateral limb of left adrenal

B Descending colon

C Left trapezius

D Spinal cord

E Coeliac artery

Sagittal contrast-enhanced CT in the arterial phase.

The adrenal glands are retroperitoneal structures which lie above the kidneys. They are found within the perirenal fascia but are separated from the kidney, as they are enclosed within their own compartment. The adrenal glands are composed of a body and two limbs (medial and lateral). The left adrenal gland can be described as having three limbs: anterior, posteromedial and posterolateral. The left adrenal gland has a slightly more variable position than the right. It tends to have a 'Y' shape on cross-sectional images, and is found behind the splenic vein, extending towards the hilum of the left kidney. The right adrenal gland tends to be more 'V' shaped on cross section, and has a more consistent position. It is found medial to the right lobe of liver, behind the inferior vena cava, with the right diaphragmatic crus to its medial side. It lies more inferior and medial compared to the left adrenal gland.

The diaphragm forms deep recesses where it attaches to the ribs – these are known as the costophrenic angles. Due to the domed shape of the diaphragm, some of the lung base extends into the costophrenic angles, and this can be seen on the same sections as the upper abdominal viscera.

The coeliac axis arises between T12 and L1 from the anterior surface of the aorta. Its initial course may be horizontal or vertically upwards. On this section, it can be seen to pass forwards in the plane of the image initially. It is found below the left lobe of the liver, and above the level of the pancreas and splenic vein. After approximately 1–2 cm, the coeliac axis divides into the common hepatic, splenic and left gastric arteries.

Ryan S, McNicholas M, Eustace SJ. Anatomy for Diagnostic Imaging, 3rd edition. Edinburgh: Saunders, 2011: 203–205.

Butler P, Mitchell AM, Ellis H. Applied Radiological Anatomy. Cambridge: Cambridge University Press, 1999: 225, 270.

Case 3.37

A Bladder dome

B Bladder neck

C Bulbar urethra

D Femoral diaphysis

E Penile urethra

Micturating cystogram, taken in an oblique position.

The male urethra runs from the internal urethral sphincter at the bladder neck, to the urethral meatus at the tip of the penis. It is divided into four parts:

- The posterior urethra is comprised of the prostatic and membranous sections
- The anterior urethra is made up of the bulbar and penile sections

The urethra is widest as it crosses through the ventral part of the prostate. This prostatic portion runs for approximately 3 cm before becoming the membranous urethra. The membranous urethra is approximately 2 cm in length and forms the narrowest segment, as it passes through the membranous urogenital diaphragm (the external sphincter).

The bulbar urethra is so called because it traverses the bulb of the penis, through the corpus spongiosum. There is a focal dilatation in the bulbar segment, which is known as the intrabulbar fossa. Lastly the penile urethra continues towards the meatus through the corpus spongiosum. This segment is relatively long and narrow, but has a small dilatation at the end, the navicular fossa.

Ryan S, McNicholas M, Eustace SJ. Anatomy for Diagnostic Imaging, 3rd edition. Edinburgh: Saunders, 2011: 231–233.

Case 3.38

A Urinary bladder

B Right superior pubic ramus

C Corpus spongiosum

D Left corpus cavernosum

E Symphysis pubis

Coronal T2-weighted pelvic MRI.

The penis is comprised of three corpora which are bound together by Buck's fascia, an extension of the deep perineal fascia. The corpora are cylindrical in shape and are made up of the corpus spongiosum on the ventral surface, and the corpora cavernosum on the dorsal surface. Within the corpus spongiosum is the penile urethra, and within the corpora cavernosum are the cavernosal arteries. The corpora appear as high signal on T2-weighted images, and intermediate signal on T1-weighted images. On contrast-enhanced imaging, they appear very vascular.

The symphysis pubis is a fibrous joint, and therefore appears dark on MRI. In this image it is seen in the midline joining the two superior pubic rami. The bladder is seen superiorly and with a high signal intensity, due to its fluid content.

Ryan S, McNicholas M, Eustace SJ. Anatomy for Diagnostic Imaging, 3rd edition. Edinburgh: Saunders, 2011: 239.

Case 3.39

A Right seminal vesical

B Rectum

C Left sacroiliac joint

D Left pubic tubercle

E Left obturator internus

Axial T2-weighted pelvic MRI.

The seminal vesicles are found posterior, and superior to the prostate gland. They are paired, sacculated structures, which run transversely behind the bladder, and store semen. They are approximately 5 cm in length, and are continuous with the ampulla of the vas deferens inferomedially, where they form the ejaculatory ducts. These pass obliquely through the prostate gland to enter the prostatic utricle.

On T2-weighted MRI, the seminal vesicles return a high signal due to their fluid contents. On T1-weighted MRI, they appear dark and will stand out from the surrounding fat, which returns a high signal. On CT, they appear as soft-tissue density structures, and have a 'bow tie' shape in between the bladder and prostate. Transrectal ultrasound imaging can be used as part of the assessment of prostatic carcinoma, and can demonstrate the seminal vesicles very clearly. With ultrasound, they appear as serpiginous tubular structures, which contain anechoic fluid.

Butler P, Mitchell AM, Ellis H. Applied Radiological Anatomy. Cambridge: Cambridge University Press, 1999: 289.

Case 3.40

A Peripheral zone prostate gland

B Lesser trochanter of right femur

C Left common femoral vein

D Transitional zone prostate gland

E Right sartorius

Axial T2-weighted pelvic MRI.

The prostate can be described as having a pyramidal shape, with its base situated superiorly against the bladder and its apex inferiorly against the urogenital diaphragm. It has an anterior wall behind the pubic symphysis, a posterior wall adjacent to the rectum and two inferolateral walls.

The prostate gland has three different glandular zones, which are nicely demonstrated on T2-weighted MRI images. There is also a fibromuscular isthmus located anterior to the urethra, containing little glandular tissue.

The peripheral zone returns a high signal on T2-weighted images, and is located posterolaterally extending towards the apex. The central and transitional zones return an intermediate signal and cannot be distinguished radiologically; both zones together are usually referred to as the central gland. They are located more superiorly within the gland and surround the urethra. The transitional zone is located within the central zone; it is a small area of tissue around the urethra at the level of the verumontanum. The ejaculatory ducts pass through the central zone to join the urethra at the verumontanum.

As part of the ageing process, the transitional zone hypertrophies and the central zone atrophies. The transitional zone is the area of the prostate affected by benign prostatic hypertrophy. Most prostate cancers, however, occur in the peripheral zone.

Ryan S, McNicholas M, Eustace SJ. Anatomy for Diagnostic Imaging, 3rd edition. Edinburgh: Saunders, 2011: 233–234.

Case 3.41

A Right sacroiliac joint

B Right uterine cornu

C Endometrial cavity filled with contrast

D Internal cervical os

E Contrast within the distal left fallopian tube

A frontal projection hysterosalpingogram.

From superior to inferior the uterus is made up of a fundus, body and cervix. It is a pear-shaped organ which is usually anteverted and anteflexed, and is located extraperitoneally between the bladder and rectum. The fallopian tubes (uterine tubes) join the uterus superolaterally at the uterine cornua, the junction of the fundus and body. The Fallopian tubes have an isthmus, ampulla and infundibulum (from medial to lateral). At the lateral end, there are the fimbriae which begin the transportation of ova towards the endometrial cavity once they are released from the ovaries.

The endometrial cavity is well demonstrated on a hysterosalpingogram, and is seen as a triangular shape on a frontal view. The anterior and posterior walls of the uterus are apposed, and therefore the endometrial cavity appears slit-like in the sagittal plane. **Figure 3.4** demonstrates the anatomy and relationships of the uterus, fallopian tubes and ovaries.

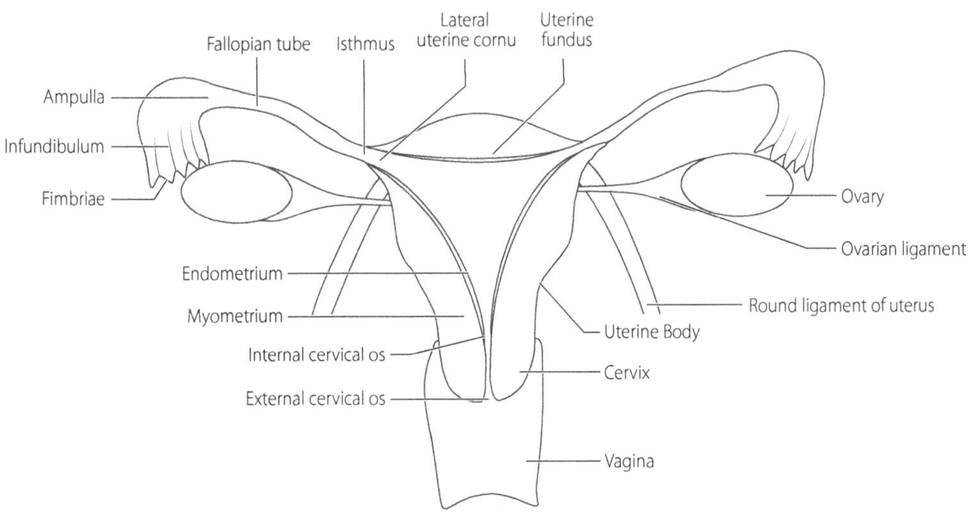

Figure 3.4 Anatomy of the uterus, fallopian tubes and ovaries.

Ryan S, McNicholas M, Eustace SJ. Anatomy for Diagnostic Imaging, 3rd edition. Edinburgh: Saunders, 2011: 240–243.

Butler P, Mitchell AM, Ellis H. Applied Radiological Anatomy. Cambridge: Cambridge University Press, 1999: 295.

Case 3.42

A Myometrium

B Right external oblique

C Left gluteus maximus

D Endometrium

E Bladder

Coronal contrast-enhanced CT of the abdomen and pelvis.

The uterus is usually anteverted and anteflexed; therefore, the uterus is seen in transverse section on this image. Enhancement of the uterus on CT is variable, but both the myometrium and endometrium can show enhancement, especially mid-cycle. This enhancement helps to differentiate the uterus from other soft-tissue structures within the pelvis, such as pelvic small bowel loops. During the secretory phase of the menstrual cycle there may be non-enhancing fluid visualised within the endometrial cavity.

The fovea of the femoral head is an ovoid depression, which marks the attachment of the ligamentum teres. This ligament is attached at its base to either side of the acetabular notch. Within the ligamentum teres runs the acetabular branch of the obturator artery, which provides the blood supply to the central part of the head of femur.

Butler P, Mitchell AM, Ellis H. Applied Radiological Anatomy. Cambridge: Cambridge University Press, 1999: 360.

Ryan S, McNicholas M, Eustace SJ. Anatomy for Diagnostic Imaging, 3rd edition. Edinburgh: Saunders, 2011: 240–247, 287.

Case 3.43

A Muscles of the anterior abdominal wall

B Endometrium

C Myometrium of posterior uterine wall

D Urine within bladder

E Vaginal stripe

Longitudinal, trans-abdominal ultrasound of the pelvis.

The endometrium appears as a hyperechoic stripe on longitudinal ultrasound images, running from the fundus to the cervix. It has a variable width throughout the menstrual cycle depending on the influence of oestrogen and progesterone. This image was obtained on day 21 of the menstrual cycle, and shows the endometrium to be 6.5 mm in thickness. During the secretory phase, the endometrium thickens and typically measures between 7–16 mm. In the periovulatory period, the endometrium may take on a striated/layered appearance which usually disappears within 48 hours of ovulation. As the endometrium proliferates it becomes thicker and more echogenic, and may demonstrate a degree of posterior acoustic enhancement due to local oedema. A thin and, hypoechoic layer can be seen immediately deep to the endometrium, which represents a relatively hypovascular layer of myometrium. This is analogous to the junctional zone seen on MRI.

The vagina is located between the urethra and rectum on transabdominal scans. On a longitudinal scan the vagina is seen as an echogenic 'stripe' which forms an acute angle with the uterine body.

Nalaboff KM. Imaging the endometrium: disease and normal variants. Radiographics 2001; 21: 1409–1424.

Ryan S, McNicholas M, Eustace SJ. Anatomy for Diagnostic Imaging, 3rd edition. Edinburgh: Saunders, 2011: 239–245.

Case 3.44

A Endometrium

B Pubis

C Myometrium

D Junctional zone

E Anal canal

Sagittal T2-weighted MRI of a female pelvis.

Uterine anatomy is well demonstrated on MRI. On T2-weighted sequences the endometrium, endocervical canal and vaginal canal all return a high signal. The serosal layer which surrounds the uterus gives a thin hypointense line around the periphery. Below this is the myometrial tissue which returns an intermediate signal. However, the deeper myometrium, found just below the endometrial layer, returns a low signal and is known as the junctional zone. This tissue is histologically similar to the remainder of the myometrium, but it is thought that its increased nuclear:cellular ratio is responsible for this low signal. The low signal junctional zone is continuous with the fibrous stroma of the cervix, which can be nicely demonstrated on sagittal images.

Ryan S, McNicholas M, Eustace SJ. Anatomy for Diagnostic Imaging, 3rd edition. Edinburgh: Saunders, 2011: 240–247.

Case 3.45

A Right round ligament

B Right external iliac vein

C Mesorectal fat

D Left inferior epigastric vessels

E Femoral head

Axial contrast-enhanced CT.

The round ligament is one of the suspensory ligaments of the uterus. It runs from the superolateral aspect of the uterus, anteriorly through the inguinal canal, and ends as its fibres become part of the tissue of the mons pubis. The round ligament acts to keep the uterus in a position of anteversion and is stretched during pregnancy, which can cause pain.

The common iliac arteries bifurcate at the level of the pelvic brim, in front of the lower sacroiliac joints. The external iliac artery then runs along the surface of psoas before passing under the inguinal ligament, where it becomes the common femoral artery. The inferior epigastric artery arises from the external iliac artery just before it passes under the inguinal ligament. It then takes a path up the internal surface of the anterior abdominal wall to enter the rectus sheath.

Hirsch HA. Atlas of Gynaecological Surgery. New York: Thieme Medical Publishers, 1997: 114.

Ryan S, McNicholas M, Eustace SJ. Anatomy for Diagnostic Imaging, 3rd edition. Edinburgh: Saunders, 2011: 226–228, 240.

Butler P, Mitchell AM, Ellis H. Applied Radiological Anatomy. Cambridge: Cambridge University Press, 1999: 282

Case 3.46

A Fetal pole

B Myometrium, anterior uterine wall

C Decidua parietalis

D Decidua capsularis

E Gestational sac

Transabdominal ultrasound of an early pregnancy, with the uterus in transverse section.

During early pregnancy, before a fetal pole can be identified, the double decidual sac sign indicates the presence of an intrauterine pregnancy. This appearance is created by the interface of the decidua capsularis and parietalis. The decidua capsularis is the tissue which has grown over the blastocyst as it implants, and contains the gestational sac as the blastocyst develops. As the gestational sac grows it pushes the decidua capsularis towards the opposite side of the endometrial cavity to come into contact with the decidua parietalis, which lines the uterine cavity. These two layers fuse together, obliterating the endometrial cavity. The double sac sign is then seen as two echogenic rings surrounding the gestational sac. **Table 3.3** summarises the key features seen on ultrasound in early pregnancy.

Table 3.3 Key features of early pregnancy seen on ultrasound

4 weeks	Gestational sac visible on transvaginal (TV) scanning
5 weeks	• Yolk sac visible by TV scanning • Gestational sac visible on transabdominal (TA) scans
5–6 weeks	Fetal pole and cardiac pulsations seen on TV scanning
7 weeks	Fetal pole and cardiac pulsations visible on TA scanning

Butler P, Mitchell AM, Ellis H. Applied Radiological Anatomy. Cambridge: Cambridge University Press, 1999: 399–401.

Case 3.47

A Fetal diaphragm

B Placenta

C Fetal globe

D Amniotic fluid

E Maternal bladder

Coronal T2-weighted MRI through a pregnant uterus.

This fetus is in a cephalic presentation with a right lateral lie. The placenta is positioned to the left and returns a moderately high signal, which allows differentiation between it and the myometrium beneath. On contrast-enhanced images, the placenta enhances avidly and early during the arterial phase. The myometrium enhances later and to a lesser degree. During the second trimester, the placenta demonstrates a heterogenous enhancement pattern, but by the third trimester, it develops into a more lobular pattern, due to the organisation of the placenta into cotyledons.

The T2-weighting means that fluid-containing structures return a high signal. Therefore, the amniotic fluid and the urine within the bladder both appear bright. The fetal globe also has a high signal on this sequence.

Prayer D. Fetal MRI. London: Springer, 2011: 407.

Case 3.48

A Coeliac axis

B Common hepatic artery

C Gastroduodenal artery

D Splenic artery

E Arterial catheter

Angiogram of the coeliac axis.

The coeliac axis is located between T12 and L1. Its usual course begins in a caudal direction, but it may pass horizontally or superiorly. It arises from the anterior surface of the aorta, and after approximately 1–2 cm divides into the common hepatic, left gastric and splenic arteries.

The common hepatic artery runs to the right, along the superior surface of the pancreatic head, to reach the hepatoduodenal ligament. Within this ligament it travels towards the porta hepatis, with the portal vein behind it, and the common bile duct and common hepatic duct just to the right. It gives off the gastroduodenal artery and then continues as the hepatic artery proper, before dividing into the right, middle and left hepatic arteries.

The left gastric artery arises superiorly, and is usually the 1st branch from the coeliac axis; it is also usually the smallest. From its origin it passes superolaterally towards the gastric cardia, where it divides into multiple branches to supply the anterior and posterior surfaces of the stomach.

The splenic artery often has a very tortuous course. It is the largest branch from the coeliac axis and travels along the superior surface of the pancreas towards the splenic hilum. Once it reaches the hilum, the splenic artery divides into superior and inferior branches. Occasionally a third (middle) branch may also be present. These then further divide to become the intrasplenic arteries; approximately 4–6 branches arise from each of the superior middle and inferior splenic arteries. **Figure 3.5** demonstrates the anatomy of the coeliac axis and its branches.

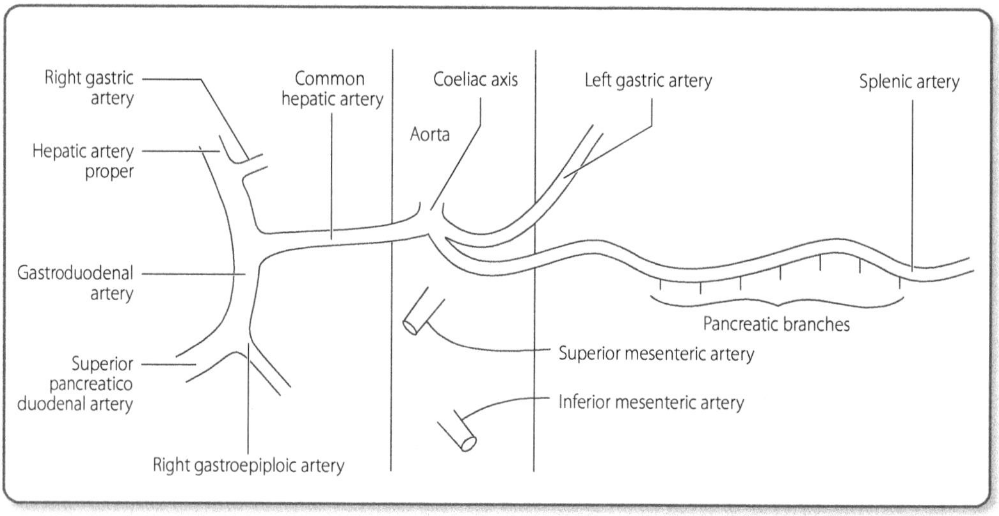

Figure 3.5 Anatomy of the coeliac axis.

Butler P, Mitchell AM, Ellis H. Applied Radiological Anatomy. Cambridge: Cambridge University Press, 1999: 225–228.

Case 3.49

A Right colic artery

B Ileocolic artery

C Superior mesenteric artery

D Ileal branch of superior mesenteric artery

E Arterial catheter within aorta

Angiogram of the superior mesenteric artery.

The superior mesenteric artery (SMA) arises at the level of L1 from the anterior surface of the abdominal aorta, approximately 1 cm below the origin of the coeliac axis. It passes anteriorly, before descending behind the pancreatic neck. Between the SMA and the aorta are the uncinate process of the pancreas, the left renal vein and the third part of duodenum. The superior mesenteric vein lies to the right of the SMA – this arrangement is important in the assessment of malrotation.

The branches of the SMA are as follows:

- **Inferior pancreaticoduodenal**: Supplies the pancreatic head and distal duodenum (D3 and D4); anastomoses with the superior pancreaticoduodenal artery allowing a collateral circulation between the coeliac axis and the SMA
- **Jejunal branches**: Four to six branches arising from the left side of the SMA. Each branch divides into two, communicating with the vessels either side to form a series of arcades. Three to six further arcades are formed, with vasa rectae arising from the last of them. The vasa rectae have a final division to supply the anterior and posterior surfaces of the small bowel
- **Ileal branches**: 9–13 branches, which arise beyond the origin of the ileocolic artery. These have a similar pattern of division to the jejunal arteries, with the formation of arcades
- **Ileocolic**: Passes inferiorly to the right, and supplies the terminal ileum, caecum and appendix, as well as part of the ascending colon. This vessel anastomoses with the last ileal artery of the SMA
- **Right colic**: Courses behind the parietal peritoneum to supply the ascending colon. It has an ascending branch which anastomoses with the middle colic artery, and a descending branch which anastomoses with the marginal artery of the ileocolic artery
- **Middle colic**: Arises inferior to the uncinate process of the pancreas, entering the transverse mesocolon. It supplies the transverse colon and usually arises as a common trunk with the right colic artery. However, these vessels may also have separate origins

The marginal artery of Drummond runs in the large bowel mesentery, alongside the colon, and is part of the system of arcades that forms an anastomosis between the SMA and inferior mesenteric artery, which allows collateral flow. There is a similar marginal artery of Dwight which runs along the small bowel – it is the vessel from which the vasa recta originate. **Figure 3.6** demonstrates the anatomy of the SMA and its branches.

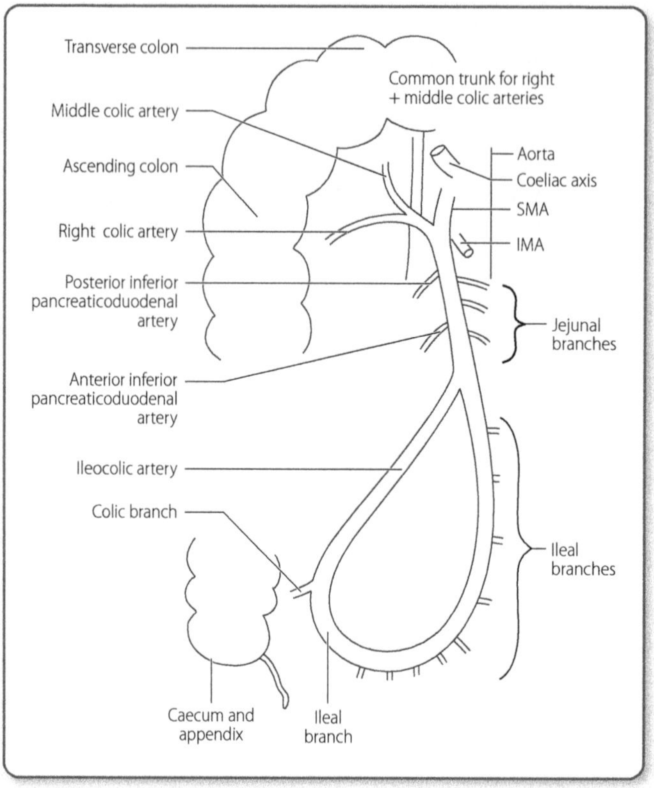

Figure 3.6 Anatomy of the superior mesenteric artery and its branches. IMA, inferior mesenteric artery; SMA, superior mesenteric artery.

Butler P, Mitchell AM, Ellis H. Applied Radiological Anatomy. Cambridge: Cambridge University Press, 1999: 230–233.

Case 3.50

A Left colic artery

B Inferior mesenteric artery

C Sigmoid artery

D Superior rectal/haemorrhoidal artery

E Marginal artery of Drummond

Angiogram of the inferior mesenteric artery.

The inferior mesenteric artery (IMA) arises at the level of L3. Its first branch is the left colic artery, which divides into ascending and descending branches after a short distance. The ascending branch forms an anastomosis with the middle colic artery and there is a further anastomosis between the descending branch and the first sigmoid artery. There are then two to three sigmoid branches. The superior rectal artery (haemorrhoidal artery) is the terminal artery of the IMA. It branches into a left and right branch, to supply the proximal rectum. These branches communicate with each other, the sigmoid arteries above and the middle and inferior rectal arteries below (which arise from the internal iliac vessels).

The marginal artery of Drummond runs parallel to the colon and connects the main arterial trunks and their arcades to one another, thereby forming a collateral blood supply. It may be absent at the splenic flexure. In the case of arterial compromise to one of the main vessels, it may be seen to hypertrophy. **Figure 3.7** demonstrates the anatomy of the IMA and its branches.

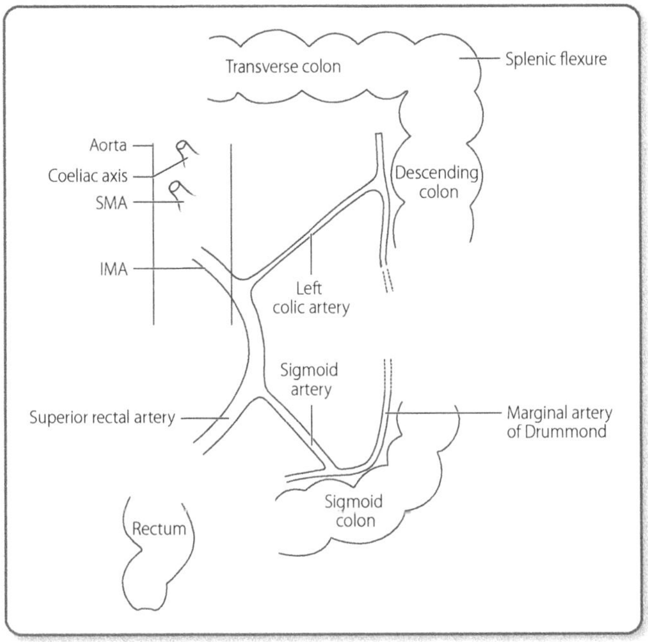

Figure 3.7 Anatomy of the inferior mesenteric artery and its branches. IMA, inferior mesenteric artery; SMA, superior mesenteric artery.

Butler P, Mitchell AM, Ellis H. Applied Radiological Anatomy. Cambridge: Cambridge University Press, 1999: 230–233.

Case 3.51

A Right renal artery

B Right common iliac artery

C Right internal iliac artery

D Left renal artery

E Left accessory renal artery

Renal MR angiogram.

The abdominal aorta has three unpaired branches and three paired branches. The renal arteries arise just distal to the origin of the superior mesenteric artery, at the level of the upper border of L2. There can be variation: multiple renal arteries are relatively common. The right renal artery tends to be straighter than the left, with a longer course, as it crosses the midline and passes posteriorly to the inferior vena cava. The renal arteries usually divide into an anterior and posterior division, which pass either side of the renal pelvis. These vessels then further divide into segmental branches (usually five), which enter the kidney via the hilum and continue between the medullary pyramids where they are referred to as interlobar arteries. As they reach the cortex they become the arcuate arteries. The arcuate arteries give rise to the interlobular arteries, and it is from here that the afferent arterioles provide the blood supply to the glomeruli.

The distal abdominal aorta divides into the common iliac arteries at the level of L4, after which it divides into the internal and external iliacs at the level of the pelvic brim, anterior to the lower sacroiliac joints. The external iliac artery is of a larger calibre than the internal iliac, and it goes on to become the common femoral artery as it passes under the inguinal ligament.

Butler P, Mitchell AM, Ellis H. Applied Radiological Anatomy. Cambridge: Cambridge University Press, 1999: 265, 272.

Case 3.52

A Right intercostal muscle

B Right lumbar vessels

C Right iliac crest

D Left diaphragmatic crus

E Left adrenal gland

Coronal contrast-enhanced CT.

The lumbar arteries are paired vessels arising from the abdominal aorta and supply the posterior abdominal wall; they are analogous to the intercostal arteries. There are usually four pairs which have their origins from the posterolateral aspect of the aorta at the levels of the 1st to 4th lumbar vertebral bodies. A 5th pair arising from the middle sacral artery is sometimes present. The lumbar arteries pass posteriorly along the sides of the vertebral bodies beneath the psoas muscles. They course around the quadratus lumborum muscles, and then cross the posterior aponeurosis of transversus abdominis. From here, they run anteriorly between transversus abdominis and internal oblique.

There are four pairs of lumbar veins which pass along the sides of the vertebral bodies and drain into the posterior aspect of the inferior vena cava (IVC). The left sided veins have a longer course than the right, and run posteriorly to the aorta to reach the IVC. The ascending lumbar veins run longitudinally in front of the transverse processes and connect the lumbar veins together. When they reach the diaphragm, the ascending lumbar veins continue as the azygous and hemiazygous veins.

Butler P, Mitchell AM, Ellis H. Applied Radiological Anatomy. Cambridge: Cambridge University Press, 1999: 272.

Case 3.53

A Right main branch of portal vein

B Portal vein

C Superior mesenteric vein

D Right iliacus

E Left lung base

Coronal contrast-enhanced T1-weighted MRI.

The portal vein arises from the confluence of the superior mesenteric and splenic veins at the level of L1/2. The portal vein drains blood from the spleen, pancreas, gallbladder and GI tract (excluding the anus). From its origin, the portal vein passes to the right behind the neck of pancreas, then behind the first part of duodenum and on towards the porta hepatis. Between the confluence and the porta, the portal vein is joined by the superior pancreaticoduodenal vein and the left and right gastric veins. Once the portal vein enters the liver at the porta hepatis it divides into right and left main branches. The branches of the hepatic artery accompany the portal veins, with the same branching pattern. The hepatic arteries, however, have a much smaller calibre than the adjacent portal veins. The cystic vein drains into the right portal vein and the paraumbilical veins into the left. The ligamentum teres (a remnant from the obliterated left umbilical vein) arises from the left portal vein and is continuous with the ligamentum venosum.

Ryan S, McNicholas M, Eustace SJ. Anatomy for Diagnostic Imaging, 3rd edition. Edinburgh: Saunders, 2011: 178–181.

Case 3.54

A Superior mesenteric vein

B Urinary bladder

C Right portal vein

D Stomach

E Ileocolic vein

Coronal contrast-enhanced abdominal MRI.

The superior mesenteric vein (SMV) forms a confluence with the splenic vein to become the portal vein. The tributaries of the superior mesenteric vein are listed below.

From the right side:
- Ileocolic vein
- Right colic vein – drains the ascending colon
- Middle colic vein – drains the transverse colon

From the left side:
- Ileal veins
- Jejunal veins

Proximally:
- Inferior pancreaticoduodenal vein
- Right gastroepiploic vein

The inferior mesenteric vein drains into the splenic vein, which takes a horizontal course behind the pancreas to join the SMV to form the portal vein. The portal vein then takes an oblique course laterally towards the porta hepatis. En route it receives the superior pancreaticoduodenal vein, as it passes behind the neck of the pancreas. Next it receives the right and left gastric veins as it passes behind the first part of duodenum. The portal vein continues in the free edge of the lesser omentum, with the common bile duct and hepatic artery anterior to it. **Figure 3.8** demonstrates the anatomy of the portal venous system

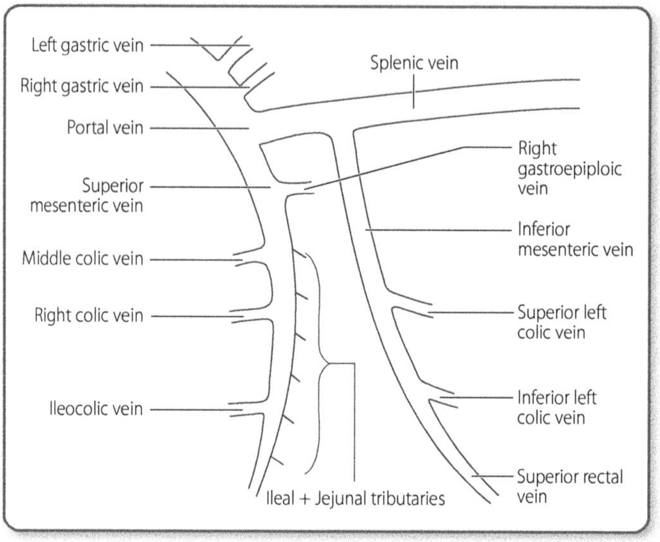

Figure 3.8 Portal venous system.

Butler P, Mitchell AM, Ellis H. Applied Radiological Anatomy. Cambridge: Cambridge University Press, 1999: 235.
Ryan S, McNicholas M, Eustace SJ. Anatomy for Diagnostic Imaging, 3rd edition. Edinburgh: Saunders, 2011: 193–196.

Case 3.55

A Azygos vein

B Hemiazygos vein

C Oesophagus

D Left ventricular wall

E Left breast – fibroglandular tissue

Axial contrast-enhanced CT.

The azygous venous system drains deoxygenated blood from the posterior thorax and abdomen into the superior vena cava (SVC). It is made up of the right-sided azygos vein, and the left-sided hemiazygos and accessory hemiazygos veins.

The azygous vein can arise either as a branch of the inferior vena cava (IVC), or as a confluence between the right ascending lumbar vein and the right subcostal vein, at the level of L2. It rises up behind the right diaphragmatic crus and follows a path anterior to the bodies of T12–5, with the aorta and thoracic duct to its left. Once it reaches the level of the pulmonary hilum it arches anteriorly over the right main bronchus, to drain into the SVC. The 'azygos arch' can occasionally be displaced laterally. It is invested in four layers of pleura to create an accessory fissure, which delineates an azygos lobe, separate from the upper lobe.

The accessory hemiazygos vein drains the 4th to 8th posterior intercostal veins and may also drain the left bronchial veins. It follows a path to the left of the vertebral column until it reaches the midthoracic level, where it crosses the midline and passes behind the aorta to drain into the azygos vein.

The hemiazygos vein arises on the left, below the diaphragm and similarly to the azygos vein can have a variable origin. It may arise from the left renal vein, or as a confluence of the left ascending lumbar and left subcostal veins. It rises on the left of the vertebral column and passes across the midline, behind the aorta at the midthoracic level, to drain into the azygos vein. **Figure 3.9** demonstrates the anatomy of the azygous venous system.

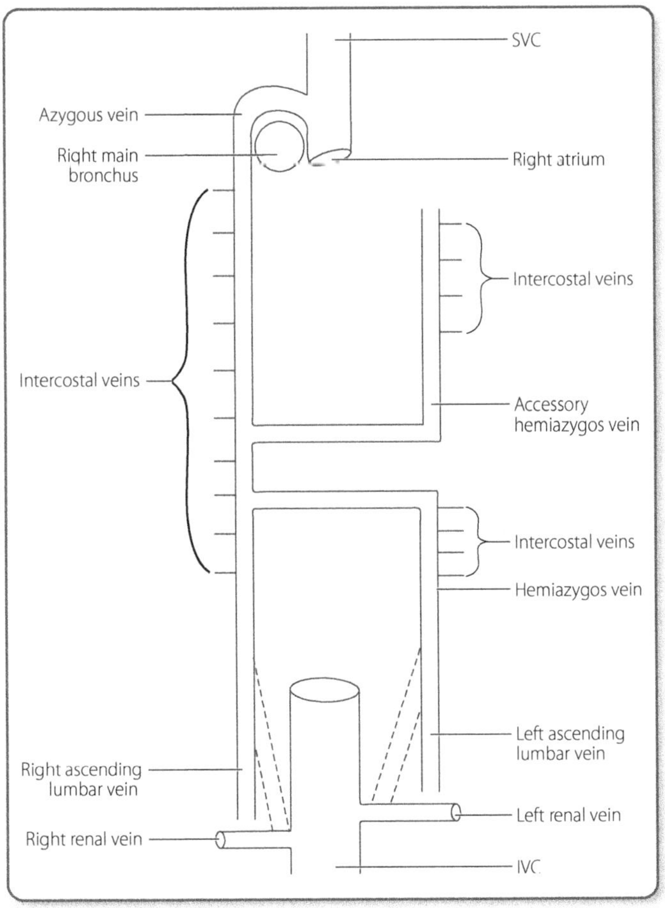

Figure 3.9 Anatomy of the azygous venous system. IVC, inferior vena cava.

Ryan S, McNicholas M, Eustace SJ. Anatomy for Diagnostic Imaging, 3rd edition. Edinburgh: Saunders, 2011: 147–149.

Case 3.56

A Azygous vein

B Right costophrenic angle

C Medullary pyramid, right lower pole of kidney

D Descending thoracic aorta

E Descending colon

Oblique coronal contrast-enhanced T1-weighted MRI.

This image demonstrates the relationship between the azygous vein and the descending aorta. The azygous vein rises from the abdomen into the thoracic cavity, to the right of the aorta and the thoracic duct and in front of the spinal column and the right posterior intercostal arteries. Its course passes just medial to the right lung, with its pleural surface adjacent to the azygous vein. When it reaches the level of T4 it takes an anterior course, arching over the hilum of the right lung, to drain into the superior vena cava.

The thoracic aorta descends in the posterior mediastinum, with the vertebral column to its right. The oesophagus is found to the right of the aorta superiorly, but as it descends it passes anterior to the aorta. The oesophagus traverses the diaphragm at the level of T10, and the aorta passes through the diaphragm at the level of T12.

The descending thoracic aorta has five branches:

1. Posterior intercostal arteries: Nine pairs, arising posteriorly, that run along the neurovascular grooves on the underside of the 3rd to 11th ribs
2. Subcostal arteries: One pair, arising posteriorly as the last branches of the thoracic aorta, that runs along the neurovascular groove of the 12th ribs
3. Bronchial arteries: Two to three, with variable origins. The two left bronchial arteries usually arise from the aorta at the level of T5 and just below the left main bronchus. The right bronchial artery usually has its origin from the third posterior intercostal artery
4. Oesophageal arteries: Four to five branches that arise anteriorly to form a network with branches from the left phrenic, left gastric and inferior thyroid arteries
5. Mediastinal branches:
   - Pericardial branches: Supply the posterior pericardium
   - Phrenic branches: Supply the posterosuperior part of the diaphragm

Ryan S, McNicholas M, Eustace SJ. Anatomy for Diagnostic Imaging, 3rd edition. Edinburgh: Saunders, 2011: 141–143.

Case 3.57

A Spermatic cord within right inguinal canal

B Crus of right corpus cavernosum

C Right inferior pubic ramus

D Anal canal

E Left gluteus maximus

Axial T2-weighted pelvic MRI.

The spermatic cord is made up of the arterial and venous supply to the testis and the lymphatics, nervous supply and vas deferens. The cord travels from the abdominal cavity to the scrotum via the inguinal canal and is covered by a tough fibrous sheath which originates from the fasciae of the anterior abdominal wall muscles. As they descend, these fascial layers become the internal and external spermatic, as well as the cremasteric, fascial layers.

The corpora cavernosa, located on the dorsal aspect of the penis, are paired cylindrical structures comprised of erectile tissue. They are fused in the sagittal plane, separated by a septum. However, at their most posterior extent they separate to form the crura. These crura are each attached to the ischiopubic rami on the inferomedial surface. On T2-weighted MRIs the corpora return a high signal, with the surrounding fascial layers appearing dark. On T1-weighted scans they are of an intermediate signal.

The anal canal begins at the level of the pelvic floor, and is angled posteriorly, at 90° to the rectum. At this level, it is encircled by the puborectal sling, which causes its angulation. It passes downwards and backwards, and is about 3cm in length. The upper two-thirds of the canal is formed by the internal sphincter. The external sphincter forms the lower two-thirds, and the two muscles therefore overlap in the middle. The inferior rectal artery supplies the lower half of the anal canal, below the level of the mucocutaneous junction, which marks the termination of the hind gut. The proximal portion is supplied by the superior rectal artery. The lymphatic drainage is similarly split, with the inferior half of the anal canal draining to the medial group of the superficial inguinal nodes, and the upper canal draining via the inferior mesenteric nodes.

The lymphatic drainage in the abdomen tends to follow the arterial supply. Lymph drains first to local nodes, and then on to regional nodal groups (lumbar, coeliac, superior and inferior mesenteric groups). These lymphatic groups drain via the intestinal and lumbar lymphatic trunks to the cisterna chyli, which in turn drains into the thoracic duct.

Ryan S, McNicholas M, Eustace SJ. Anatomy for Diagnostic Imaging, 3rd edition. Edinburgh: Saunders, 2011: 207–208, 225–226, 239.

Butler P, Mitchell AM, Ellis H. Applied Radiological Anatomy. Cambridge: Cambridge University Press, 1999: 221–222, 274–275.

Case 3.58

A Spleen

B Upper pole of left kidney, cortex

C Abdominal aorta

D Right common iliac artery

E Normal variant: Left-sided inferior vena cava

Coronal abdominal CT in the arterial phase.

A left-sided inferior vena cava (IVC) is a normal variant which occurs in approximately 0.2–0.5% of people. In this situation, the confluence of the iliac veins is found behind the left common iliac artery and the IVC ascends from here, on the left side of the abdominal aorta. Typically, once it receives the left renal vein, it crosses anterior to the aorta, towards the right hand side. At this point, it receives the right renal vein and resumes a normal course.

This example demonstrates the typical course taken by a left-sided IVC, crossing in front of the aorta once the left renal vein has been received. The arterial phase of this study should help you to identify this anomaly, as the contrast has not yet reached the venous system.

Branchereau A, Jacobs M. Unexpected Challenges in Vascular Surgery. Heidelberg: Springer, 2005: 46.

Chapter 4

Musculoskeletal system

Lower limb

Case 4.1

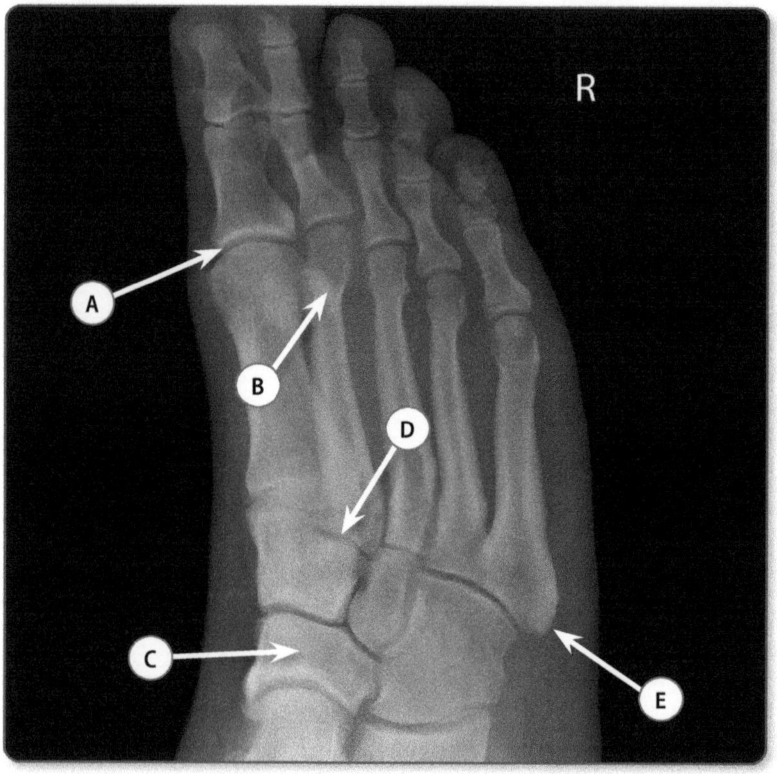

Case 4.1

QUESTION		WRITE YOUR ANSWER HERE
A	Name the structure labelled A.	
B	Name the structure labelled B.	
C	Name the structure labelled C.	
D	Name the structure labelled D.	
E	What attaches here?	

Case 4.2

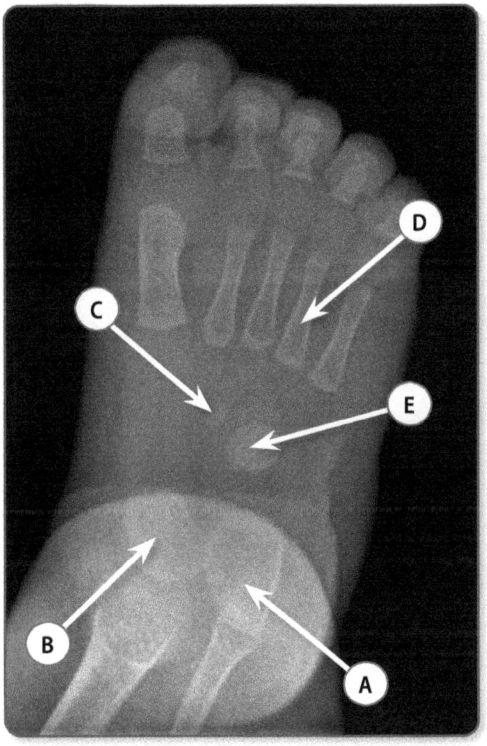

Case 4.2

QUESTION		WRITE YOUR ANSWER HERE
A	Name the structure labelled A.	
B	Name the structure labelled B.	
C	Name the structure labelled C.	
D	Name the structure labelled D.	
E	Name the structure labelled E.	

Case 4.3

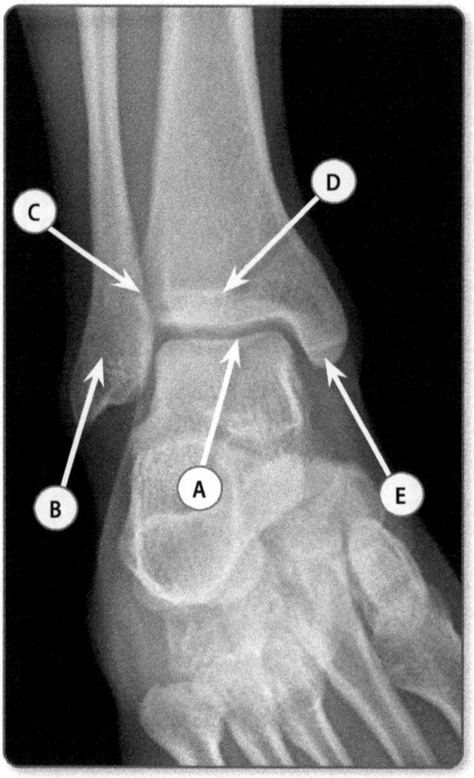

Case 4.3

QUESTION		WRITE YOUR ANSWER HERE
A	Name the structure labelled A.	
B	Name the structure labelled B.	
C	Name the structure labelled C.	
D	Name the structure labelled D.	
E	Name the structure labelled E.	

Case 4.4

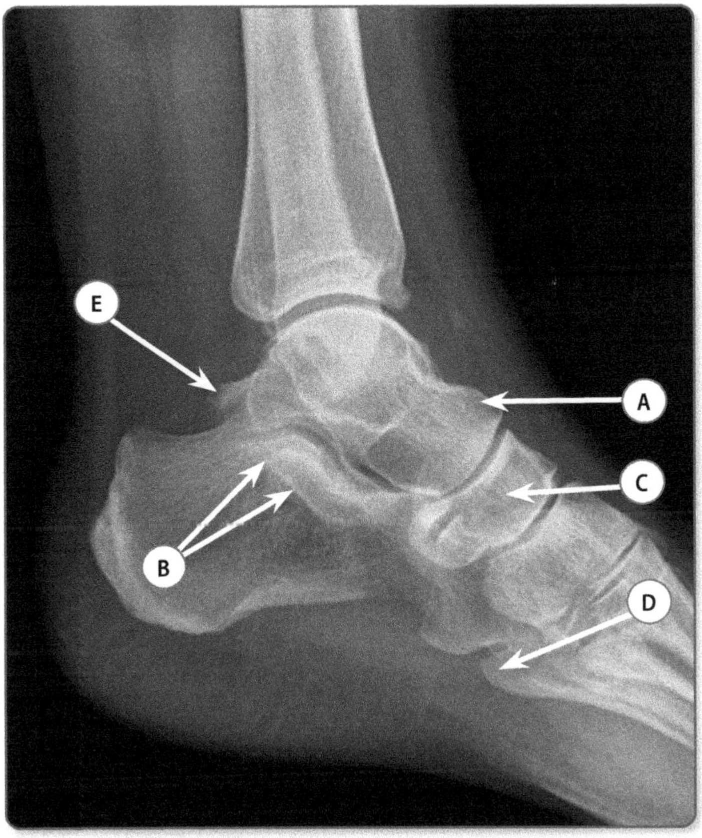

Case 4.4		
QUESTION		WRITE YOUR ANSWER HERE
A	Name the structure labelled A.	
B	Name the structure labelled B.	
C	Name the structure labelled C.	
D	Name the structure labelled D.	
E	Name the structure labelled E.	

Case 4.5

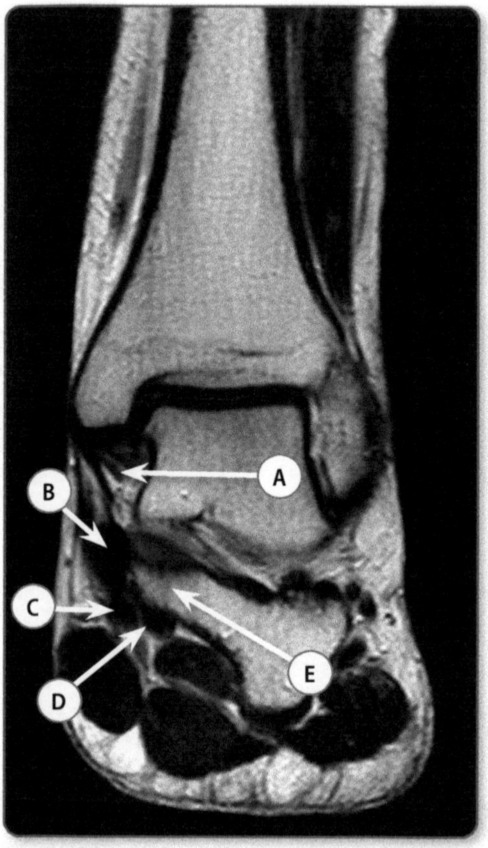

Case 4.5

QUESTION		WRITE YOUR ANSWER HERE
A	Name the structure labelled A.	
B	Name the structure labelled B.	
C	Name the structure labelled C.	
D	Name the structure labelled D.	
E	Name the structure labelled E.	

Case 4.6

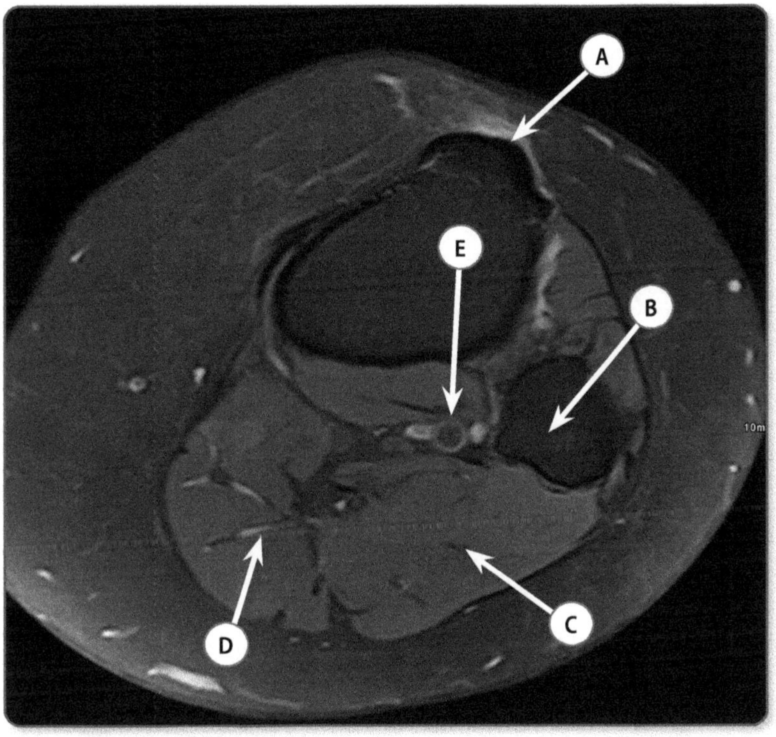

Case 4.6

	QUESTION	WRITE YOUR ANSWER HERE
A	What attaches to this structure?	
B	Name the structure labelled B.	
C	Name the structure labelled C.	
D	Name the structure labelled D.	
E	Name the structure labelled E.	

Case 4.7

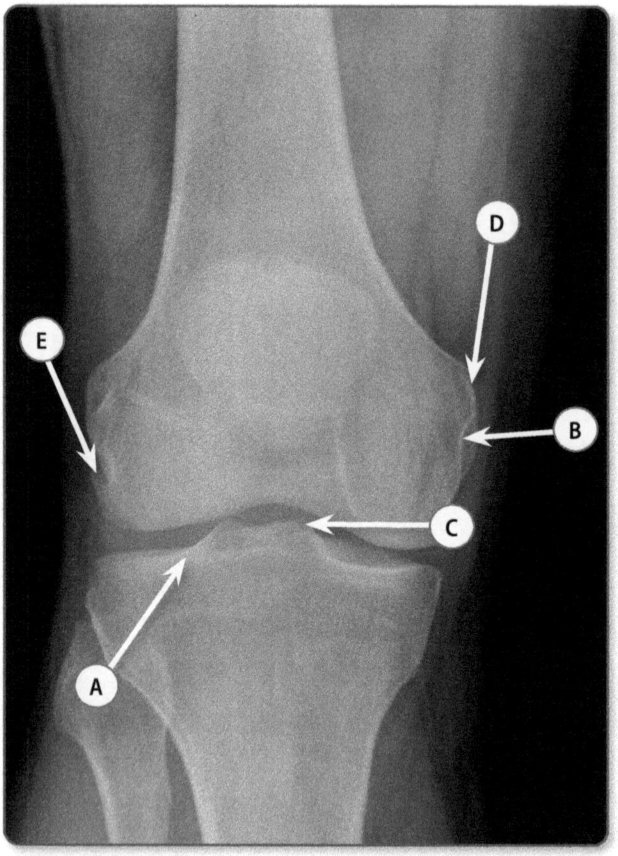

Case 4.7

QUESTION		WRITE YOUR ANSWER HERE
A	Name the structure labelled A.	
B	Name the structure labelled B.	
C	Name the structure labelled C.	
D	Name the structure labelled D.	
E	Name the structure labelled E.	

Case 4.8

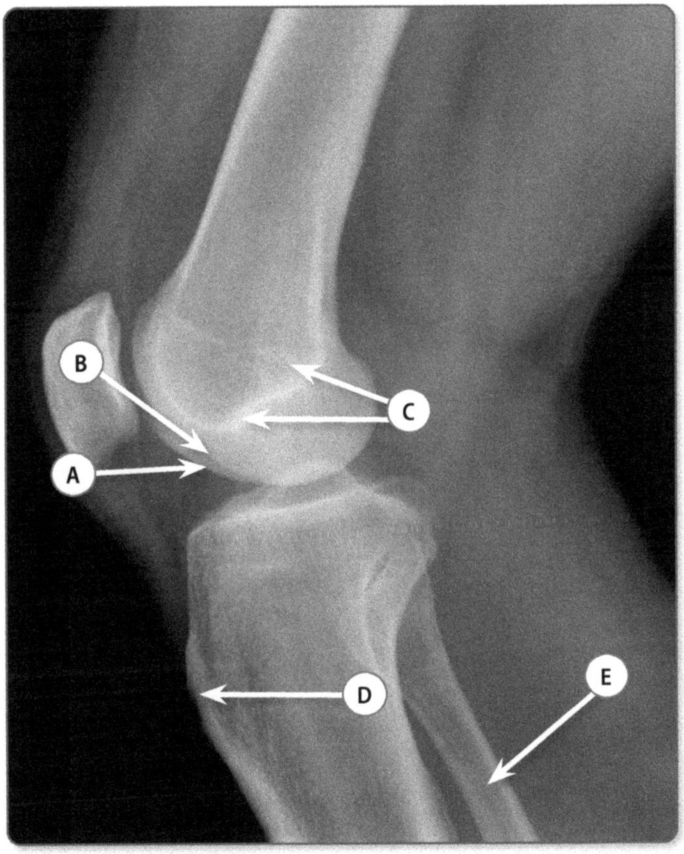

Case 4.8

QUESTION		WRITE YOUR ANSWER HERE
A	Name the structure labelled A.	
B	Name the structure labelled B.	
C	Name the structure labelled C.	
D	Name the structure labelled D.	
E	Name the structure labelled E.	

Case 4.9

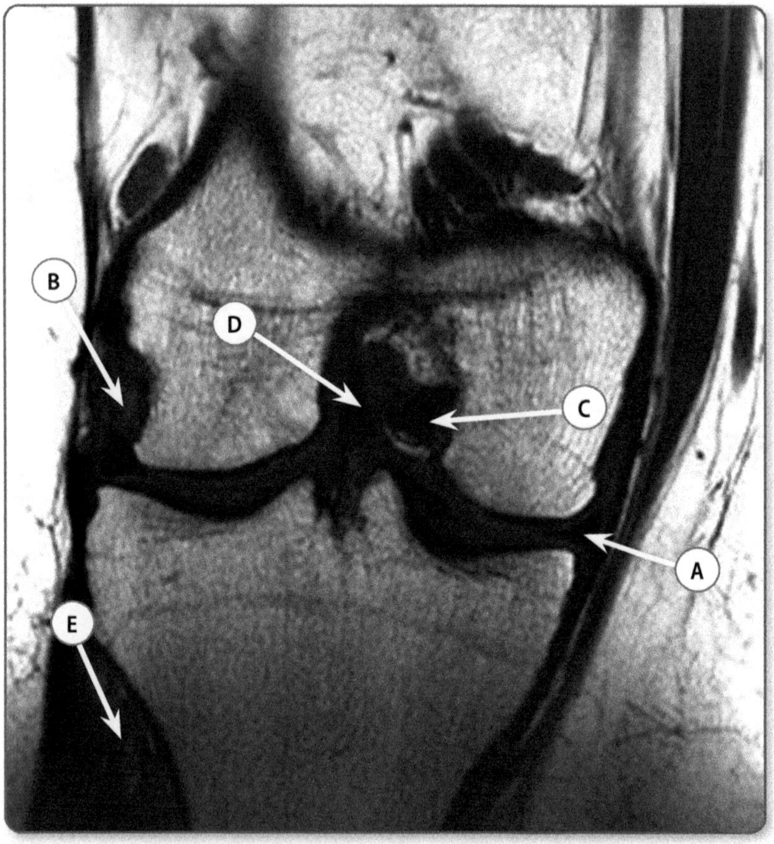

Case 4.9

QUESTION		WRITE YOUR ANSWER HERE
A	Name the structure labelled A.	
B	Name the structure labelled B.	
C	Name the structure labelled C.	
D	Name the structure labelled D.	
E	Name the structure labelled E.	

Case 4.10

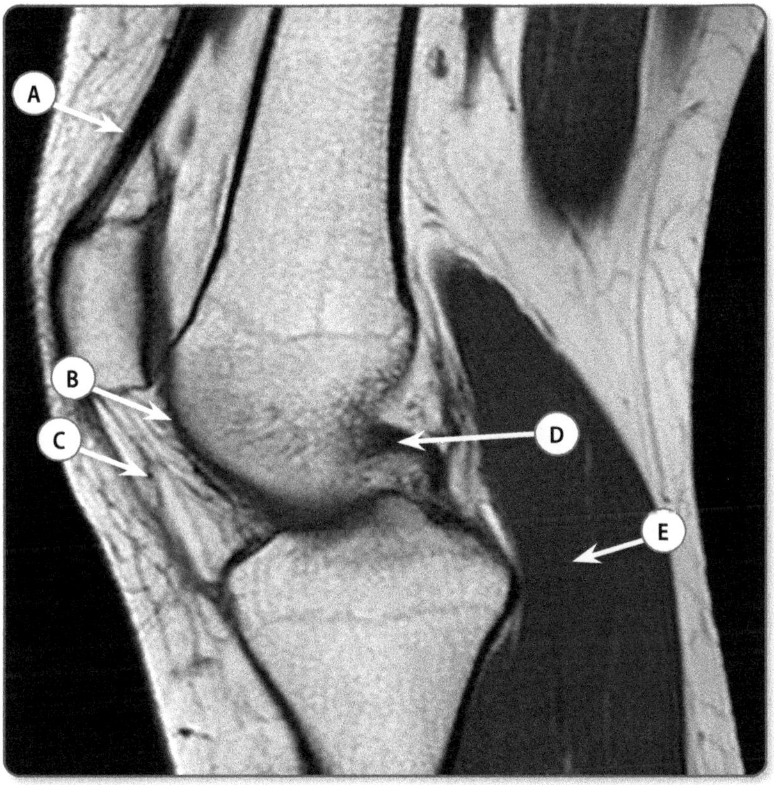

Case 4.10

QUESTION		WRITE YOUR ANSWER HERE
A	Name the structure labelled A.	
B	Name the structure labelled B.	
C	Name the structure labelled C.	
D	Name the structure labelled D.	
E	Name the structure labelled E.	

Case 4.11

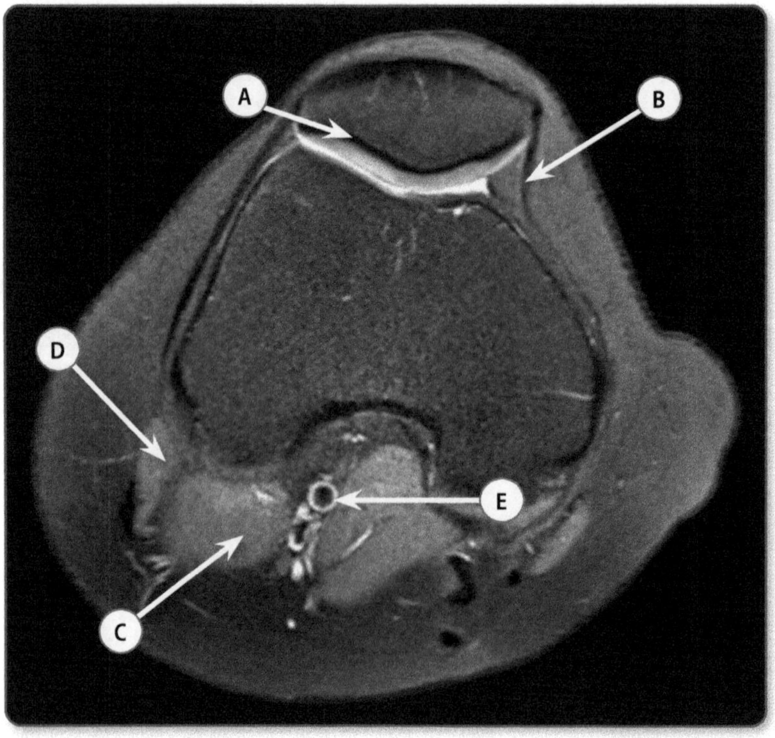

Case 4.11

QUESTION		WRITE YOUR ANSWER HERE
A	Name the structure labelled A.	
B	Name the structure labelled B.	
C	Name the structure labelled C.	
D	Name the structure labelled D.	
E	Name the structure labelled E.	

Case 4.12

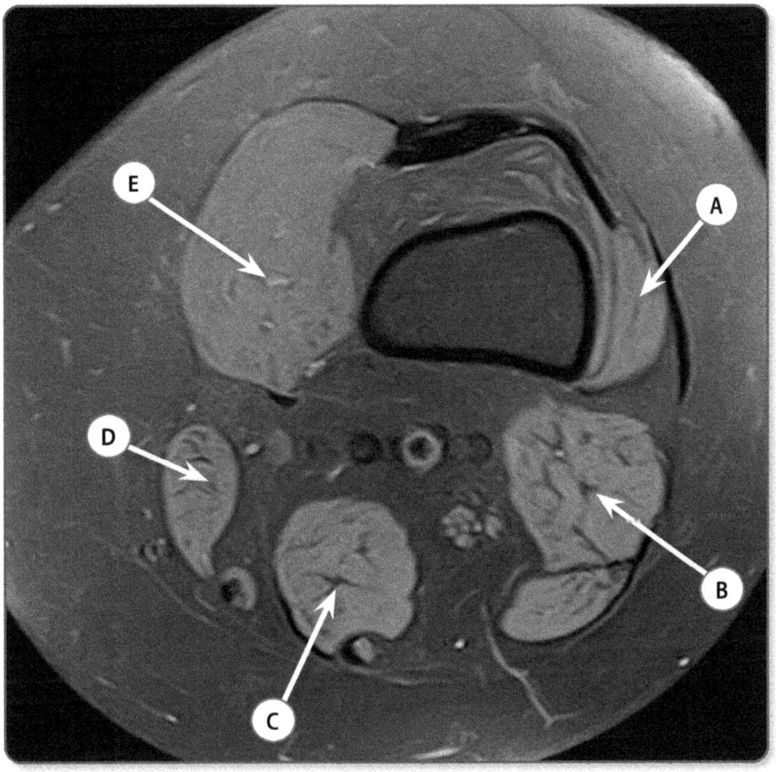

Case 4.12

QUESTION		WRITE YOUR ANSWER HERE
A	Name the structure labelled A.	
B	Name the structure labelled B.	
C	Name the structure labelled C.	
D	Name the structure labelled D.	
E	Name the structure labelled E.	

Case 4.13

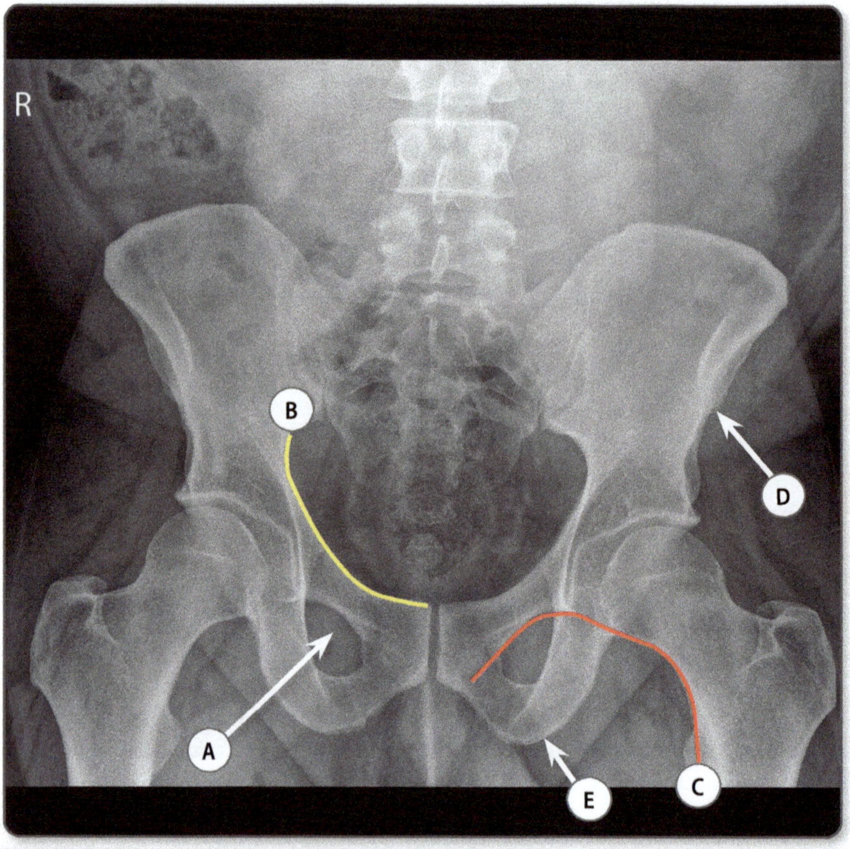

Case 4.13

QUESTION		WRITE YOUR ANSWER HERE
A	Name the structure labelled A.	
B	Name this pelvic line.	
C	Name this pelvic line.	
D	Name the muscle tendon that attaches to this structure.	
E	Name the muscle tendon that attaches to this structure.	

Case 4.14

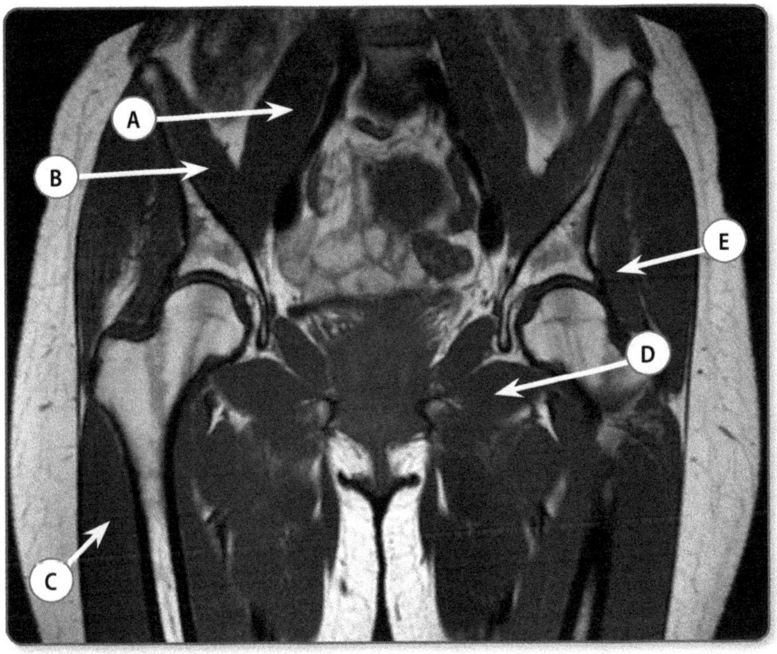

Case 4.14

QUESTION		WRITE YOUR ANSWER HERE
A	Name the structure labelled A.	
B	Name the structure labelled B.	
C	Name the structure labelled C.	
D	Name the structure labelled D.	
E	Name the structure labelled E.	

Case 4.15

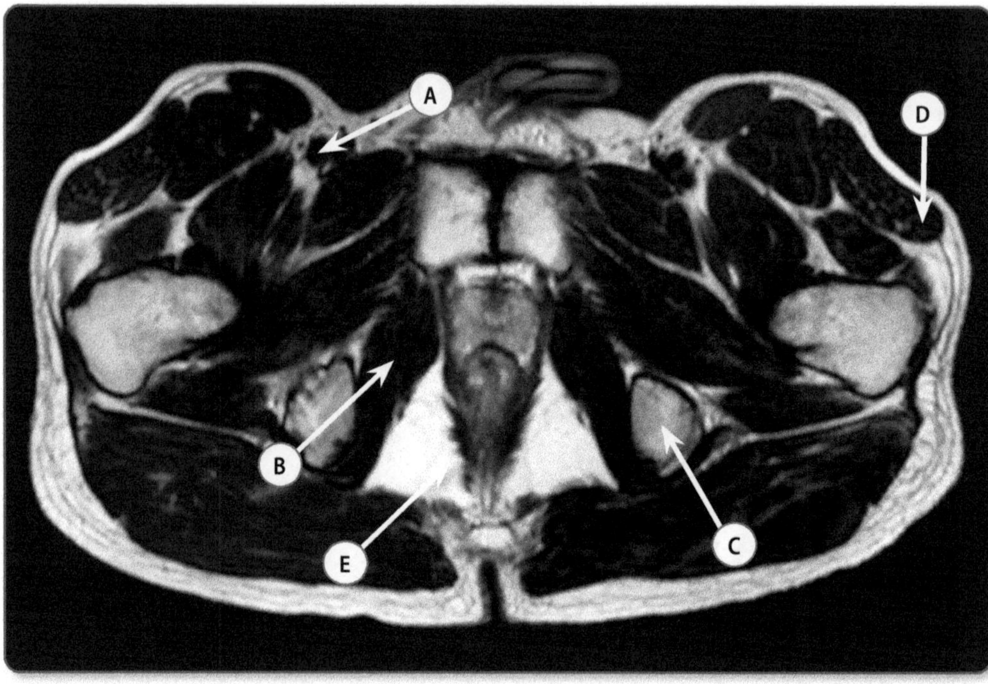

Case 4.15

QUESTION		WRITE YOUR ANSWER HERE
A	Name the structure labelled A.	
B	Name the structure labelled B.	
C	Name the structure labelled C.	
D	Name the structure labelled D.	
E	Name the structure labelled E.	

Case 4.16

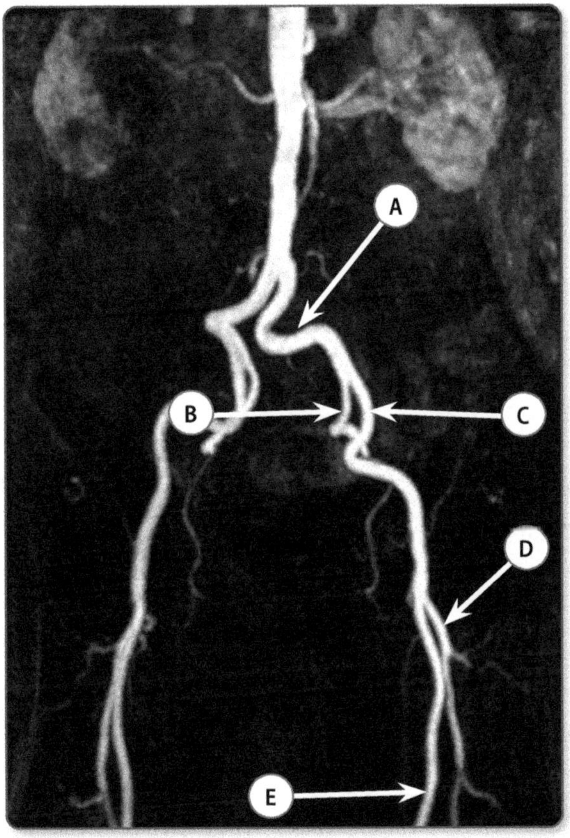

Case 4.16

QUESTION		WRITE YOUR ANSWER HERE
A	Name the structure labelled A.	
B	Name the structure labelled B.	
C	Name the structure labelled C.	
D	Name the structure labelled D.	
E	Name the structure labelled E.	

Case 4.17

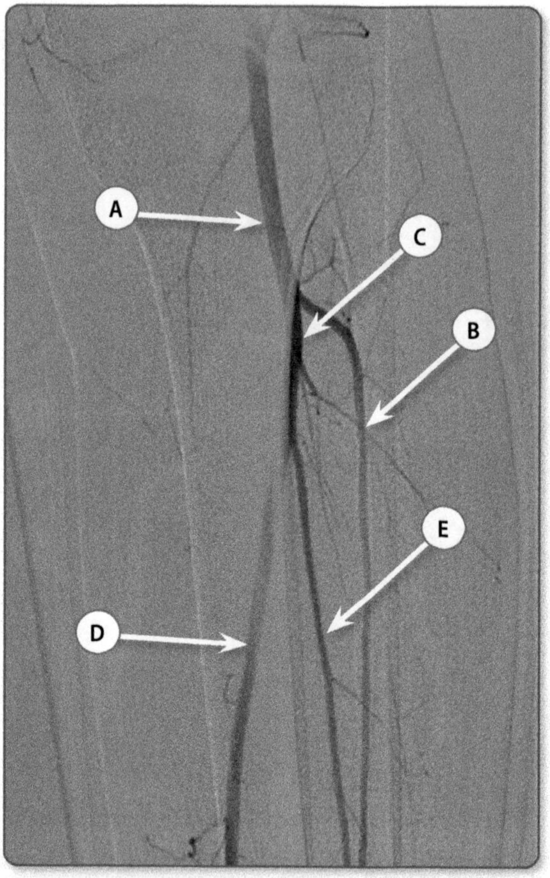

Case 4.17

QUESTION		WRITE YOUR ANSWER HERE
A	Name the structure labelled A.	
B	Name the structure labelled B.	
C	Name the structure labelled C.	
D	Name the structure labelled D.	
E	Name the structure labelled E.	

Case 4.18

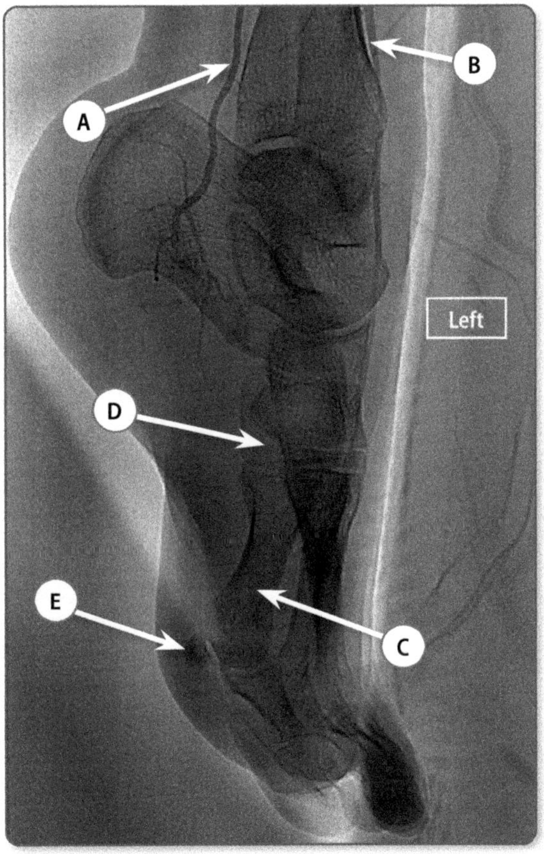

Case 4.18

QUESTION		WRITE YOUR ANSWER HERE
A	Name the structure labelled A.	
B	Name the structure labelled B.	
C	Name the structure labelled C.	
D	Name the structure labelled D.	
E	Name the structure labelled E.	

Spine

Case 4.19

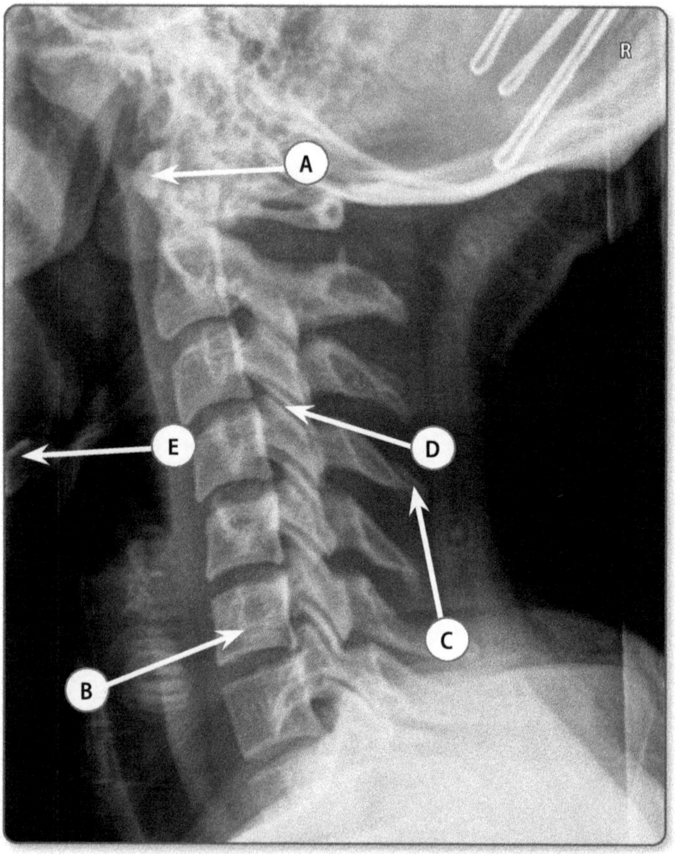

Case 4.19

QUESTION		WRITE YOUR ANSWER HERE
A	Name the structure labelled A.	
B	Name the structure labelled B.	
C	Name the structure labelled C.	
D	Name the structure labelled D.	
E	Name the structure labelled E.	

Case 4.20

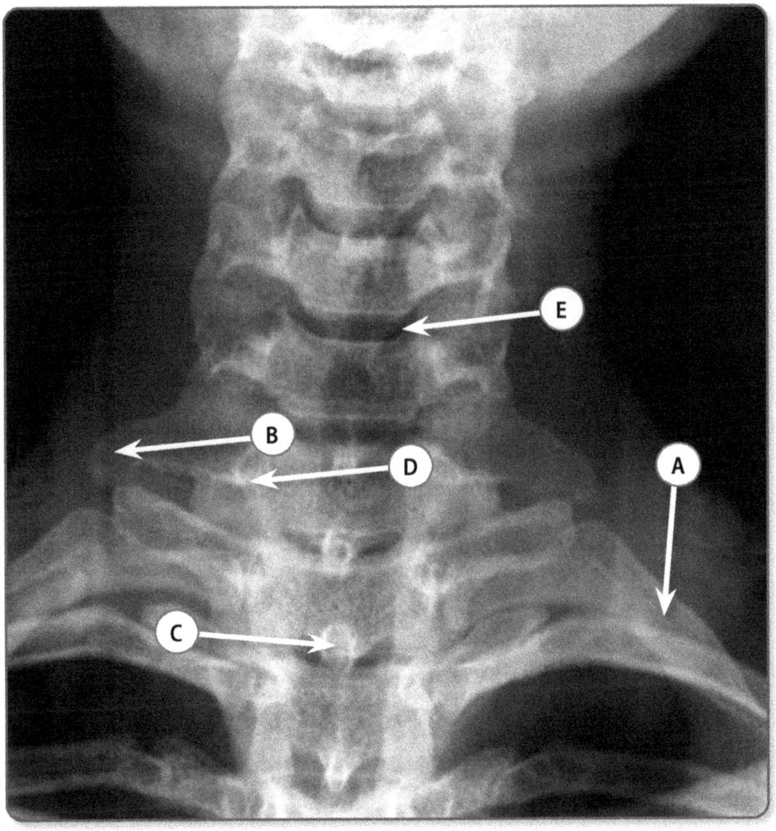

Case 4.20		
QUESTION		WRITE YOUR ANSWER HERE
A	Name the structure labelled A.	
B	Name the structure labelled B.	
C	Name the structure labelled C.	
D	Name the structure labelled D.	
E	Name the structure labelled E.	

Case 4.21

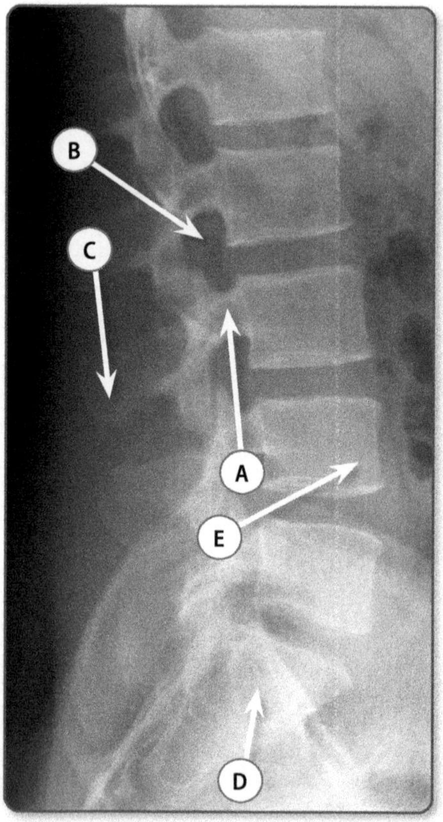

Case 4.21

QUESTION		WRITE YOUR ANSWER HERE
A	Name the structure labelled A.	
B	Name the structure labelled B.	
C	Name the structure labelled C.	
D	Name the structure labelled D.	
E	Name the structure labelled E.	

Case 4.22

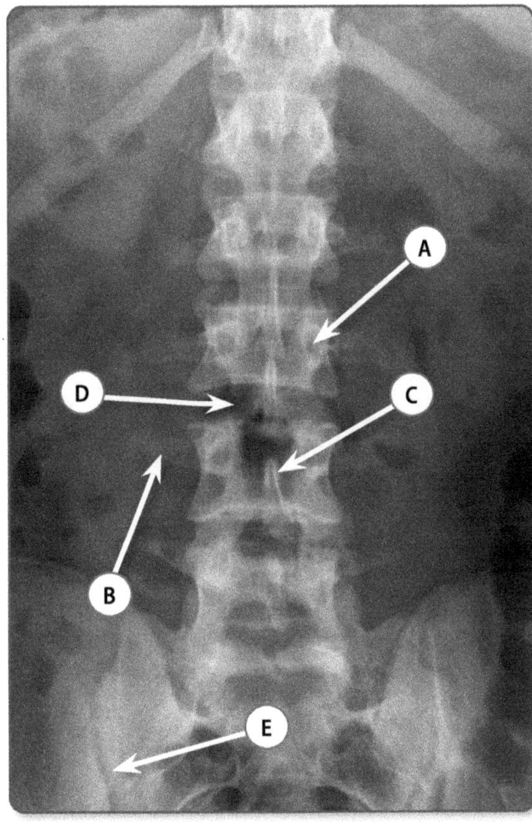

Case 4.22

QUESTION		WRITE YOUR ANSWER HERE
A	Name the structure labelled A.	
B	Name the structure labelled B.	
C	Name the structure labelled C.	
D	Name the structure labelled D.	
E	Name the structure labelled E.	

Case 4.23

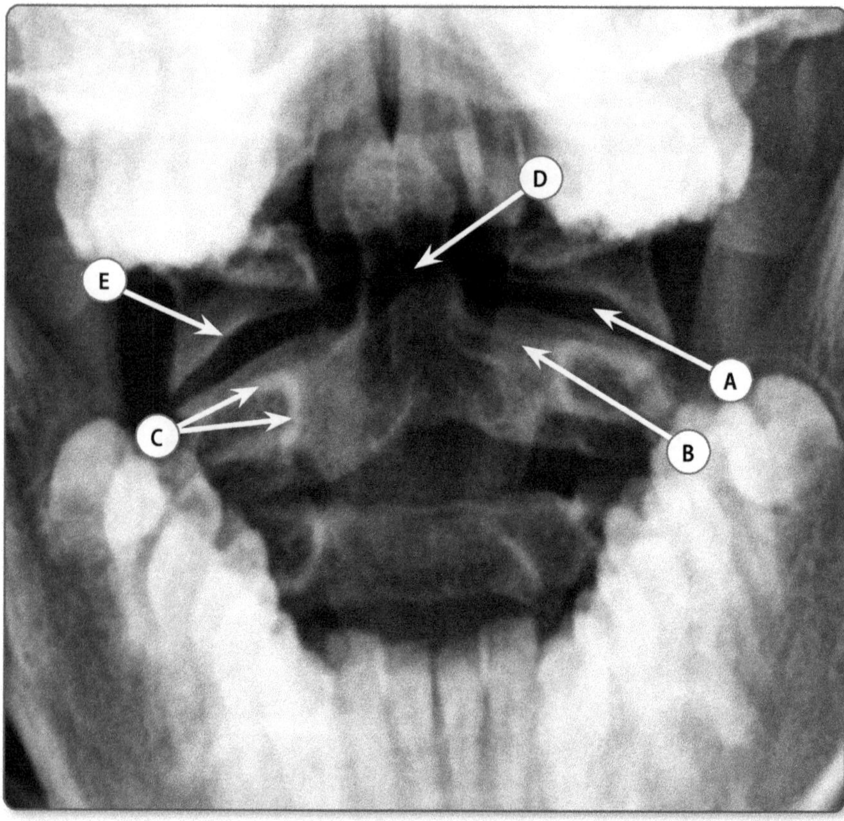

Case 4.23

QUESTION		WRITE YOUR ANSWER HERE
A	Name the structure labelled A.	
B	Name the structure labelled B.	
C	Name the structure labelled C.	
D	Name the structure labelled D.	
E	Name the structure labelled E.	

Case 4.24

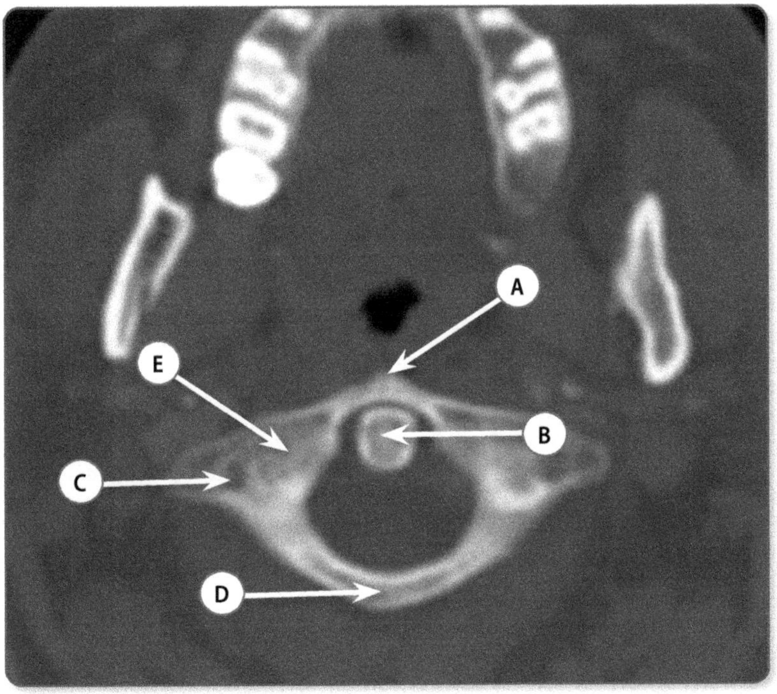

Case 4.24

QUESTION		WRITE YOUR ANSWER HERE
A	Name the structure labelled A.	
B	Name the structure labelled B.	
C	Name the structure labelled C.	
D	Name the structure labelled D.	
E	Name the structure labelled E.	

Case 4.25

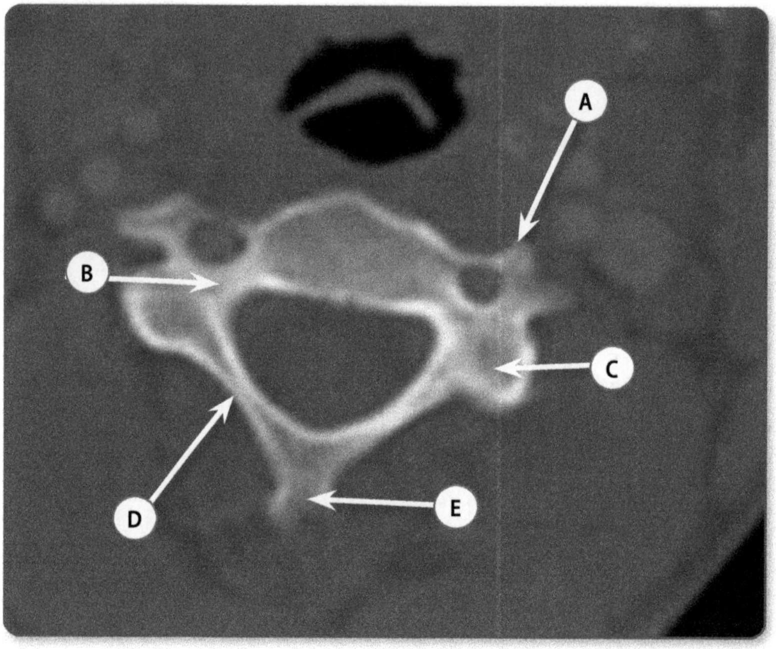

Case 4.25

QUESTION		WRITE YOUR ANSWER HERE
A	Name the structure labelled A.	
B	Name the structure labelled B.	
C	Name the structure labelled C.	
D	Name the structure labelled D.	
E	Name the structure labelled E.	

Case 4.26

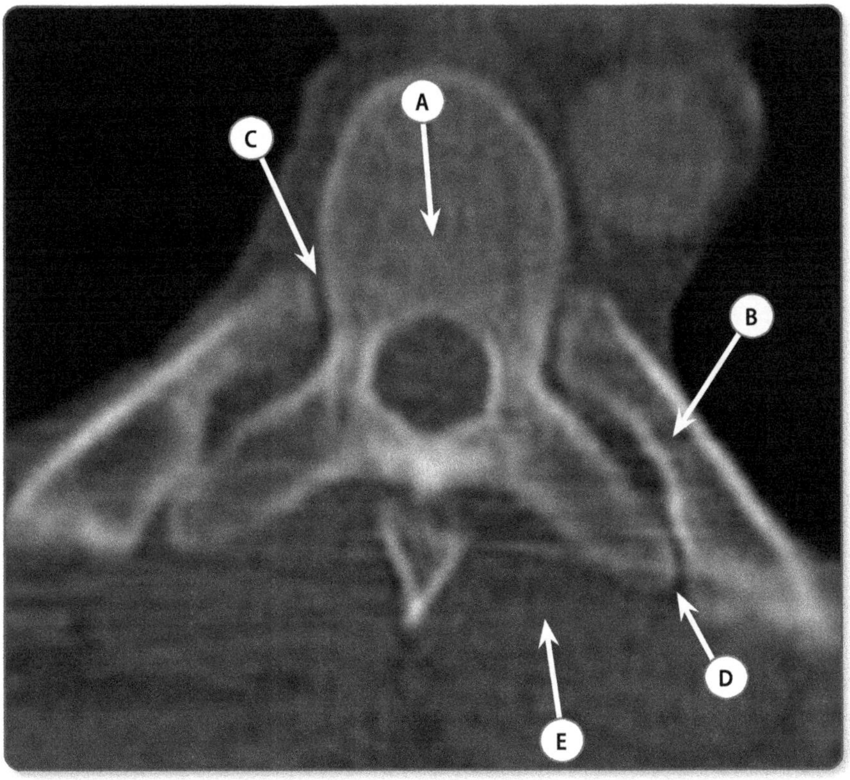

Case 4.26

QUESTION		WRITE YOUR ANSWER HERE
A	Name the structure labelled A.	
B	Name the structure labelled B.	
C	Name the structure labelled C.	
D	Name the structure labelled D.	
E	Name the structure labelled E.	

Case 4.27

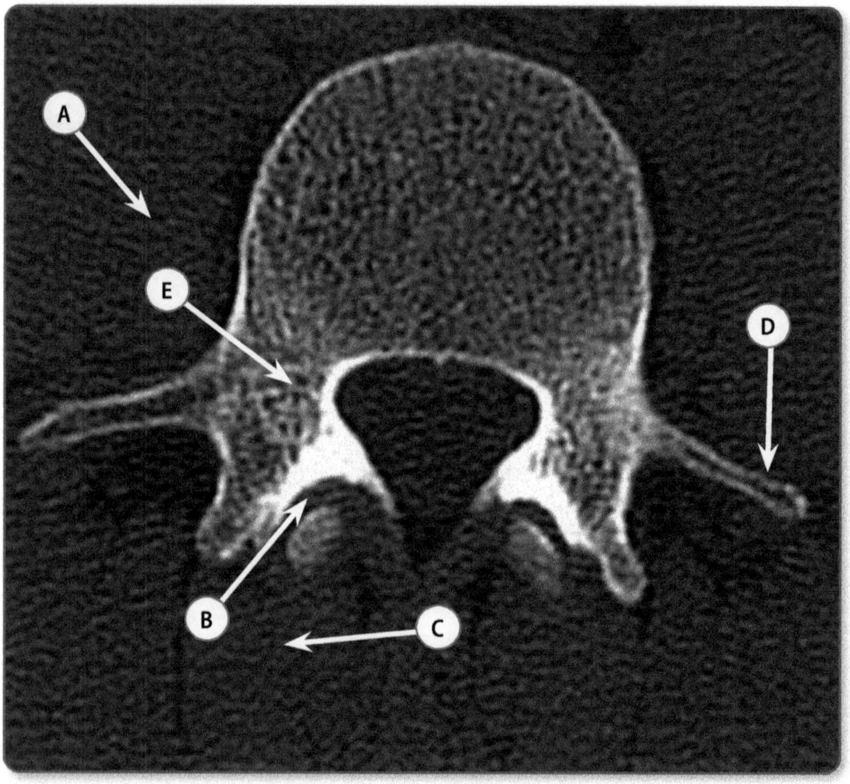

Case 4.27

QUESTION		WRITE YOUR ANSWER HERE
A	Name the structure labelled A.	
B	Name the structure labelled B.	
C	Name the structure labelled C.	
D	Name the structure labelled D.	
E	Name the structure labelled E.	

Case 4.28

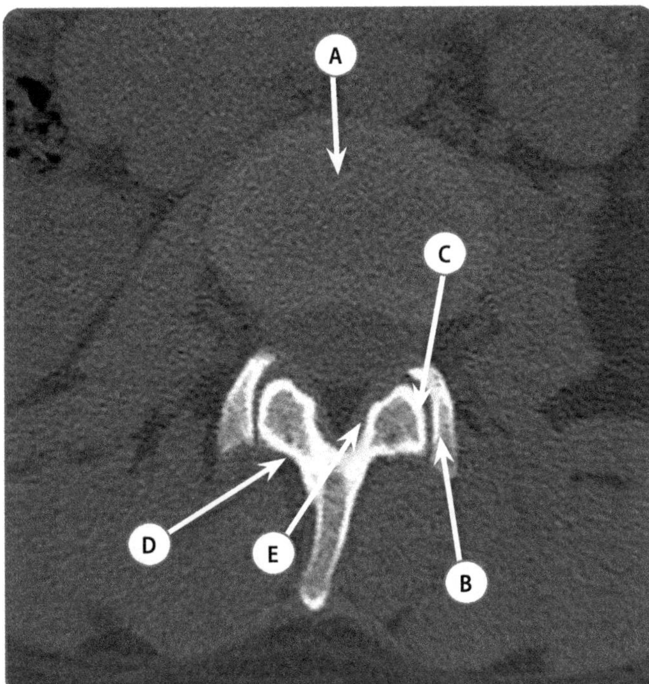

Case 4.28

QUESTION		WRITE YOUR ANSWER HERE
A	Name the structure labelled A.	
B	Name the structure labelled B.	
C	Name the structure labelled C.	
D	Name the structure labelled D.	
E	Name the structure labelled E.	

Case 4.29

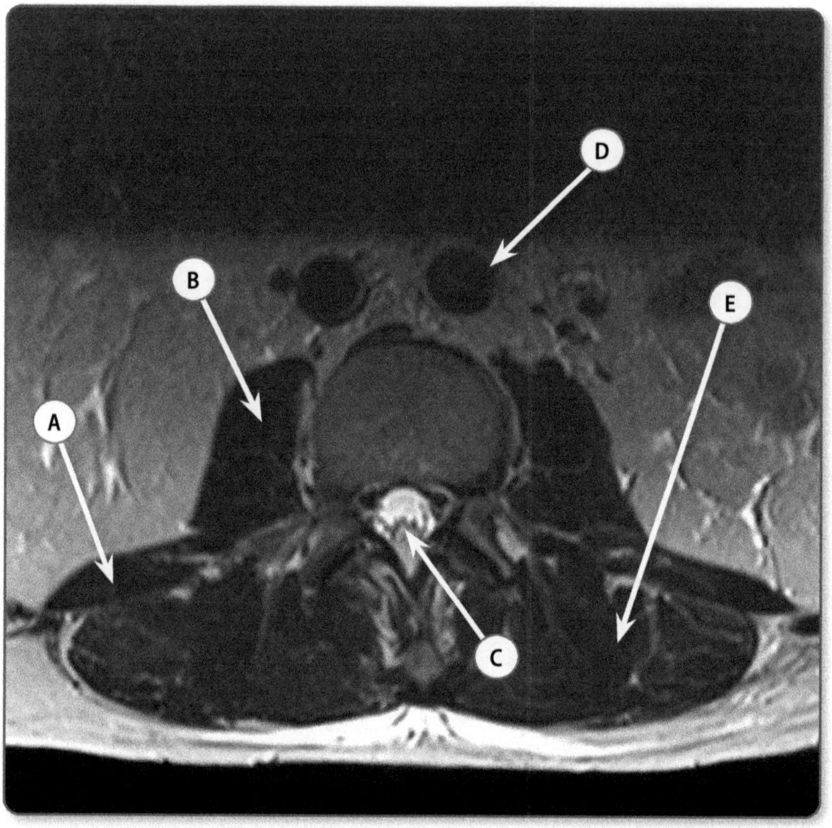

Case 4.29

QUESTION		WRITE YOUR ANSWER HERE
A	Name the structure labelled A.	
B	Name the structure labelled B.	
C	Name the structure labelled C.	
D	Name the structure labelled D.	
E	Name the structure labelled E.	

Case 4.30

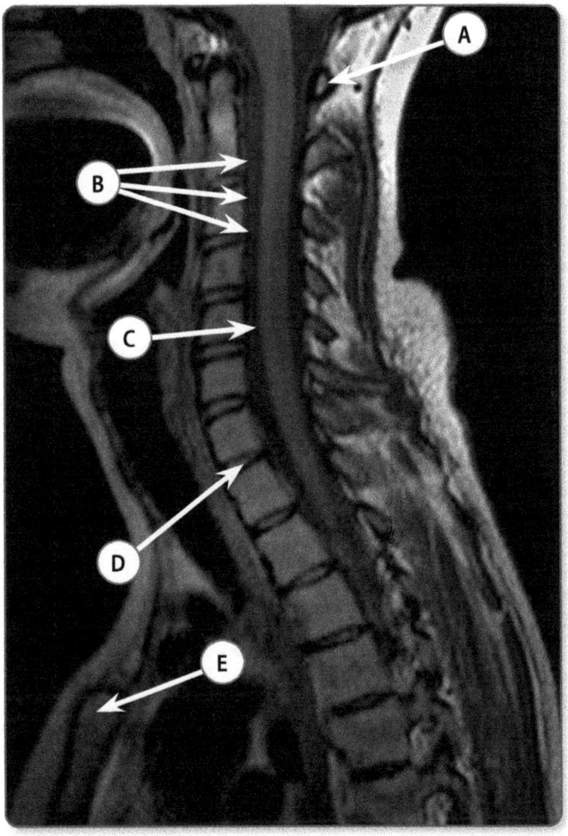

Case 4.30

QUESTION		WRITE YOUR ANSWER HERE
A	Name the structure labelled A.	
B	Name the structure labelled B.	
C	Name the structure labelled C.	
D	Name the structure labelled D.	
E	Name the structure labelled E.	

Case 4.31

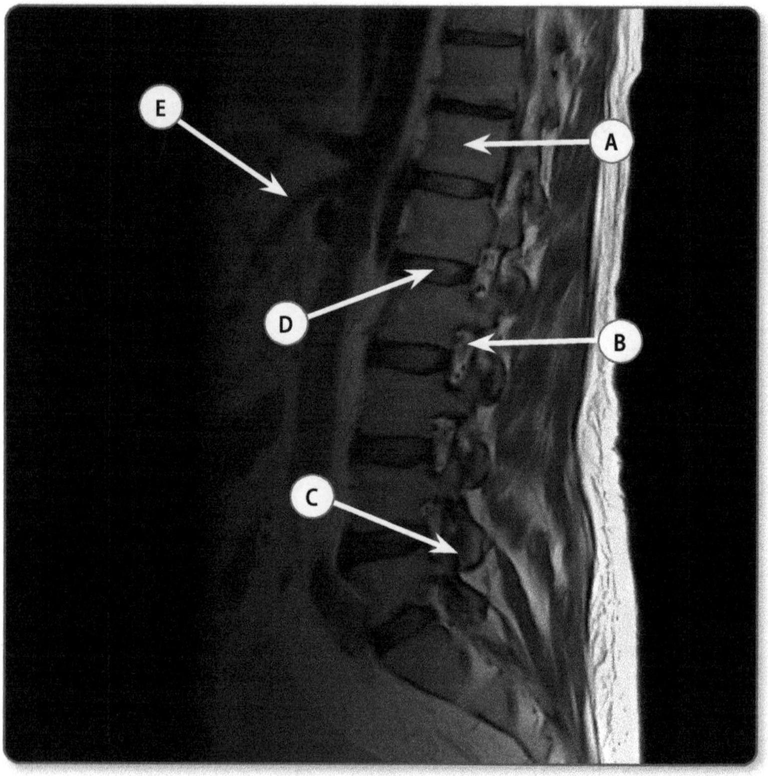

Case 4.31

	QUESTION	WRITE YOUR ANSWER HERE
A	Name the structure labelled A.	
B	Name the structure labelled B.	
C	Name the structure labelled C.	
D	Name the structure labelled D.	
E	Name the structure labelled E.	

Case 4.32

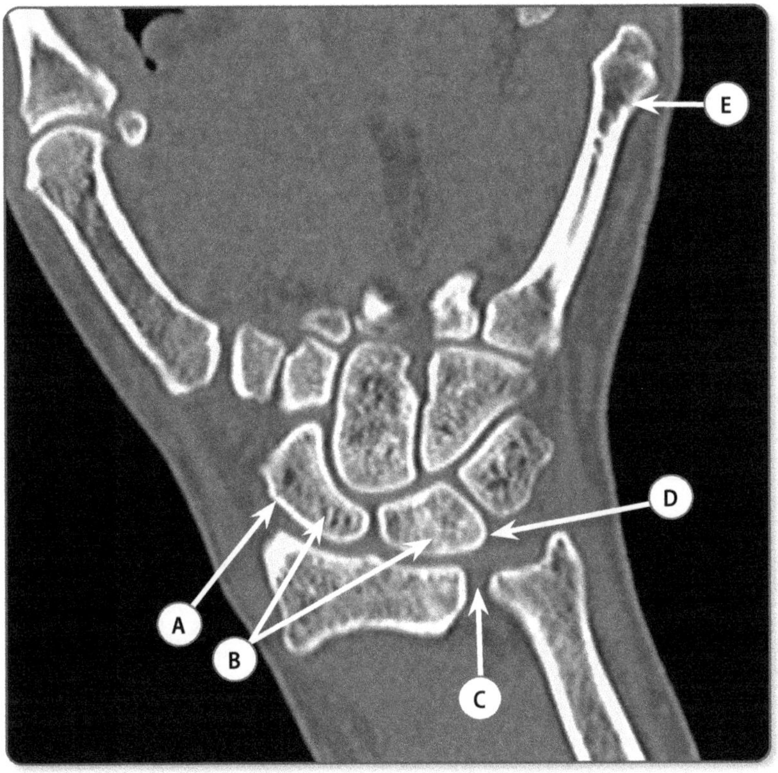

Case 4.32

QUESTION		WRITE YOUR ANSWER HERE
A	Name the structure labelled A.	
B	What ligament joins these two structures?	
C	Name the structure labelled C.	
D	Name the structure labelled D.	
E	Name the structure labelled E.	

Case 4.33

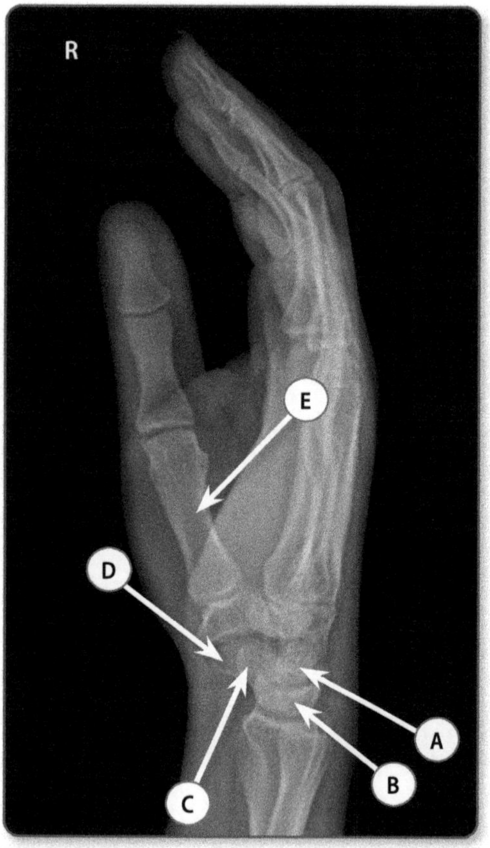

Case 4.33

QUESTION		WRITE YOUR ANSWER HERE
A	Name the structure labelled A.	
B	Name the structure labelled B.	
C	Name the structure labelled C.	
D	Name the structure labelled D.	
E	Name the structure labelled E.	

Case 4.34

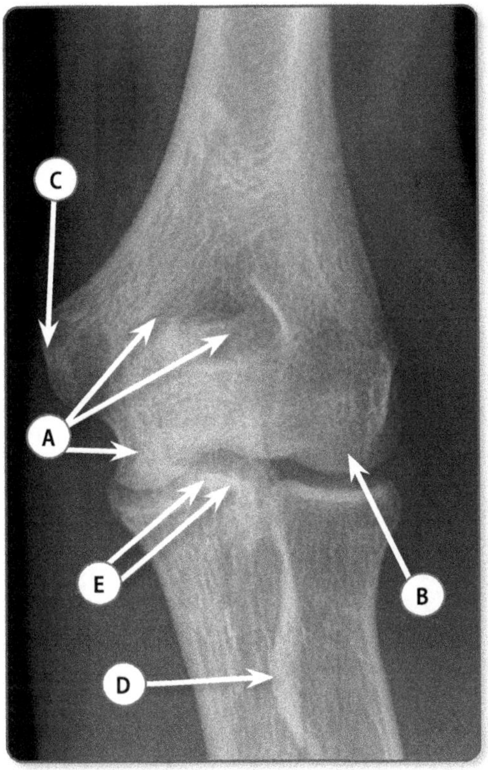

Case 4.34

QUESTION		WRITE YOUR ANSWER HERE
A	Name the structure labelled A.	
B	Name the structure labelled B.	
C	Name the structure labelled C.	
D	Name the structure labelled D.	
E	Name the structure labelled E.	

Case 4.35

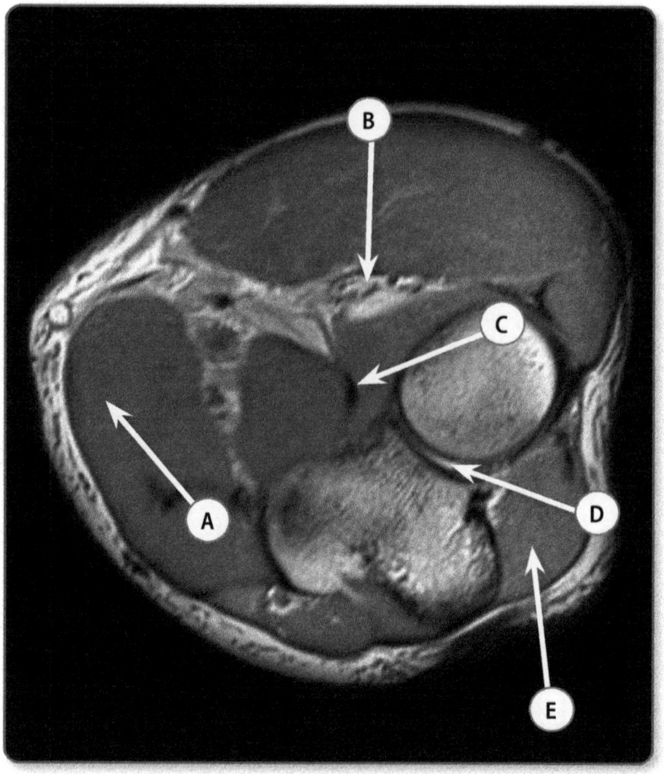

Case 4.35

QUESTION		WRITE YOUR ANSWER HERE
A	Name the structure labelled A.	
B	Name the structure labelled B.	
C	Name the structure labelled C.	
D	Name the structure labelled D.	
E	Name the structure labelled E.	

Case 4.36

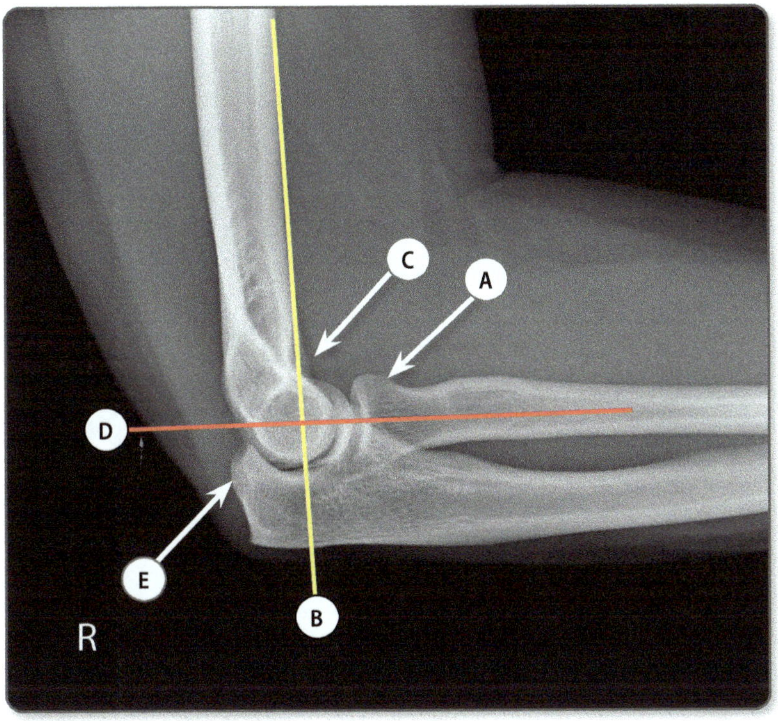

Case 4.36

QUESTION		WRITE YOUR ANSWER HERE
A	Name the structure labelled A.	
B	Name the line labelled B.	
C	Name the structure labelled C.	
D	Name the line labelled D.	
E	What attaches to this structure?	

Case 4.37

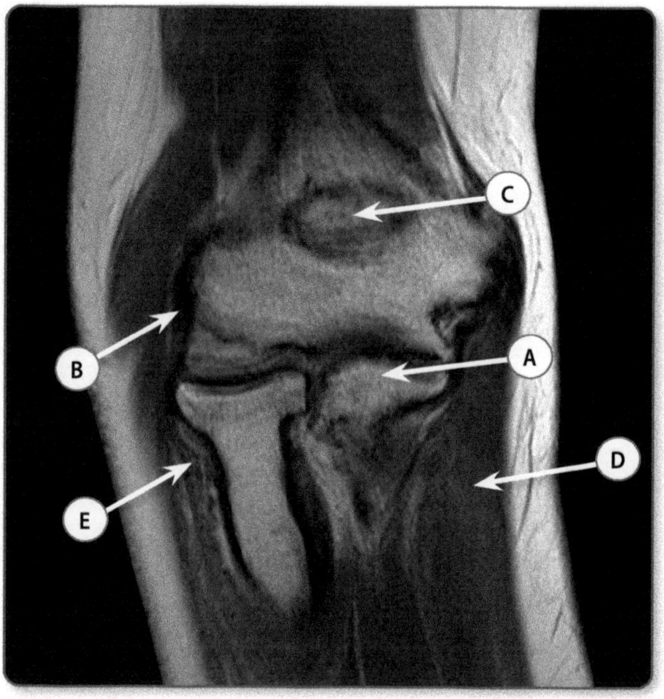

Case 4.37		
QUESTION		WRITE YOUR ANSWER HERE
A	Name the structure labelled A.	
B	Name the structure labelled B.	
C	Name the structure labelled C.	
D	Name the structure labelled D.	
E	Name the structure labelled E.	

Case 4.38

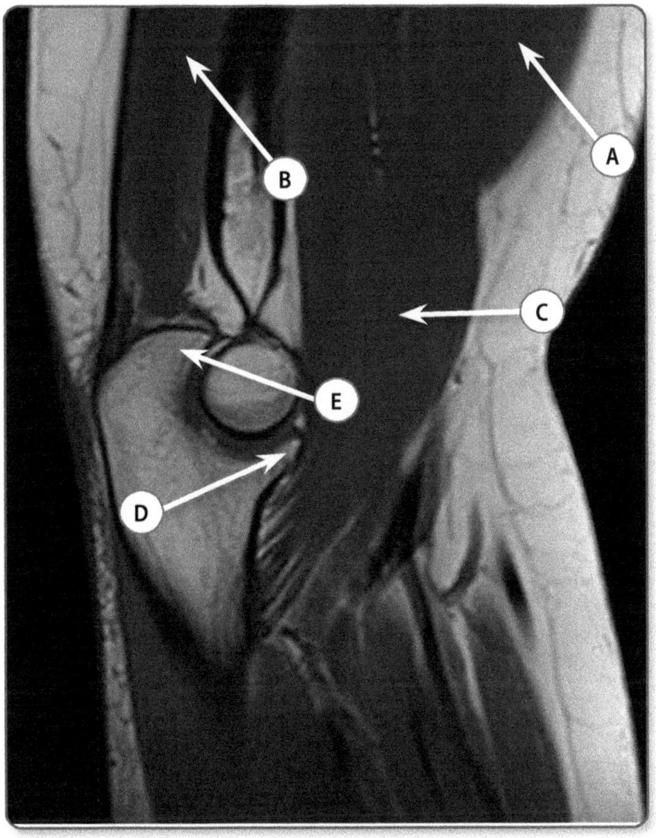

Case 4.38

QUESTION		WRITE YOUR ANSWER HERE
A	Name the structure labelled A.	
B	Name the structure labelled B.	
C	Name the structure labelled C.	
D	Name the structure labelled D.	
E	Name the structure labelled E.	

Case 4.39

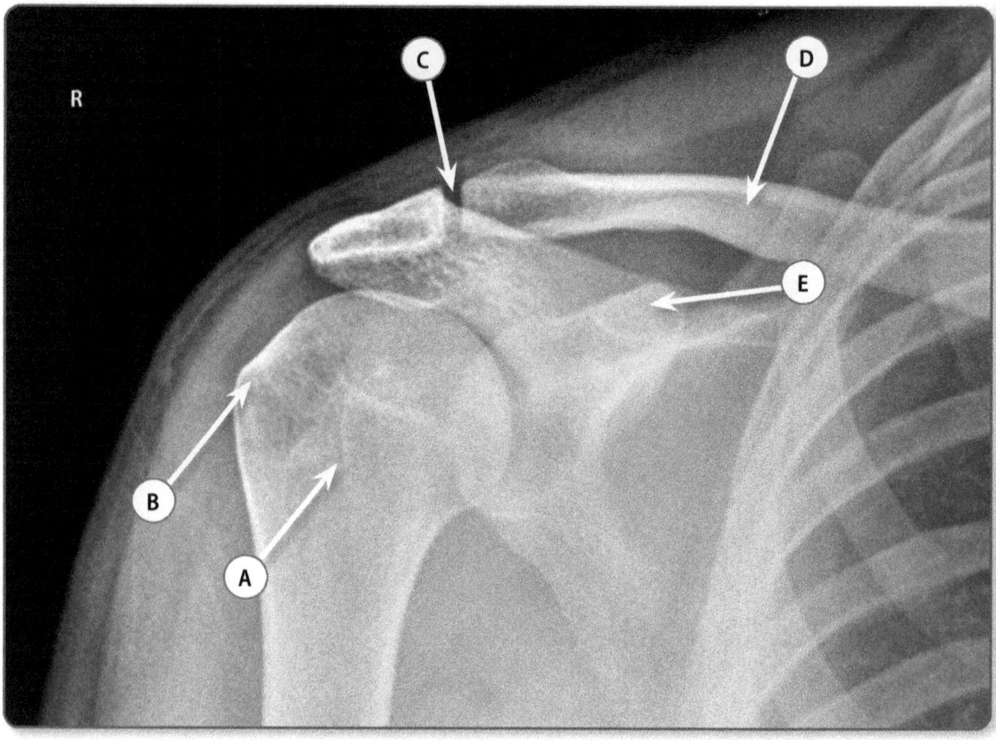

Case 4.39

QUESTION		WRITE YOUR ANSWER HERE
A	Name the structure labelled A.	
B	Name the structure labelled B.	
C	Name the structure labelled C.	
D	Name the structure labelled D.	
E	Name the structure labelled E.	

Case 4.40

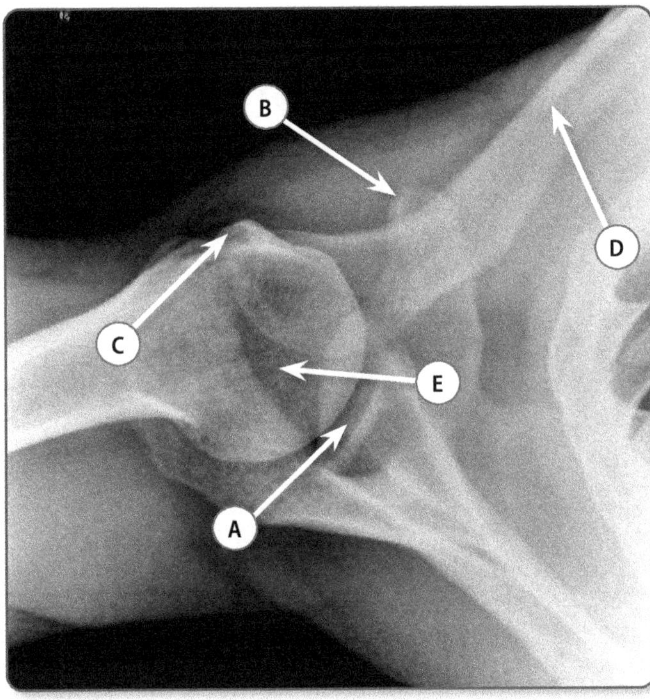

Case 4.40

QUESTION		WRITE YOUR ANSWER HERE
A	Name the structure labelled A.	
B	Name the structure labelled B.	
C	Name the structure labelled C.	
D	Name the structure labelled D.	
E	Name the structure labelled E.	

Case 4.41

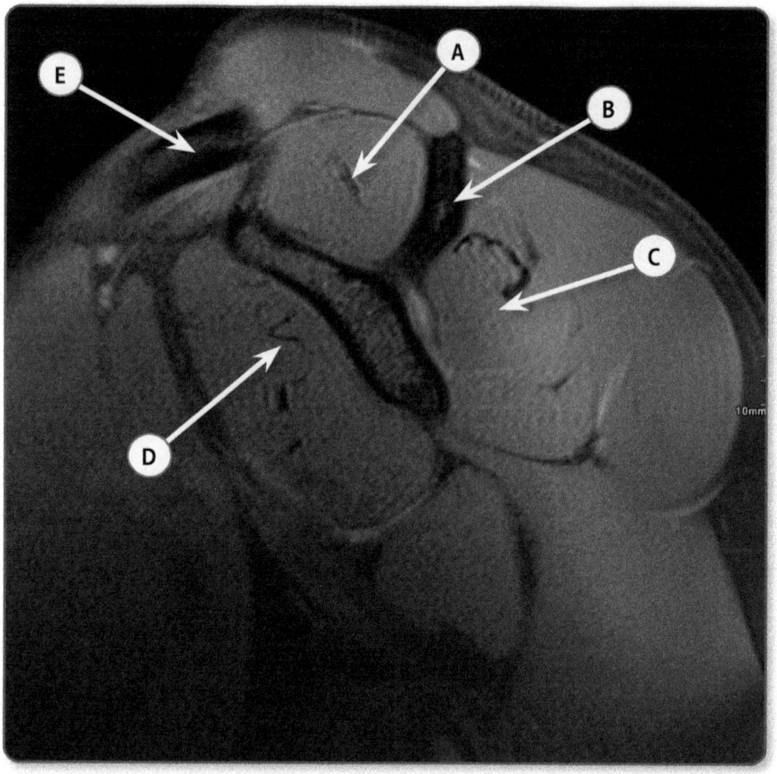

Case 4.41

QUESTION		WRITE YOUR ANSWER HERE
A	Name the structure labelled A.	
B	Name the structure labelled B.	
C	Name the structure labelled C.	
D	Name the structure labelled D.	
E	Name the structure labelled E.	

Case 4.42

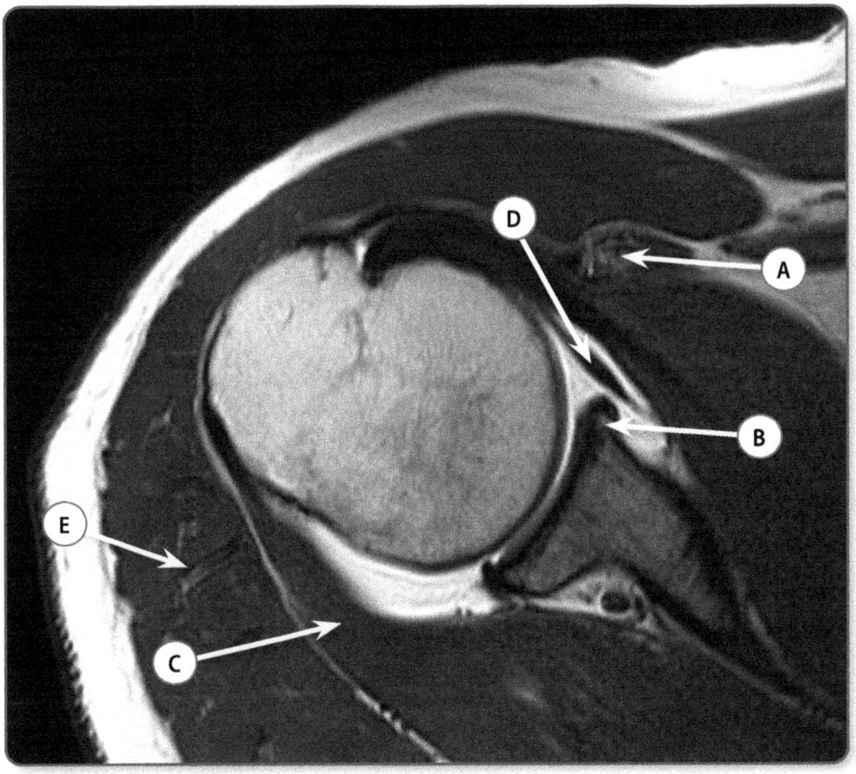

Case 4.42

QUESTION		WRITE YOUR ANSWER HERE
A	Name the structure labelled A.	
B	Name the structure labelled B.	
C	Name the structure labelled C.	
D	Name the structure labelled D.	
E	Name the structure labelled E.	

Case 4.43

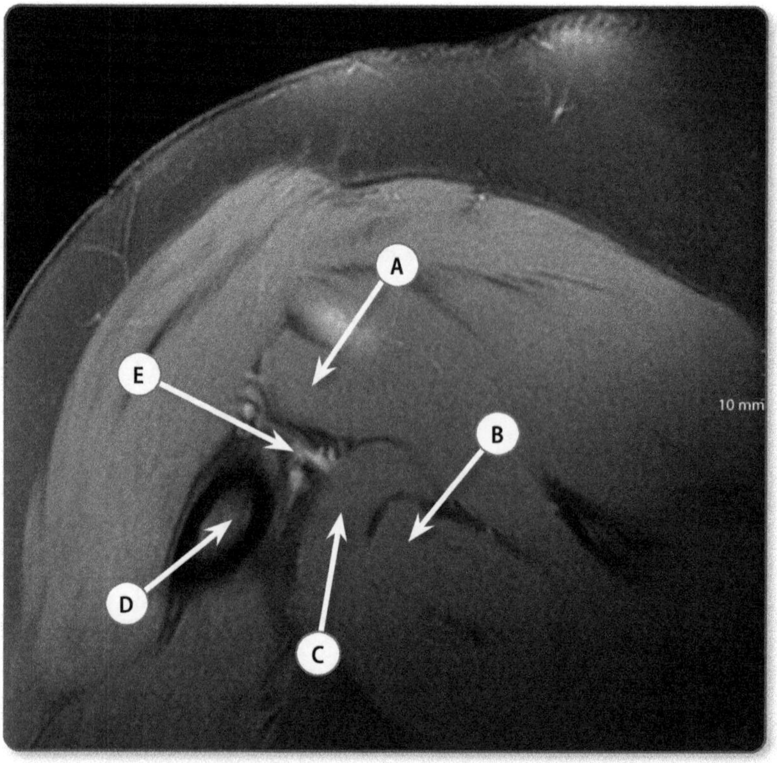

Case 4.43

QUESTION		WRITE YOUR ANSWER HERE
A	Name the structure labelled A.	
B	Name the structure labelled B.	
C	Name the structure labelled C.	
D	Name the structure labelled D.	
E	Name the structure labelled E.	

Case 4.44

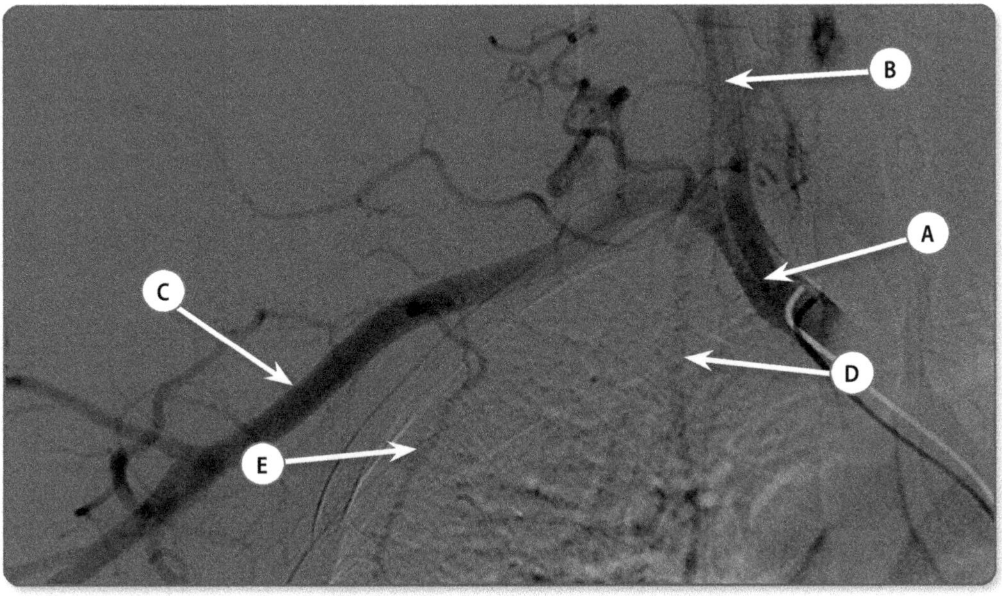

Case 4.44

QUESTION		WRITE YOUR ANSWER HERE
A	Name the structure labelled A.	
B	Name the structure labelled B.	
C	Name the structure labelled C.	
D	Name the structure labelled D.	
E	Name the structure labelled E.	

Case 4.45

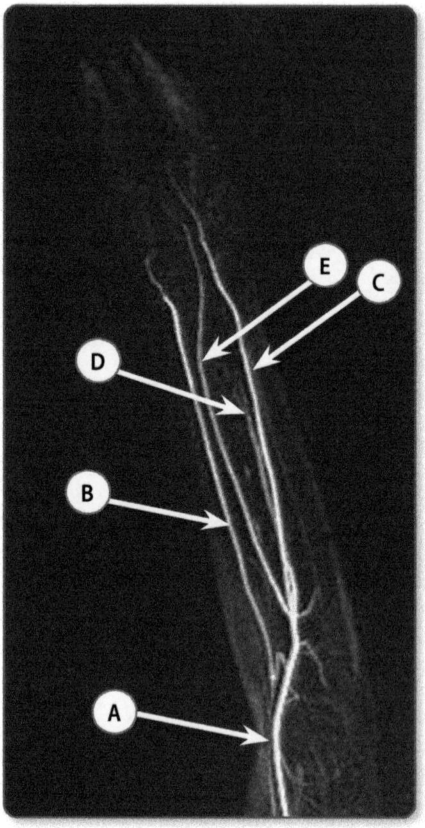

Case 4.45

QUESTION		WRITE YOUR ANSWER HERE
A	Name the structure labelled A.	
B	Name the structure labelled B.	
C	Name the structure labelled C.	
D	Name the structure labelled D.	
E	Name the structure labelled E.	

Answers

Case 4.1

A First metatarsophalangeal joint

B Second metatarsal neck

C Navicular bone

D Second tarsometatarsal joint

E Peroneal brevis tendon

X-ray of foot (right)

First metatarsophalangeal joint: This is the most common site for gout, a type of crystal arthropathy.

Second metatarsal neck: This is a common site for stress fracture (also called 'march fractures') along with 3rd and 4th metatarsal neck. Stress fractures can be difficult to spot with only subtle periosteal reaction and is an examination favourite for plain film assessments including the Fellowship of the Royal College of Radiologists (FRCR) Part 2B rapids.

Navicular bone: Navicular bone is not a commonly fractured bone, but it is a common site for avascular necrosis (osteonecrosis) in the foot. Avascular necrosis (AVN) of navicular in children is also called Kohler disease while that of adult is called Mueller–Weiss syndrome.

Second tarsometatarsal joint: Malalignment of this joint is a key finding for Lisfranc injury. There are other findings associated with Lisfranc injury and you should be familiar with them. It can result in significant morbidity and can be difficult to spot.

Peroneal brevis tendon: Attachments to bony protuberances often appear in FRCR part 1 examination and base/styloid of the 5th metatarsal bone is a common site for this type of question. Avulsion fracture at this site is common in dancers and tennis players and called pseudo-Jones fracture.

Weir J, Abrahams P, Spratt JD, et al. Imaging Atlas of Human Anatomy, 6th edition. UK: Elsevier, 2021:218.

Butler P, Mitchell AWM, Healy JC. Applied Radiological Anatomy, 2nd edition. Cambridge: Cambridge University Press, 2012:354–355.

Case 4.2

A Right calcaneus

B Right talus

C Right lateral cuneiform

D Shaft of the right 4th metatarsal

E Right cuboid

Anteroposterior radiograph of the foot (child).

Identifying the tarsal bones on the radiograph of a child is challenging as they ossify at different times. Consequently, the normal relationships between the tarsal bones are not always visible to help to identify them.

The calcaneus, the talus and cuboid begin to ossify during fetal life. So, in the radiograph of the foot of the normal child, these three bones will always be present (note that the cuboid ossification may be delayed until 3 weeks).

Of the cuneiforms, the lateral appears first (4–20 months) followed by the medial cuneiform (2 years of age). The intermediate cuneiform ossifies last (3 years of age).

Weir J, Abrahams P. Imaging Atlas of Human Anatomy, 4th edition. Edinburgh: Mosby, 2010:215.

Butler P, Mitchell AM, Ellis H. Applied Radiological Anatomy. Cambridge: Cambridge University Press, 1999:372–376.

Case 4.3

A Dome of the right talus (trochlear surface of talus)

B Right lateral malleolus (distal fibula)

C Right distal tibiofibular joint

D Distal epiphyseal scar of the right tibia

E Right medial malleolus

Anteroposterior radiograph of the ankle.

The articular surfaces of the ankle joint are:

- The lower tibia
- The inner surface of the medial malleolus of the tibia
- The medial surface of the lateral malleolus of the fibula
- The trochlear surface of the talus

On radiographs of long bones in adults, a radio-dense band can be seen at the junction of the epiphysis and the metaphysis. This is called the epiphyseal scar.

The inferior tibiofibular joint (syndesmosis) is formed by the convex medial surface of the distal fibula and the concave lateral surface of the distal tibia. It is reinforced by the interosseous ligament and the anterior and posterior tibiofibular ligaments.

Weir J, Abrahams P. Imaging Atlas of Human Anatomy, 4th edition. Edinburgh: Mosby, 2010:212.

Ryan S, McNicholas M, Eustace SJ. Anatomy for Diagnostic Imaging, 3rd edition. Edinburgh: Saunders, 2010:300–304.

Butler P, Mitchell AM, Ellis H. Applied Radiological Anatomy. Cambridge: Cambridge University Press, 1999:378.

Case 4.4

A Head of talus

B Sustentaculum tali of the calcaneus

C Navicular

D Base of 5th metatarsal

E Os trigonum

Lateral radiograph of the ankle.

The talus is composed of a body, a head and a neck. The body lies between the tibia and the calcaneum. The head is the anterior, rounded portion of the bone and the neck is the constriction between the body and head.

The posterior surface of the body of talus narrows to a pointed tubercle called the posterior process. Sometimes the process is represented as a separate bone. This is a normal anatomical variant called os trigonum. This normal variant is present in this image. Note that in the examination, you may be asked to name the anatomical variant present on an image but not necessarily labelled.

The inferior surface of the talus has two articular surfaces. They are separated by a deep groove, the sulcus tali. Both these facets articulate with portions of the calcaneum. Part of the anterior facet articulates with the sustentaculum tali which projects from the medial side of the calcaneum.

The navicular lies between the talus and the cuneiform bones. It is described as boat shaped. The posterior surface of the navicular articulates with the head of talus.

The base of the 5th metatarsal can be seen on a lateral ankle radiograph. Its lateral surface has a prominent tubercle which projects backwards and laterally.

Weir J, Abrahams P. Imaging Atlas of Human Anatomy, 4th edition. Edinburgh: Mosby, 2010:212.

Ryan S, McNicholas M, Eustace SJ. Anatomy for Diagnostic Imaging, 3rd edition. Edinburgh: Saunders, 2010:300–304.

Butler P, Mitchell AM, Ellis H. Applied Radiological Anatomy. Cambridge: Cambridge University Press, 1999:378.

Case 4.5

A The medial collateral ligament (deltoid ligament)

B Tibialis posterior tendon

C Flexor digitorum longus

D Flexor hallucis longus tendon

E Calcaneus (sustentaculum tali)

Coronal image of the ankle.

The deltoid ligament has five components: the anterior and posterior tibiotalar, the tibiocalcaneal, the tibiospring and the tibionavicular ligaments. The part of the deltoid ligament that is routinely visualised on coronal images is the deep part that arises from the posterior margin of the medial malleolus and attaches to the medial aspect of the talus.

The flexor retinaculum extends from the medial malleolus to the calcaneus and plantar fascia. The deep flexor muscles of the posterior compartment of the calf pass beneath the flexor retinaculum. They are surrounded by their synovial sheaths, the tibial nerve and the posterior tibial artery. 'Tom Dick and Harry' is a widely used mnemonic for remembering the position of these tendons. The calcaneus is the largest of the tarsal bones and has several features that can be identified. In this image, the sustentaculum tali is labelled which lies on the medial side of the bone, below the middle talar facet. When an arrow points at a large, easily identifiable bone, consider whether you are asked to name a specific feature within the bone. Failure to do so may lead to unnecessary loss of marks.

Weir J, Abrahams P. Imaging Atlas of Human Anatomy, 4th edition. Edinburgh: Mosby, 2010:206.

Ryan S, McNicholas M, Eustace SJ. Anatomy for Diagnostic Imaging, 3rd edition. Edinburgh: Saunders, 2010:293–299.

Butler P, Mitchell AM, Ellis H. Applied Radiological Anatomy. Cambridge: Cambridge University Press, 1999:377.

Case 4.6

A Patellar tendon

B Left fibula

C Left lateral head of gastrocnemius

D Left medial head of gastrocnemius

E Left popliteal artery

MR knee left.

Tibial tuberosity: The patellar tendon (also known as the patellar ligament) attaches here and thus forms an important part of the extensor mechanism of the knee joint.

Fibula: Makes a ring structure with the tibia so make sure to check for a fracture elsewhere if there is one.

Lateral head of the gastrocnemius: Primary plantar flexor along with the medial head of the gastrocnemius. Note that there is a normal variant where the lateral head is missing.

Medial head of the gastrocnemius: Clinically, this is the location of Baker's cyst (which will not be given in FRCR part 1 as the examination should only test you on normal images) which arises between the medial head of the gastrocnemius and semimembranosus tendons.

Popliteal artery: There are a few clues to tell you this is the popliteal artery rather than vein. First, it is round and not collapsed, second it has prominent flow void and lastly it is situated lateral to the popliteal vein (which can be seen slit like and collapsed medially). If you are not sure, you can just put 'popliteal vessel' to get half a mark.

Weir J, Abrahams P, Spratt JD, et al. Imaging Atlas of Human Anatomy, 6th edition. UK: Elsevier, 2021:230.

Butler P, Mitchell AWM, Healy JC. Applied Radiological Anatomy, 2nd edition. Cambridge: Cambridge University Press, 2012:344.

Case 4.7

A Lateral tibial plateau of the right knee

B Medial femoral epicondyle of the right femur

C Medial tibial spine of the right tibia

D Adductor tubercle of the right femur

E Popliteal groove of the right femur

Plain frontal radiograph of the knee.

The articular surfaces of the knee joint that are visible on the anteroposterior radiograph consist of the condyles of the femur and the flat upper surfaces of the tibial condyles (tibial plateau).

Between the articular facets of the proximal tibia lies the intercondylar eminence which is surmounted on either side by the tibial spines (medial and lateral). Anterior and posterior to the intercondylar eminence are the attachments of the anterior and posterior cruciate ligaments and the menisci.

The linea aspera is a ridge of bone in the posterior surface of the femur. Distally, the linea aspera is prolonged by two ridges. The medial ridge ends in the adductor tubercle. The tendon of the adductor magnus inserts there.

The popliteal groove is a landmark in the lateral condyle of the femur between the epicondyle and the articular margin. Its anterior end gives origin to popliteus. When the knee is fully flexed, popliteus helps to 'lock' the knee by lodging into the posterior end of this grove.

In radiographs of the limbs, when laterality is indicated by a marker on the radiograph, it is better to indicate which limb it is after the structure. For example: 'Adductor tubercle of the left femur' rather than 'left adductor tubercle'.

Weir J, Abrahams P. Imaging Atlas of Human Anatomy, 4th edition. Edinburgh: Mosby, 2010:210.

Ryan S, McNicholas M, Eustace SJ. Anatomy for Diagnostic Imaging, 3rd edition. Edinburgh: Saunders, 2010:295.

Butler P, Mitchell AM, Ellis H. Applied Radiological Anatomy. Cambridge: Cambridge University Press, 1999:366.

Case 4.8

A Medial condyle of the right femur

B Lateral condyle of the right femur

C Intercondylar fossa of the right femur

D Right tibial tuberosity

E Diaphysis of the right fibula

Lateral radiograph of the knee.

In a lateral radiograph of the knee, the femoral condyles are superimposed. If asked to differentiate between the medial and the lateral femoral condyles, use the size of the condyles and the lateral femoral notch to help do this.

The medial condyle is larger and projects more inferiorly.

The lateral femoral notch (also known as lateral condylopatellar sulcus) forms a shallow groove in the middle of the lateral femoral condyle.

Make sure the specific parts of the long bones are named rather than just naming the bone, e.g. diaphysis of fibula instead of fibula.

Weir J, Abrahams P. Imaging Atlas of Human Anatomy, 4th edition. Edinburgh: Mosby, 2010:210.

Ryan S, McNicholas M, Eustace SJ. Anatomy for Diagnostic Imaging, 3rd edition. Edinburgh: Saunders, 2010:295.

Butler P, Mitchell AM, Ellis H. Applied Radiological Anatomy. Cambridge: Cambridge University Press, 1999:366.

Case 4.9

A Medial meniscus

B Popliteus tendon

C Posterior cruciate ligament

D Anterior cruciate ligament

E Tibialis anterior

Coronal MRI of the knee.

The knee joint is a synovial joint which consists of two condylar femorotibial components and a saddle-shaped patellofemoral component. On a plain film, the fibula can be used to distinguish between the medial and lateral femoral condyles/epicondyles. When given a coronal MRI like this one where the fibula is not seen, remember that the lateral condyle is flatter ('lat-flat').

The menisci of the knee joint are C-shaped semilunar rings of fibrocartilage found between the articular surfaces of the femur with the tibia. In cross-section, these structures appear triangular.

Again, we see the popliteal groove of the lateral femoral condyle and the tendon of the popliteus.

The anterior and posterior cruciate ligaments are intrasynovial and extracapsular. They are seen in this level in the intercondylar notch of the femur where the posterior cruciate ligament lies medially and the anterior cruciate ligament laterally.

The tibialis anterior originates in the upper two-thirds of the lateral surface of the tibia and inserts into the medial cuneiform and the 1st metatarsal. It acts to dorsiflex and invert the foot.

Weir J, Abrahams P. Imaging Atlas of Human Anatomy. Edinburgh: Mosby, 2003:224–225.

Ryan S, McNicholas M, Eustace SJ. Anatomy for Diagnostic Imaging, 3rd edition. Edinburgh: Saunders, 2010:296.

Butler P, Mitchell AM, Ellis H. Applied Radiological Anatomy. Cambridge: Cambridge University Press, 1999:367–369.

Case 4.10

A Quadriceps tendon

B Articular cartilage of the medial femoral condyle

C Infrapatellar fat pad (Hoffa's fat pad)

D Posterior cruciate ligament

E Medial head of gastrocnemius

Sagittal MRI of the knee.

Extension of the knee joint occurs through contraction of the quadriceps. The force is translated through the quadriceps tendon, the patella and the patella tendon to the tibia.

The posterior cruciate ligament is primarily responsible for resisting posterior translation of the tibia. It arises from the inner aspect of the medial femoral condyle. It runs posteriorly to attach in a midline depression in the posterior margin of the tibial plateau. Note that the posterior cruciate ligament is composed of two subdivisions: a dominant anterolateral bundle and a small posteromedial band.

The insertion of the posterior cruciate ligament provides a clue as to which femoral condyle is seen in this image. Therefore, when asked to identify the articular cartilage of the femoral condyle, you can confidently label it as medial condyle to score maximum points.

The infrapatellar fat pad (Hoffa's fat pad) is cylindrical in shape and is intracapsular. Disease in this region is not uncommon and therefore it is an area routinely visualised and reviewed on an MRI of the knee.

The gastrocnemius is the largest and most superficial of the calf muscles. It has two heads which arise from the medial and lateral condyles. It crosses the knee and ankle joints to insert via the Achilles tendon into the calcaneum. Again, make sure that it is identified as the medial head of gastrocnemius to gain maximum points.

Weir J, Abrahams P. Imaging Atlas of Human Anatomy. Edinburgh: Mosby, 2003:227.

Ryan S, McNicholas M, Eustace SJ. Anatomy for Diagnostic Imaging, 3rd edition. Edinburgh: Saunders, 2010:297.

Butler P, Mitchell AM, Ellis H. Applied Radiological Anatomy. Cambridge: Cambridge University Press, 1999:367–369.

Case 4.11

A Lateral articular facet of the patella

B Medial retinaculum

C Lateral head of gastrocnemius

D Biceps femoris

E Popliteal artery

Axial T2-weighted fat sat MRI at the level of the patellofemoral articulation.

The articular surface of the patella has two facets: the lateral and the medial. The lateral articular facet is larger than the medial. Knowing this fact is key to identifying the other structures correctly.

The medial patellar retinaculum is part of the aponeurosis of vastus medialis. It runs between the patella and the medial condyle of the tibia and forms the anteromedial aspect of the fibrous capsule of the knee joint. This capsule is strengthened posteriorly by the two heads of gastrocnemius and by the oblique popliteal ligament. Laterally, it is strengthened by the iliotibial tract.

The biceps femoris is part of the hamstrings. Distally, it crosses the knee joint on the lateral side to insert on to the head of the fibula.

Weir J, Abrahams P. Imaging Atlas of Human Anatomy, 4th edition. Edinburgh: Mosby, 2010:228.

Ryan S, McNicholas M, Eustace SJ. Anatomy for Diagnostic Imaging, 3rd edition. Edinburgh: Saunders, 2010:298.

Butler P, Mitchell AM, Ellis H. Applied Radiological Anatomy. Cambridge: Cambridge University Press, 1999:367–369.

Case 4.12

A Left vastus lateralis muscle

B Left biceps femoris muscle

C Left semimembranosus muscle

D Left sartorius muscle

E Left vastus medialis muscle

MR knee left.

This case demonstrates nicely that there are many muscles to remember for the MSK anatomy! (Often the worse nightmare for poor radiology ST1s). Keep practising identifying the quadriceps and hamstring muscles.

Quadriceps are the key extensors of the leg and consist of four muscles (hence the 'quad' in the name): Rectus femoris, vastus medialis, vastus lateralis and vastus intermedius.

Hamstring muscles extend the hip joint and flex the knee joint. They include the semimembranosus, semitendinosus and biceps femoris muscles.

Sartorius muscle is neither a part of the quadriceps nor hamstring. It is a long and small muscle that mainly flexes both the hip and knee joints synergistically with other muscles.

You can tell which side is lateral or medial in this case by the layout of the muscles as well as the fact that the vastus medialis is bulkier than the vastus lateralis.

Weir J, Abrahams P, Spratt JD, et al. Imaging Atlas of Human Anatomy, 6th edition. UK: Elsevier, 2021:229.

Butler P, Mitchell AWM, Healy JC. Applied Radiological Anatomy, 2nd edition. Cambridge: Cambridge University Press, 2012:337.

Case 4.13

A Right obturator foramen

B Iliopectineal line

C Shenton line

D Left sartorius

E Left hamstrings

X-ray of pelvis.

Obturator foramen: Obturator nerve, artery and vein exit the pelvis through this foramen into the medial compartment of the thigh. Trace a ring around it to look for pubic rami fractures!

Iliopectineal line: This line marks the inner margin of the pelvic ring and disruption indicates anterior acetabular or superior pubic ramus fracture.

Shenton line: Disruption of this line may indicate neck of femur fracture or developmental dysplasia of hip.

Sartorius attaches to anterior inferior iliac spine, while **hamstrings** insert into the ischial tuberosity. Avulsion fracture of the ischial tuberosity can happen in athletic adolescent patients. Muscle attachments are frequently asked in FRCR part 1, so be sure to revise them.

Weir J, Abrahams P, Spratt JD, et al. Imaging Atlas of Human Anatomy, 6th edition. UK: Elsevier, 2021:188.

Butler P, Mitchell AWM, Healy JC. Applied Radiological Anatomy, 2nd edition. Cambridge: Cambridge University Press, 2012:319.

Case 4.14

A Right psoas

B Right iliacus

C Right vastus lateralis

D Left obturator externus

E Left gluteus minimus

Coronal MRI of the hips.

The psoas arises from the transverse processes, vertebral bodies and intervertebral discs of T12–L5. The iliacus arises from the iliac fossa. Both muscles insert on the lesser trochanter of the femur.

The vastus lateralis is the most lateral of the quadriceps and is seen in this image lateral to the femur.

The obturator externus is an adductor of the thigh. It arises from the outer surface of the obturator membrane and inserts onto the greater trochanter of the femur.

The gluteus minimus arises from the ileus to insert in the greater trochanter of the femur. It medially rotates the thigh.

Weir J, Abrahams P. Imaging Atlas of Human Anatomy, 4th edition. Edinburgh: Mosby, 2010:165–167.

Ryan S, McNicholas M, Eustace SJ. Anatomy for Diagnostic Imaging, 3rd edition. Edinburgh: Saunders, 2010:290.

Butler P, Mitchell AM, Ellis H. Applied Radiological Anatomy. Cambridge: Cambridge University Press, 1999:290.

Case 4.15

A Right femoral artery

B Right obturator internus

C Left ischium

D Left tensor fasciae latae

E Right ischioanal fossa

Axial MRI of the pelvis at the level of the neck of femur.

The external iliac artery passes into the anterior part of the thigh beneath the inguinal ligament. Its name changes at this point to the femoral artery. In this image, we can identify the femoral vein medial to the artery and the femoral nerve lateral to the femoral artery (mnemonic NAVY).

Obturator internus arises from the internal surface of obturator membrane and the posterior bony margins of obturator foramen. It inserts in the medial surface of the greater trochanter of femur.

The tensor fasciae latae arises from the anterior part of the iliac crest and the fascia lata, by which it is enveloped. It becomes continuous with the iliotibial tract.

The ischioanal fossa is wedge-shaped and filled with fat. It is crossed by the inferior rectal nerve and artery. It has Alcock's canal in its lateral wall which contains the internal pudendal vessels and the pudendal nerve.

Weir J, Abrahams P. Imaging Atlas of Human Anatomy, 4th edition. Edinburgh: Mosby, 2010:162–164.

Ryan S, McNicholas M, Eustace SJ. Anatomy for Diagnostic Imaging, 3rd edition. Edinburgh: Saunders, 2010:291.

Butler P, Mitchell AM, Ellis H. Applied Radiological Anatomy. Cambridge: Cambridge University Press, 1999:355.

Case 4.16

A Left common iliac artery

B Left internal iliac artery

C Left external iliac artery

D Left profunda femoris

E Left superficial femoral artery

MR angiography of the pelvis and proximal lower limbs.

The aorta divides into the two common iliac arteries at the level of the fourth lumbar vertebral body. The common iliac artery divides into the external and internal iliac arteries. The blood supply to the lower limb derives from the external iliac artery and its branches.

The external iliac artery becomes the common femoral artery when it crosses the inguinal ligament, midway between the anterior superior iliac spine and the pubic symphysis.

The profunda femoris arises 3.5 cm distal to the inguinal ligament and has six branches: the medial and lateral circumflex artery and four penetrating arteries. After the profunda is given off, the femoral artery is referred to as the superficial femoral artery.

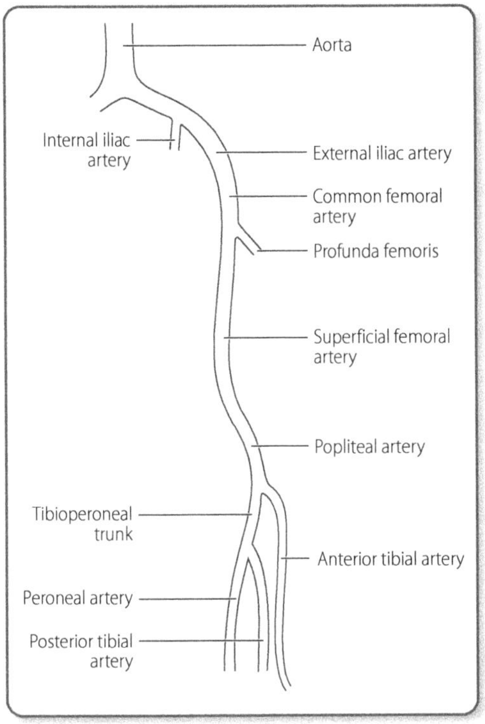

Figure 4.1 Arterial supply to the lower limb.

Figure 4.1 summarises the arterial supply to the lower limb.

Weir J, Abrahams P. Imaging Atlas of Human Anatomy, 4th edition. Edinburgh: Mosby, 2010:187.

Ryan S, McNicholas M, Eustace SJ. Anatomy for Diagnostic Imaging, 3rd edition. Edinburgh: Saunders, 2010:306–312.

Butler P, Mitchell AM, Ellis H. Applied Radiological Anatomy. Cambridge: Cambridge University Press, 1999:386.

Case 4.17

A Popliteal artery

B Anterior tibial artery

C Tibioperoneal trunk

D Posterior tibial artery

E Peroneal artery

Catheter angiogram of the left lower limb.

The superficial femoral artery becomes the popliteal artery after passing through the adductor hiatus of the adductor magnus tendon. Five genicular branches are given off in the popliteal fossa.

The popliteal artery ends by dividing into the anterior tibial artery and the tibioperoneal trunk. The anterior tibial artery pierces the interosseous membrane and runs into the anterior compartment of the leg.

The tibioperoneal trunk divides into the peroneal artery (which runs close to the fibula) and the posterior tibial artery (which runs in the posterior compartment).

Weir J, Abrahams P. Imaging Atlas of Human Anatomy, 4th edition. Edinburgh: Mosby, 2010:217.

Ryan S, McNicholas M, Eustace SJ. Anatomy for Diagnostic Imaging, 3rd edition. Edinburgh: Saunders, 2010:310.

Butler P, Mitchell AM, Ellis H. Applied Radiological Anatomy. Cambridge: Cambridge University Press, 1999:387.

Case 4.18

A Left posterior tibial artery

B Left anterior tibial artery

C Left 1st metatarsal

D Left medial cuneiform

E Sesamoid bones in left flexor hallucis brevis

Angiogram of the foot.

The posterior tibial artery descends in the posterior compartment between tibialis posterior and soleus. It passes behind the medial malleolus, deep to the flexor retinaculum. It divides into the medial and lateral plantar arteries.

The anterior tibial artery descends in the anterior compartment of the leg on the anterior surface of the interosseous membrane. It crosses the anterior aspect of the ankle joint between the tendons of tibialis anterior and extensor hallucis longus. In the foot, it is called the dorsalis pedis.

Weir J, Abrahams P. Imaging Atlas of Human Anatomy, 4th edition. Edinburgh: Mosby, 2010:217.

Ryan S, McNicholas M, Eustace SJ. Anatomy for Diagnostic Imaging, 3rd edition. Edinburgh: Saunders, 2010:306–312.

Butler P, Mitchell AM, Ellis H. Applied Radiological Anatomy. Cambridge: Cambridge University Press, 1999:386.

Case 4.19

A Anterior arch of the atlas

B Vertebral body of C6

C Spinous process of C4

D C3–C4 facet joint

E Hyoid bone

Lateral C-spine radiograph.

There are seven cervical vertebrae. The atlas (C1) does not have a body. It has a lateral mass on each side, an anterior and a posterior arch. The anterior arch of the atlas has a tubercle on its anterior surface and a facet posteriorly for articulation with the odontoid process.

Identifying a vertebral body and spinous process may appear straightforward but it is easy to lose marks by forgetting to number them. Numbering can be done by identifying the axis (C2) and counting from there. The axis has the odontoid process projecting upwards from its body.

The hyoid is a U-shaped bone which lies below the floor of the mouth anterior to the C3 vertebral body. It consists of a body and four processes: two great cornua (singular cornu) and two lesser cornua. The great cornua project backwards from the lateral limits of the body and have a tubercle at the posterior end. The lesser cornua project upwards and backwards at the junction of the body of the hyoid with the great cornua.

Weir J, Abrahams P. Imaging Atlas of Human Anatomy, 4th edition. Edinburgh: Mosby, 2010:57.

Butler P, Mitchell AM, Ellis H. Applied Radiological Anatomy. Cambridge: Cambridge University Press, 1999:315–316.

Case 4.20

A Left first rib

B Right transverse process of C7

C Spinous process of T1

D Right pedicle of C7

E Left uncovertebral joint C5–C6

Anteroposterior C-spine radiograph.

From C3 to C7 the vertebral bodies progressively increase in size from superior to inferior. On each side of the superior aspect of the vertebral body is the uncinate process: a bony ridge projecting superiorly from the lateral margin. The uncinate process articulates with a bevelled notch on the posterolateral surface of the vertebra above. This is called the uncovertebral joint.

The transverse processes of a cervical vertebra are short and end laterally with an anterior and a posterior tubercle. The transverse processes enclose the foramen transversarium with transmits the vertebral artery, accompanying veins and sympathetic nerves. The foramen transversarium of C7 may be absent. If present, it is small and usually only transmits vertebral veins (not the vertebral artery).

Weir J, Abrahams P. Imaging Atlas of Human Anatomy. Edinburgh: Mosby, 2003:56.

Butler P, Mitchell AM, Ellis H. Applied Radiological Anatomy. Cambridge: Cambridge University Press, 1999:315–316.

Case 4.21

A Pedicle of L3

B Inferior vertebral notch of L2 (exit foramen of the L2 nerve root)

C Spinous process of L3

D Sacrum

E Vertebral body of L4

Lateral lumbar spine radiograph.

The fifth lumbar vertebra is atypical. It has a wedge-shaped body which is taller anteriorly. The junction between L5 and S1 is inclined to the horizon at an angle between 25° and 55° in the supine position and between 8° and 12° in the erect position.

Identification of the labelled lumbar vertebral body is done on the assumption that segmentation is normal with five free lumbar vertebrae. Another assumption would be that the first vertebral body that does not articulate with a rib is L1. An image of a spine which has abnormal segmentation is unlikely to feature in an examination so it would be safe to number the vertebrae based on these assumptions. In fact, the only way to be certain which vertebra is labelled is to count from the top when imaging of the whole spine is available.

Note how the height of the intervertebral discs increases progressively from superior to inferior. The lumbosacral disc however is smaller than the other lumbar discs (usually <10 mm in height).

Weir J, Abrahams P. Imaging Atlas of Human Anatomy, 4th edition. Edinburgh: Mosby, 2010:59.

Butler P, Mitchell AM, Ellis H. Applied Radiological Anatomy. Cambridge: Cambridge University Press, 1999:318–320.

Case 4.22

A Left pedicle of L3

B Right transverse process of L4

C Spinous process of L4

D L3–L4 intervertebral disc space

E Right sacroiliac joint

Anteroposterior lumbar radiograph.

There are normally five free lumbar vertebrae. The L3 is the largest.

Projecting posteriorly are the pedicles which connect to the laminae to form the spinal canal.

The articular processes arise from the junction of the pedicles and the laminae. The superior facets are concave. They face backwards and medially. They articulate with the inferior process of the vertebra above. The inferior articular facets are convex and face forwards and laterally.

Weir J, Abrahams P. Imaging Atlas of Human Anatomy, 4th edition. Edinburgh: Mosby, 2010:59.

Butler P, Mitchell AM, Ellis H. Applied Radiological Anatomy. Cambridge: Cambridge University Press, 1999:318–320.

Case 4.23

A Left atlantoaxial joint

B Left lateral mass of the axis (C2)

C Right pedicle of the axis (C2)

D Odontoid peg

E Right lateral mass of the atlas (C1)

Dens views (open mouth).

This radiograph is performed through an open mouth. It shows an anteroposterior projection of the atlantoaxial joint. The lateral masses of the atlas have a superior and inferior articular facet each. The superior articular facets articulate with the occipital condyles to form the atlanto-occipital joints. The inferior articular facets articulate with the axis in the atlantoaxial joint.

Weir J, Abrahams P. Imaging Atlas of Human Anatomy, 4th edition. Edinburgh: Mosby, 2010:57.

Butler P, Mitchell AM, Ellis H. Applied Radiological Anatomy. Cambridge: Cambridge University Press, 1999:312.

Case 4.24

A Anterior tubercle of the atlas

B Odontoid peg

C Right foramen transversarium of the axis

D Posterior arch of the atlas

E Right lateral mass of the atlas

Axial CT image of the atlantoaxial joint.

We have already seen the atlas and the axis in the lateral CT spine radiograph and the open mouth dens views. Here, we see the odontoid peg and its relation to the anterior arch of the atlas. This relationship is maintained by the transverse ligament which attaches to the lateral masses of C1.

In this axial view, we see the tubercles on the arches of the atlas. The anterior tubercle projects from the anterior surface of the anterior arch. It is a blunt midline projection. The posterior tubercle is a midline projection on the posterior surface of the posterior arch. It represents the spinous process of the atlas and is an attachment of the ligamentum nuchae.

The atlas has transverse processes that arise from two roots. The anterior root projects from the lateral mass and the posterior route from the posterior arch. The tips of these transverse processes are square and have no tubercles.

Weir J, Abrahams P. Imaging Atlas of Human Anatomy, 4th edition. Edinburgh: Mosby, 2010:61.

Ryan S, McNicholas M, Eustace SJ. Anatomy for Diagnostic Imaging, 3rd edition. Edinburgh: Saunders, 2010:93.

Butler P, Mitchell AM, Ellis H. Applied Radiological Anatomy. Cambridge: Cambridge University Press, 1999:312.

Case 4.25

A Anterior tubercle of the left transverse process

B Right pedicle

C Left articular pillar

D Right lamina

E Bifid spinous process

Axial CT image of the fifth cervical vertebra.

From C3 to C7 the vertebrae are broadly similar. They have small and oval bodies. The transverse processes are short and end laterally with an anterior and posterior tubercle. The tubercles are connected by the intertubercular lamellae. The transverse processes enclose the foramen transversarium which transmits the vertebral artery from C6 and above.

The pillars (or articular masses) are dense, rhomboid-shaped structures bounded by the anterior and posterior facets. The laminae are posteromedial extensions of the articular masses and form the posteromedial aspects of the spinal canal.

The spinous processes in the cervical spine are small and bifid with the exception of the C7.

Weir J, Abrahams P. Imaging Atlas of Human Anatomy, 4th edition. Edinburgh: Mosby, 2010:61.

Ryan S, McNicholas M, Eustace SJ. Anatomy for Diagnostic Imaging, 3rd edition. Edinburgh: Saunders, 2010:92.

Butler P, Mitchell AM, Ellis H. Applied Radiological Anatomy. Cambridge: Cambridge University Press, 1999:315.

Case 4.26

A Thoracic vertebral body

B Neck of the rib (left)

C Right costovertebral joint

D Left costotransverse joint

E Left erector spinae

Axial CT image at the level of a thoracic vertebral body.

The thoracic vertebrae have roughly heart-shaped bodies. Their pedicles project directly backwards. The laminae are wide and flat bars of bone. Their superior margins overlap the inferior margins of the laminae of the vertebrae above. That means that the posterior margin of the vertebral canal at the lumbar spine is closed. The transverse processes project backwards and laterally from the junction of body and pedicles.

Close to the tip of the transverse process, on the anterior surface, there is an oval articular facet that articulates with a facet on the tubercle of the corresponding rib. This is the costotransverse joint.

From T2 to T10 the vertebrae have a superior and inferior demifacet for articulation with the head of the corresponding rib on each side. T1 has a complete facet superiorly and a demifacet inferiorly. T11 and T12 have a single and complete facet on each side.

Note that the spinous process pictured in this image belongs to the vertebra above. If the question asks which vertebral body is shown, this fact must be taken into account.

Weir J, Abrahams P. Imaging Atlas of Human Anatomy, 4th edition. Edinburgh: Mosby, 2010:55–63.

Ryan S, McNicholas M, Eustace SJ. Anatomy for Diagnostic Imaging, 3rd edition. Edinburgh: Saunders, 2010:113–114.

Butler P, Mitchell AM, Ellis H. Applied Radiological Anatomy. Cambridge: Cambridge University Press, 1999:315.

Case 4.27

A Left psoas

B Right facet joint

C Right erector spinae

D Left transverse process of the lumbar vertebra

E Right pedicle of the lumbar vertebra

Axial CT image of the lumbar spine through a vertebral body.

There are three main groups of back muscles:

1. Superficial extrinsic muscles
2. Intermediate extrinsic muscles
3. Deep intrinsic muscles

The superficial extrinsic muscles are associated with the upper limb and include the trapezius and the latissimus dorsi. The intermediate extrinsic muscles provide accessory respiratory movements and include the serratus anterior.

The deep intrinsic muscles are further divided into three groups:

1. Deep layer (interspinales and intertransversarii)
2. Intermediate layer (collectively known as transversospinalis)
3. Superficial layer (collectively known as erector spinae)

Weir J, Abrahams P. Imaging Atlas of Human Anatomy, 4th edition. Edinburgh: Mosby, 2010:62.

Ryan S, McNicholas M, Eustace SJ. Anatomy for Diagnostic Imaging, 3rd edition. Edinburgh: Saunders, 2010:95.

Butler P, Mitchell AM, Ellis H. Applied Radiological Anatomy. Cambridge: Cambridge University Press, 1999:319.

Case 4.28

A Lumbar Intervertebral disc

B Left inferior articular process of the vertebral body above (L3)

C Left superior articular process of the vertebral body below (L4)

D Right lamina

E Ligamentum flavum

CT image of the lumbar spine through the L4/L5 intervertebral disc space.

This axial image passes through the intervertebral foramen of L4/L5. The foramen is seen as a gap between the body and the posterior vertebral elements. Note that the anterior border of the vertebral canal at this slice is the intervertebral disc and not the vertebral body.

At this level we see the facet joint which is an articulation between the inferior articular process of L4 and the superior articular process of L5. Note that the inferior articular facet of L4 lies anteriorly and faces posteriorly.

In this image, we can identify the ligamentum flavum. The ligamentum flavum unites the laminae of adjacent vertebra by passing from the anterior surface of the lamina above to the posterior surface of the lamina below. It is very elastic.

Weir J, Abrahams P. Imaging Atlas of Human Anatomy, 4th edition. Edinburgh: Mosby, 2010:62.

Ryan S, McNicholas M, Eustace SJ. Anatomy for Diagnostic Imaging, 3rd edition. Edinburgh: Saunders, 2010:98.

Case 4.29

A Right quadratus lumborum muscle

B Right psoas major muscle

C Cauda equine nerve roots

D Left common iliac artery

E Left erector spinae group

MR lumbar spine.

Paraspinal muscles are important for keeping the spine stable which in itself is important for preventing degenerative disc disease. Sign up to a gym membership and start exercising! Note that the spinal cord has split into cauda equina nerve roots. Remember to always check for vessels and surrounding soft tissues for any incidental pathologies.

Psoas major muscle: The psoas muscle is enclosed by the psoas fascia where psoas abscess or haematoma can track along (in retrofascial space, not retroperitoneal space).

Quadratus lumborum muscle: In addition to lateral flexion and extension of the spine, this muscle is thought to allow precise control of the diaphragm for singing.

Erector spinae group: This is actually a group of three different muscles – spinalis, longissimus and iliocostalis. It is the most power extensor (as implied by the name 'erector') of the spine.

Cauda equina nerve roots: These are nerve roots distal to conus medullaris and literally means 'horse tail' due to the appearance. Cauda equina compression is a surgical emergency and one of most litigious conditions for delayed diagnosis so do not miss it!

Weir J, Abrahams P, Spratt JD, et al. Imaging Atlas of Human Anatomy, 6th edition. UK: Elsevier, 2021:59.

Butler P, Mitchell AWM, Healy JC. Applied Radiological Anatomy, 2nd edition. Cambridge: Cambridge University Press, 2012:83, 88.

Case 4.30

A Posterior arch of the atlas

B Posterior longitudinal ligament

C Spinal cord in the spinal canal

D Intervertebral disc C7–T1

E Manubrium

Sagittal T1-weighted image MRI of the spine.

The spinal cord extends from the foramen magnum to the conus medullaris which usually lies at the level of L1/L2. It lies in the spinal canal surrounded by cerebrospinal fluid.

Intervertebral discs lie between vertebral bodies. They are composed of a nucleus pulposus (a gelatinous core) and an outer ring of concentric fibres of fibrous tissues called annulus fibrosus.

The vertebral canal is lined anteriorly by the posterior longitudinal ligament which covers the posterior surface of vertebral bodies and intervertebral discs. Posteriorly, the spinal canal is lined by the ligamentum flavum which joins adjacent laminae.

Weir J, Abrahams P. Imaging Atlas of Human Anatomy, 4th edition. Edinburgh: Mosby, 2010:62.

Ryan S, McNicholas M, Eustace SJ. Anatomy for Diagnostic Imaging, 3rd edition. Edinburgh: Saunders, 2010:99.

Case 4.31

A T12 vertebral body

B L2 neural exit foramen

C L4/L5 facet joint

D Nucleus pulposus of the L1/L2 disc

E Superior mesenteric artery

MR lumbar spine.

Notice that they have used a collimator to block signals from the abdominal cavity. Many centres do not do this and so it is also important to look at the abdomen and pelvis.

Superior mesenteric artery: Downward course of the SMA distinguishes it from the straighter course of the coeliac trunk above.

T12 vertebral body: It is important to assess for the vertebral body height, alignment and marrow signal in spine MR studies. T12 vertebral body is a frequently fractured bone due to insufficiency fractures in elderly.

L2 neural exit foramen: While this is likely the left exit foramen as you can see the abdominal aorta and its mesenteric branches, it is not possible to confirm this with certainty. Knowing when to be vague is a skill needed to do well in the FRCR part 1.

L4/L5 facet joint: Facet joints are synovial articulations of the posterior arch. They are frequently involved in low back pain due to arthropathy and in severe cases may even cause spinal canal stenosis!

Nucleus pulposus of the L1/L2 disc: Central part of the intervertebral discs with high water content which decreases with age ('desiccation').

Weir J, Abrahams P, Spratt JD, et al. Imaging Atlas of Human Anatomy, 6th edition. UK: Elsevier, 2021:60.

Butler P, Mitchell AWM, Healy JC. Applied Radiological Anatomy, 2nd edition. Cambridge: Cambridge University Press, 2012:83–85.

Case 4.32

A Scaphoid

B Scapholunate ligament

C Distal radio-ulnar joint

D Lunate

E Fifth metacarpal neck

CT wrist left.

Scaphoid: Scaphoid fractures are common and can lead to avascular necrosis of the proximal part due to the arterial supply entering distally. This can cause significant functional impairment if missed. Therefore, repeat radiograph, CT or MRI (depending on local policy) is warranted if there is high index of suspicion.

Fifth metacarpal neck: This is the most common site of metacarpal fractures resulting from a direct blow with clenched fist, and as such also called the boxer's fracture.

Distal radio-ulnar joint: One can measure ulnar variance where positive variance is when ulna is >2.5 mm beyond radius at this joint, and negative when ulna is <2.5 mm than radius. Positive variance is associated with ulnar impaction syndrome while negative variance is associated with Kienbock disease.

Lunate: This is another carpal bone which is susceptible to avascular necrosis (osteonecrosis), known as Kienbock disease.

Scapholunate ligament: This is a ligament worth learning about as it is frequently asked in FRCR2A/2B. Injury to this ligament results in scapholunate dissociation (scapholunate interval >3–4 mm) causing carpal instability. Appearance is called Terry–Thomas sign (also known as David Letterman or Madonna sign).

Weir J, Abrahams P, Spratt JD, et al. Imaging Atlas of Human Anatomy, 6th edition. UK: Elsevier, 2021:71.

Butler P, Mitchell AWM, Healy JC. Applied Radiological Anatomy, 2nd edition. Cambridge: Cambridge University Press, 2012:307–308.

Case 4.33

A Right capitate

B Right lunate

C Right pisiform

D Right scaphoid

E Right 1st metacarpal

Lateral radiograph of the wrist.

The lunate is the key bone to understand this projection. The proximal surface of the lunate is convex and articulates with the distal radius. The distal surface of the lunate is concave and articulates with the capitate.

In a true lateral radiograph of the wrist, the most palmar carpal bone cortex belongs to the scaphoid. The palmar cortex of the pisiform lies between the palmar cortex of the scaphoid and the palmar cortex of the capitate.

Weir J, Abrahams P. Imaging Atlas of Human Anatomy, 4th edition. Edinburgh: Mosby, 2010:74.

Ryan S, McNicholas M, Eustace SJ. Anatomy for Diagnostic Imaging, 3rd edition. Edinburgh: Saunders, 2010:271.

Butler P, Mitchell AM, Ellis H. Applied Radiological Anatomy. Cambridge: Cambridge University Press, 1999:344–345.

Case 4.34

A Olecranon of the left ulna

B Capitellum of the left humerus

C Medial epicondyle of the left humerus

D Left radial tuberosity

E Coronoid process of the left ulna

Anteroposterior radiograph of the right elbow.

The distal humerus has articular surfaces for the radial head and olecranon fossa of the ulna. These are called the capitellum (interchangeable with capitulum) and trochlea respectively. Two other features of the distal humerus are the coronoid fossa and the olecranon fossa. The coronoid fossa lies anterior and superior to the trochlea, and the olecranon fossa lies posteriorly.

The radial head is cylindrical and sits on a narrower radial neck. The radial tuberosity is medial and is the point of attachment for the biceps brachii.

The olecranon of the ulna is hook-shaped with a concavity, the trochlear fossa. The olecranon is the point of attachment for the triceps muscle.

The coronoid process is the point of attachment for brachialis, the wrist flexors, and pronator teres.

If you are given a paediatric film, you may be asked the age at which one of the secondary centres of ossification appears. The mnemonic to use is CRITOL:

- Capitellum: 1 year
- Radial head: 5 years
- Internal epicondyle: 5 years

- Trochlea: 11 years
- Olecranon: 12 years
- Lateral epicondyle: 13 years

These figures vary slightly between textbooks. Fusion occurs in late teenage years.

Weir J, Abrahams P. Imaging Atlas of Human Anatomy, 4th edition. Edinburgh: Mosby, 2010:71–72.

Ryan S, McNicholas M, Eustace SJ. Anatomy for Diagnostic Imaging, 3rd edition. Edinburgh: Saunders, 2010:254.

Butler P, Mitchell AM, Ellis H. Applied Radiological Anatomy. Cambridge: Cambridge University Press, 1999:341–342.

Case 4.35

A Flexor carpi ulnaris

B Radial nerve

C Biceps tendon

D Proximal radioulnar joint

E Anconeus

Axial MRI of the elbow joint at the level of the proximal radioulnar joint.

There are two joints between the radius and the ulna: the superior and inferior radioulnar joints. The shafts are also united by an interosseous membrane.

The flexor carpi ulnaris is one of the superficial flexors in the forearm. It flexes the wrist joint and abducts the hand. The superficial group in the flexor compartment of the forearm is made of five muscles that fan out like the digits of a hand. From medial to lateral, these muscles are:

- Pronator teres
- Flexor carpi radialis
- Palmaris longus
- Flexor digitorum superficialis
- Flexor carpi ulnaris

The anconeus is a small muscle on the posterior aspect of the elbow joint. Its proximal attachment is the lateral epicondyle of the humerus. It inserts distally on the posterior aspect of the olecranon. It acts as an extensor of the forearm.

Note the position of the biceps tendon and the radial nerve at this level. In the arm, the radial nerve travels deep to the lateral head of the triceps. It pierces the intermuscular septum and comes to lie between the brachialis and brachioradialis it passes into the forearm from the anterior aspect of the elbow.

Weir J, Abrahams P. Imaging Atlas of Human Anatomy, 4th edition. Edinburgh: Mosby, 2010:84.

Ryan S, McNicholas M, Eustace SJ. Anatomy for Diagnostic Imaging, 3rd edition. Edinburgh: Saunders, 2010:266.

Case 4.36

A Radial head

B Anterior humeral line

C Anterior fat pad

D Radiocapitellar line

E Triceps brachii tendon

X-ray of elbow (right).

Radial head: Radial head fractures are most common elbow fractures in adult patients. They can be occult on plain radiographs so look at secondary signs such as raised fat pads or displaced lines.

Anterior humeral line: This is a line drawn along the anterior edge of the humerus and should intersect the middle third of the capitellum. This is an important line for paediatric elbow radiographs as misalignment is suggestive of supracondylar fracture (the most common elbow fracture in paediatric patients).

Anterior fat pad: Visible anterior fat pads can be seen in normal patients as in this case. Raised anterior fat pad is a useful secondary sign which indicates elbow joint effusion and suggestive of intra-articular fracture. Visible posterior fat pad is always abnormal and will not be tested in part 1.

Radiocapitellar line: This is a line drawn along the middle of radial neck which should bisect the capitellum. This is another line that is useful in paediatric setting as it indicates radial head dislocation.

Triceps brachii: This big muscle is the main extensor of the elbow joint and insert into the proximal olecranon.

Weir J, Abrahams P, Spratt JD, et al. Imaging Atlas of Human Anatomy, 6th edition. UK: Elsevier, 2021:67.

Butler P, Mitchell AWM, Healy JC. Applied Radiological Anatomy, 2nd edition. Cambridge: Cambridge University Press, 2012:297–298.

Case 4.37

A Coronoid process of the ulna

B Radial collateral ligament

C Olecranon fossa

D Flexor carpi radialis

E Supinator

Coronal MRI of the elbow joint.

The elbow joint incorporates three articulations: the humeroulnar, the humeroradial and the proximal radioulnar.

The articular surfaces are:

- Humerus: Capitellum laterally and trochlea medially
- Radius: The upper surface of the head of radius and the ulnar notch
- Ulna: The trochlear fossa and radial notch.

The radial and ulnar collateral ligaments are thickenings of the capsule that provide support. Another important ligament of the elbow to be aware of is the annular ligament. It is attached on the anterior and posterior edges of the radial notch of the ulna and surrounds the head of radius which rotates within it.

The radial collateral ligament is attached proximally to the lateral epicondyle of the humerus and distally to the annular ligament. The ulnar collateral ligament is attached proximally to the medial epicondyle and distally, to the medial side of the olecranon and the coronoid process of the ulna.

Two muscles are labelled on this image: on the lateral and medial side. Medially, there is the flexor carpi radialis, a superficial flexor in the forearm which flexes the wrist joint and adducts the hand. On the lateral side, there is the supinator which inserts into the neck and shaft of radius.

Weir J, Abrahams P. Imaging Atlas of Human Anatomy, 4th edition. Edinburgh: Mosby, 2010:83.

Ryan S, McNicholas M, Eustace SJ. Anatomy for Diagnostic Imaging, 3rd edition. Edinburgh: Saunders, 2010:265.

Case 4.38

A Biceps

B Triceps tendon

C Brachialis

D Coronoid process

E Olecranon process

Sagittal MRI of the elbow (ulnar side).

Biceps is composed of a long head and a short head. Distally, the two muscle bellies share a single tendon insertion on the bicipital tuberosity of the radius. The muscle flexes the elbow joint and supinates the forearm. It also helps to flex the shoulder joint.

Brachialis lies deep to the biceps on the anterior aspect of the humerus. It arises from the lower half of the humerus and inserts by a short tendon into the coronoid process of the ulna.

Triceps is a large muscle on the posterior aspect of the arm. It has three heads: the long, lateral and medial. In the mid-arm, the three heads unite to form a common tendon which inserts on the posterosuperior aspect of the olecranon.

Be sure to indicate whether a structure is a tendon or a muscle as failure to do so may lead to unnecessary loss of marks. Tendons are dark linear structures on MRI. Remember that a tendon connects a muscle to a bone while a ligament connects two bones.

Weir J, Abrahams P. Imaging Atlas of Human Anatomy, 4th edition. Edinburgh: Mosby, 2010: 82.

Ryan S, McNicholas M, Eustace SJ. Anatomy for Diagnostic Imaging, 3rd edition. Edinburgh: Saunders, 2010:265.

Case 4.39

A Surgical neck of the right humerus

B Greater tuberosity of the right humerus

C Right acromioclavicular joint

D Right clavicle

E Coracoid process of the right scapula

Anteroposterior radiograph of right shoulder.

The head of the humerus is hemispherical and it articulates with the glenoid fossa of the scapula. The anatomical neck of the humerus is formed by the boundary of the joint capsule. It separates the head of the humerus from the greater and lesser tuberosity. Note the position of the greater and lesser tuberosity on this projection and compare it with the axial projection. Between the tuberosities lies the bicipital groove for the long head of biceps.

The part of the shaft just below the tuberosities is called the surgical neck due to the tendency of the humerus to fracture at this point.

Weir J, Abrahams P. Imaging Atlas of Human Anatomy, 4th edition. Edinburgh: Mosby, 2010:68–69.

Butler P, Mitchell AM, Ellis H. Applied Radiological Anatomy. Cambridge: Cambridge University Press, 1999:334.

Case 4.40

A Glenoid fossa of the left scapula

B Coracoid process of the left scapula

C Lesser tuberosity of the left humerus

D Left clavicle

E Head of the left humerus

Axial radiograph of the shoulder.

Two articulations are visible on this radiograph: the glenohumeral joint and the acromioclavicular joint. Note the appearance of the humeral tubercles and the coracoid process. This is a good example of an image where wrongly identifying one structure will lead to wrongly identifying the rest. The key to identifying the structures on a shoulder radiograph is to identify which projection is given. It is important to appreciate the relations of the bony landmarks on different projections. A good starting point is to identify the coracoid process which points anteriorly.

The standard plain radiographic views of the shoulder are the anteroposterior and axial projections. The other important projections are the transscapular view (y-view) and Striker's view, which is acquired with the beam angled through the axilla to provide anatomical detail of the posterior aspect of the humeral head.

Weir J, Abrahams P. Imaging Atlas of Human Anatomy, 4th edition. Edinburgh: Mosby, 2010:68.

Ryan S, McNicholas M, Eustace SJ. Anatomy for Diagnostic Imaging, 3rd edition. Edinburgh: Saunders, 2010:252.

Butler P, Mitchell AM, Ellis H. Applied Radiological Anatomy. Cambridge: Cambridge University Press, 1999:336.

Case 4.41

A Left supraspinatus muscle

B Spine of the left scapula

C Left infraspinatus muscle

D Left subscapularis muscle

E Left clavicle

MR arthrogram shoulder left.

The rotator cuff anatomy is an examination favourite so make sure to drill it into your head. It is clinically important as rotator cuff injuries are common and can cause significant shoulder pain and weakness. Increasing age and manual labour occupations are known risk factors. It consists of four muscles as follows:

Supraspinatus: This is the main muscle responsible for the first 15° of shoulder abduction. It is often the rotator cuff muscle to be injured, either from a sports injury or degeneration. High-riding humeral head or calcific degeneration might be seen in a shoulder radiograph.

Infraspinatus: Responsible for external rotation of the shoulder joint along with teres minor.

Teres minor: Can be difficult to distinguish the border between the infraspinatus and teres minor muscles, but thankfully it is not as clinically relevant. Look for a thin fat plane between the two muscles. It would be unfair to ask to tell teres minor apart in this case example.

Subscapularis: Acts to internally rotate and adduct the shoulder joint.

Scapular spine: An easy way to remember the rotator cuff muscles is to first identify that Y shape made by the scapular body and spine on a sagittal slice. The locations of the muscles then tell you the name!

Weir J, Abrahams P, Spratt JD, et al. Imaging Atlas of Human Anatomy, 6th edition. UK: Elsevier, 2021:76.

Butler P, Mitchell AWM, Healy JC. Applied Radiological Anatomy, 2nd edition. Cambridge: Cambridge University Press, 2012:287–288.

Case 4.42

A Coracoid process

B Anterior glenoid labrum

C Infraspinatus

D Middle glenohumeral ligament

E Deltoid

Axial MRI of the shoulder at the level of the glenohumeral joint.

The coracoid process is a useful landmark to help to identify the orientation of this image. It lies anteriorly. The glenoid process of the scapula articulates with the head of humerus and is easily identifiable by its shape. The articular surface of the glenoid is deepened by the labrum: a rim of fibrous tissue.

The muscles of the rotator cuff are discussed in the previous question. Note that in an axial image, at the level where the glenoid is at its widest, the rotator cuff muscle anteriorly is the subscapularis and posteriorly is the infraspinatus.

The capsule is attached to the epiphyseal line of the glenoid and the humerus except inferiorly, where it forms the axillary pouch by expanding on the medial aspect of the neck of humerus. There are three anterior thickenings of the capsule, the three glenohumeral ligaments. They pass from the upper part of the glenoid to the lesser tuberosity and the inferior part of the head of humerus.

Weir J, Abrahams P. Imaging Atlas of Human Anatomy, 4th edition. Edinburgh: Mosby, 2010:79.

Ryan S, McNicholas M, Eustace SJ. Anatomy for Diagnostic Imaging, 3rd edition. Edinburgh: Saunders, 2010:261–263.

Case 4.43

A Right teres minor

B Right teres major

B Right long head of the triceps

D Right humerus

E Right quadrangular space

Figure 4.2 shows MR arthrogram shoulder right.

This is a hard question. Key to solving this question is to identify that the fat containing space (coloured green) is in fact the quadrangular (also known as quadrilateral) space. This space is important clinically as it contains the axillary nerve and posterior circumflex humeral artery which can be injured in quadrangular space syndrome or trauma. Once you have identified this space, you just need to remember the four borders.

Medial border: Long head of triceps brachii muscle, which is important for elbow extension and shoulder abduction stabilisation.

Lateral border: Surgical neck of humerus, a common site for fractures.

Superior border: Teres minor muscle, a part of the rotator cuff.

Inferior border: Teres major muscle, which acts to internally rotate, extend and adduct the shoulder joint.

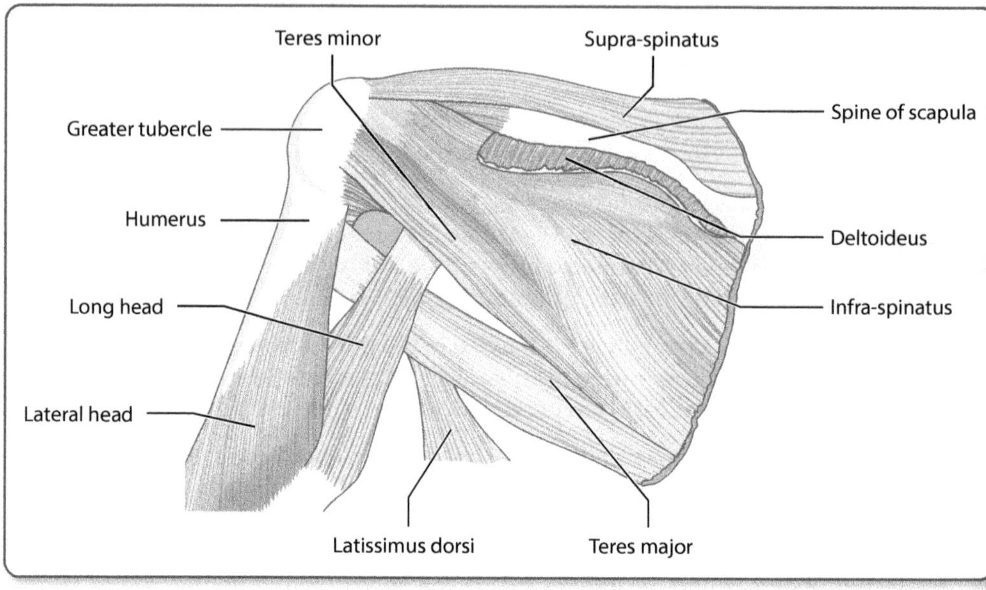

Figure 4.2 MR arthrogram shoulder right.

Weir J, Abrahams P, Spratt JD, et al. Imaging Atlas of Human Anatomy, 6th edition. UK: Elsevier, 2021:77.

Butler P, Mitchell AWM, Healy JC. Applied Radiological Anatomy, 2nd edition. Cambridge: Cambridge University Press, 2012:284–289.

Illustration from Gray's anatomy. Available in public domain on Wikimedia Commons. https://commons.wikimedia.org/wiki/Category:Gray%27s_Anatomy_plates (Last accessed 15 April 2024)

Case 4.44

A Right subclavian artery

B Right common carotid artery

C Right axillary artery

D Right superior (internal) thoracic artery

E Right lateral thoracic artery

Subclavian catheter angiogram.

The subclavian artery gives off six branches which supply the chest wall and the shoulder. The mnemonic SALSA is used to remember these branches:

*S*uperior thoracic artery (also called internal thoracic artery)

*A*cromiothoracic trunk

*L*ateral thoracic artery

*S*ubscapular artery

*A*nterior and posterior humeral artery

The subclavian artery becomes the axillary artery at the outer border of the first rib.

The arterial supply of the upper limb is summarised in **Figure 4.3**.

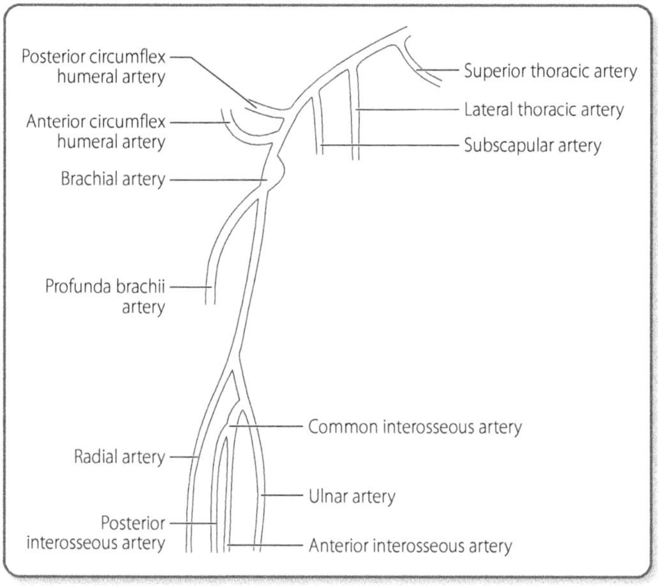

Figure 4.3 Arterial supply to the upper limb.

Weir J, Abrahams P. Imaging Atlas of Human Anatomy, 4th edition. Edinburgh: Mosby, 2010:76.

Ryan S, McNicholas M, Eustace SJ. Anatomy for Diagnostic Imaging, 3rd edition. Edinburgh: Saunders, 2010:278.

Butler P, Mitchell AM, Ellis H. Applied Radiological Anatomy. Cambridge: Cambridge University Press, 1999:384.

Case 4.45

A Brachial artery

B Radial artery

C Ulnar artery

D Posterior interosseous artery

E Anterior interosseous artery

Brachial MR angiogram.

The brachial artery begins at the lower end of teres major. It gives off a profunda brachii which arises medially. It then gives off a nutrient artery to the humerus, muscular branches and branches to the elbow joint.

Within the antecubital fossa, approximately at the level of the radial head, the brachial artery divides into the radial and ulnar artery. The radial artery lies deep to brachioradialis. The ulnar artery is larger and deeper. It gives off the common intraosseous artery, which divides into the anterior and posterior intraosseous arteries.

Weir J, Abrahams P. Imaging Atlas of Human Anatomy, 4th edition. Edinburgh: Mosby, 2010:76.

Ryan S, McNicholas M, Eustace SJ. Anatomy for Diagnostic Imaging, 3rd edition. Edinburgh: Saunders, 2010:278.

Butler P, Mitchell AM, Ellis H. Applied Radiological Anatomy. Cambridge: Cambridge University Press, 1999:384.

Chapter 5

Practice paper 1

Case 5.1

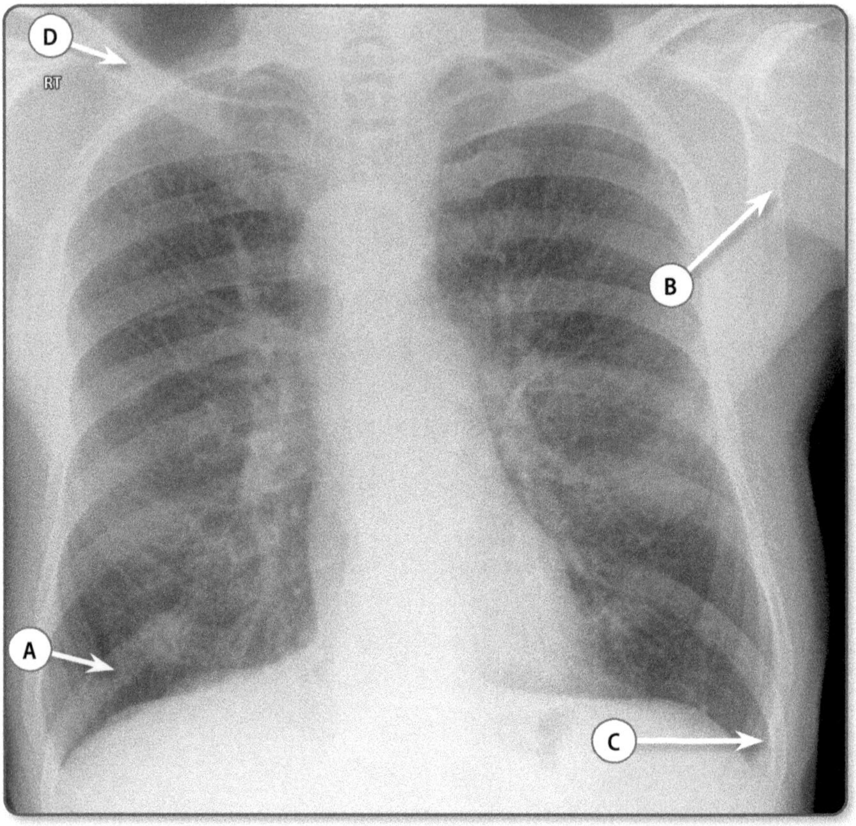

Case 5.1

QUESTION		WRITE YOUR ANSWER HERE
A	Name the structure labelled A.	
B	Name the structure labelled B.	
C	Name the structure labelled C.	
D	Name the structure labelled D.	
E	Name the normal variant present in this case.	

Case 5.2

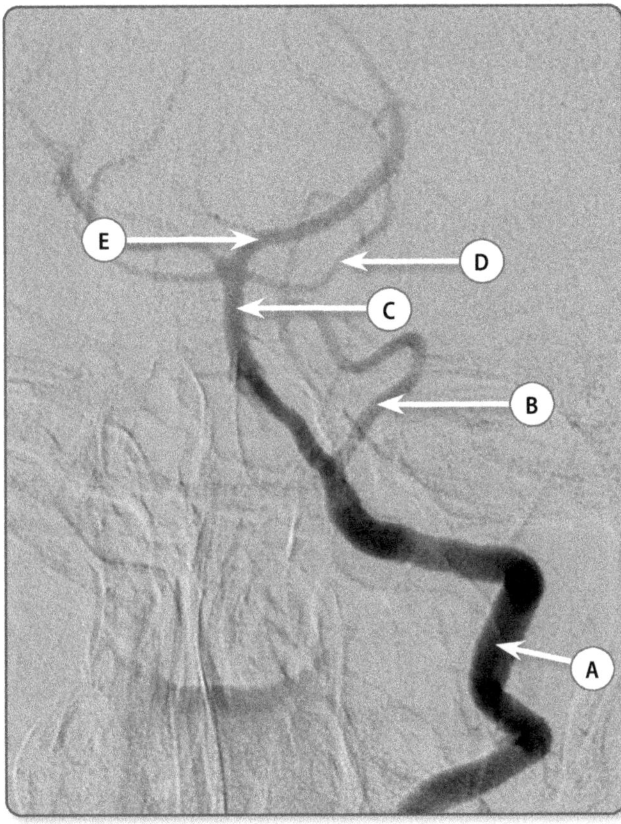

Case 5.2

QUESTION		WRITE YOUR ANSWER HERE
A	Name the structure labelled A.	
B	Name the structure labelled B.	
C	Name the structure labelled C.	
D	Name the structure labelled D.	
E	Name the structure labelled E.	

Case 5.3

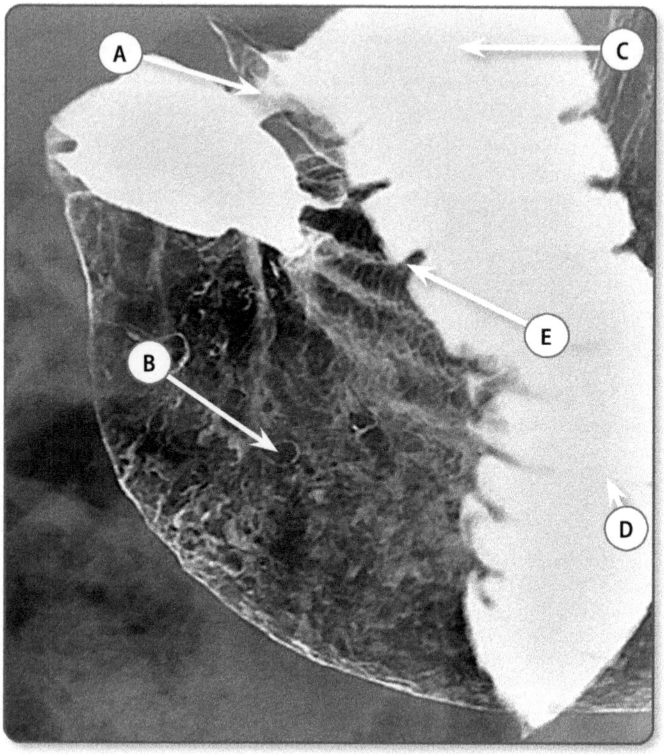

Case 5.3

QUESTION		WRITE YOUR ANSWER HERE
A	Name the structure labelled A.	
B	Name the structure labelled B.	
C	Name the structure labelled C.	
D	Name the structure labelled D.	
E	Name the structure labelled E.	

Case 5.4

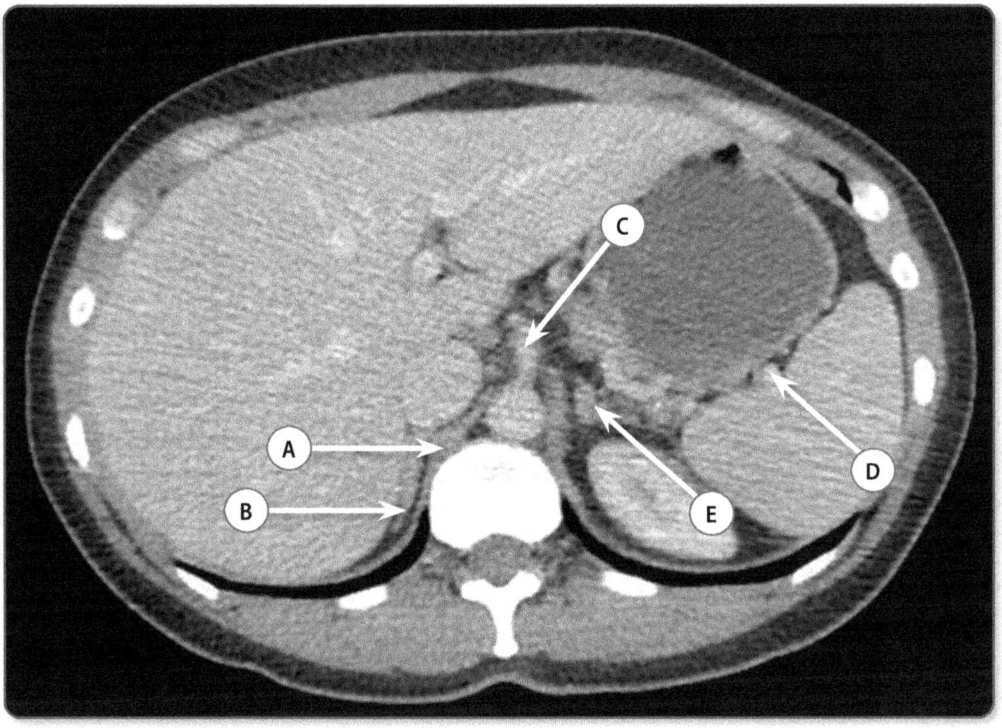

Case 5.4		
QUESTION		WRITE YOUR ANSWER HERE
A	Name the structure labelled A.	
B	Name the structure labelled B.	
C	Name the structure labelled C.	
D	Name the structure labelled D.	
E	Name the structure labelled E.	

Case 5.5

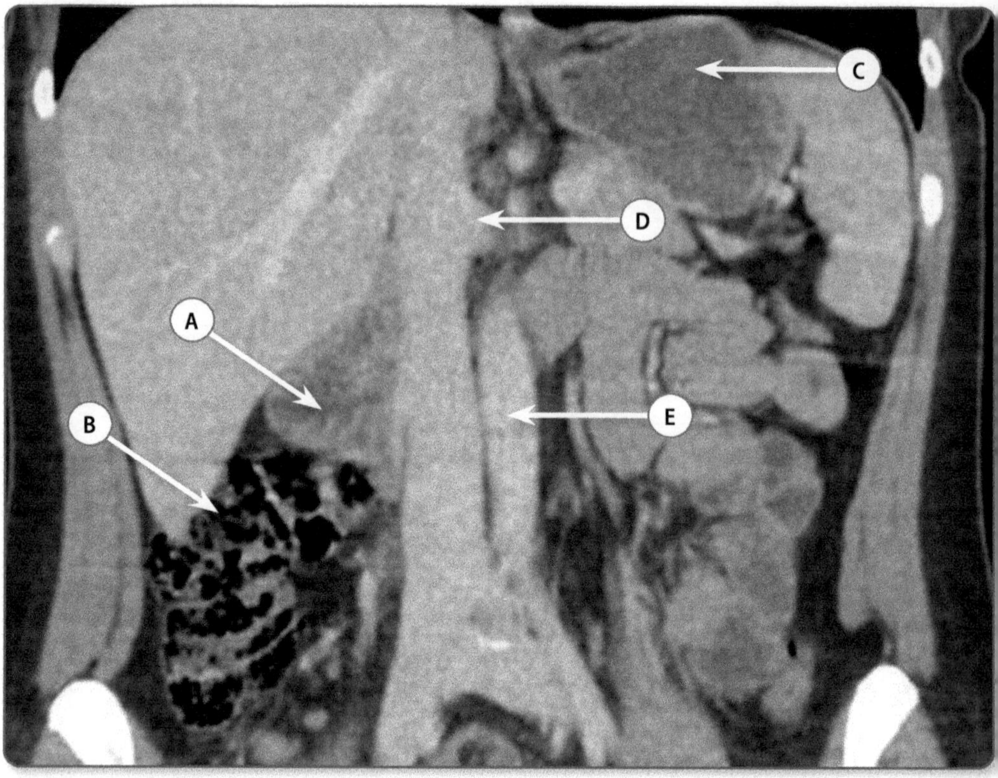

Case 5.5

QUESTION		WRITE YOUR ANSWER HERE
A	Name the structure labelled A.	
B	Name the structure labelled B.	
C	Name the structure labelled C.	
D	Name the structure labelled D.	
E	Name the structure labelled E.	

Case 5.6

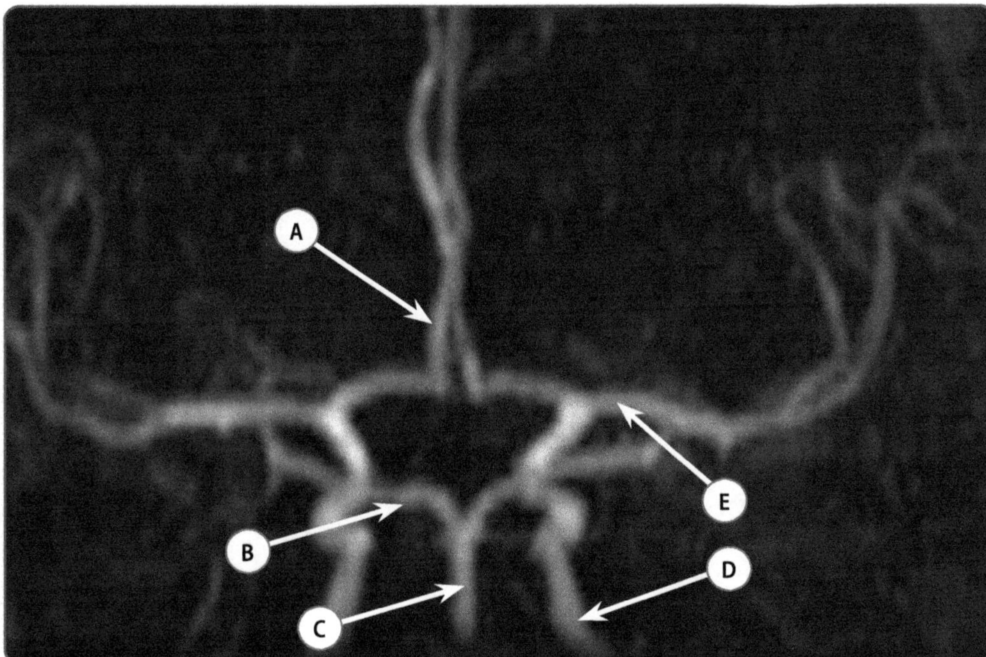

Case 5.6

QUESTION		WRITE YOUR ANSWER HERE
A	Name the structure labelled A.	
B	Name the structure labelled B.	
C	Name the structure labelled C.	
D	Name the structure labelled D.	
E	Name the structure labelled E.	

Case 5.7

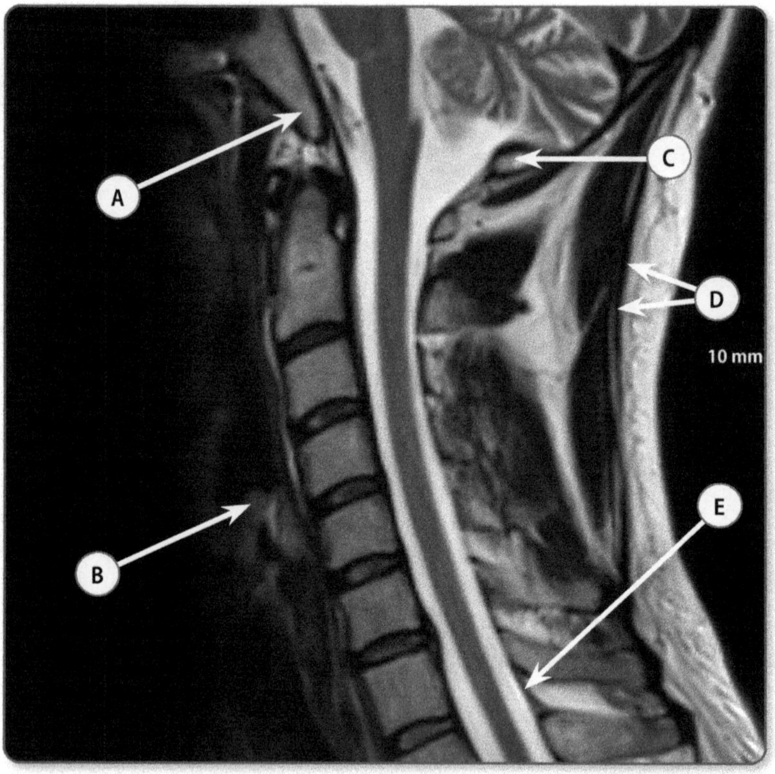

Case 5.7

QUESTION		WRITE YOUR ANSWER HERE
A	Name the structure labelled A.	
B	Name the structure labelled B.	
C	Name the structure labelled C.	
D	Name the structure labelled D.	
E	Name the structure labelled E.	

Case 5.8

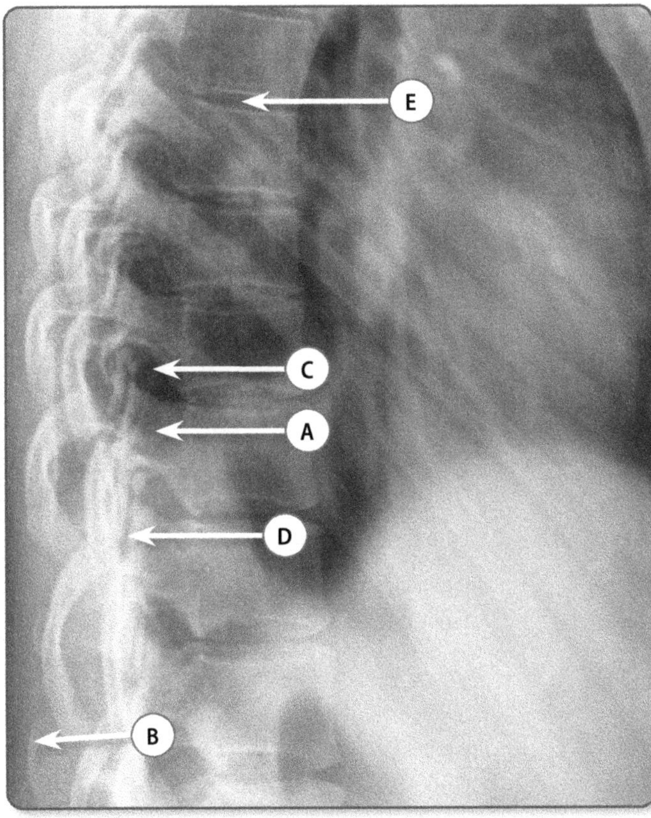

Case 5.8

QUESTION		WRITE YOUR ANSWER HERE
A	Name the structure labelled A.	
B	Name the structure labelled B.	
C	Name the structure labelled C.	
D	Name the structure labelled D.	
E	Name the structure labelled E.	

Case 5.9

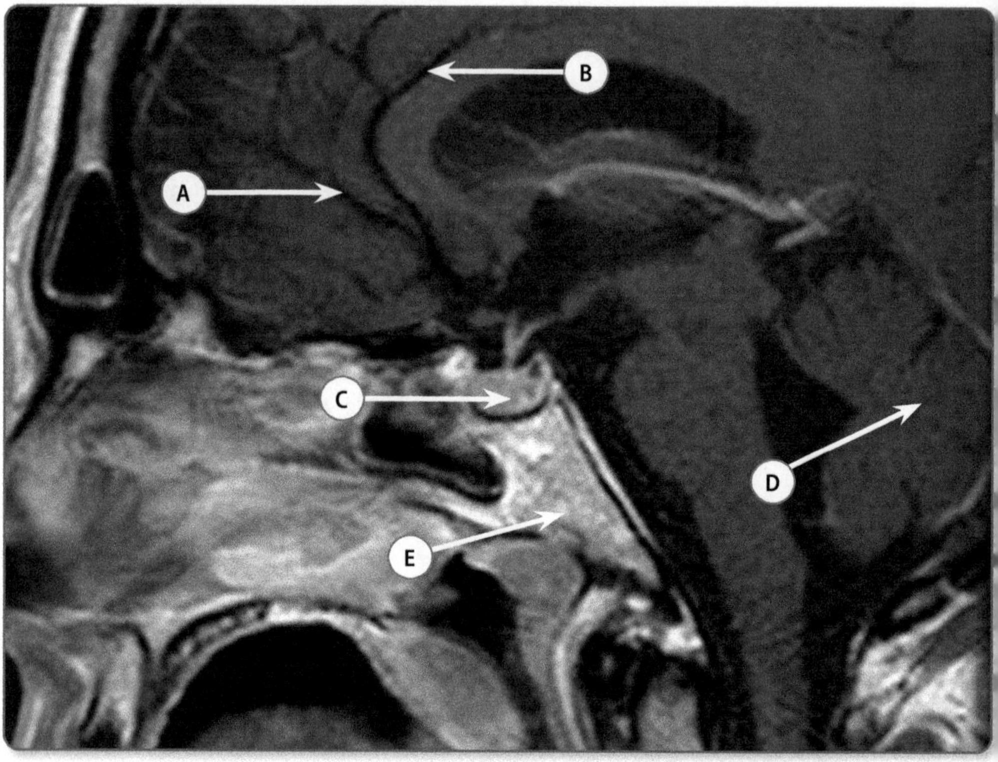

Case 5.9

QUESTION		WRITE YOUR ANSWER HERE
A	Name the structure labelled A.	
B	Name the structure labelled B.	
C	Name the structure labelled C.	
D	Name the structure labelled D.	
E	Name the structure labelled E.	

Case 5.10

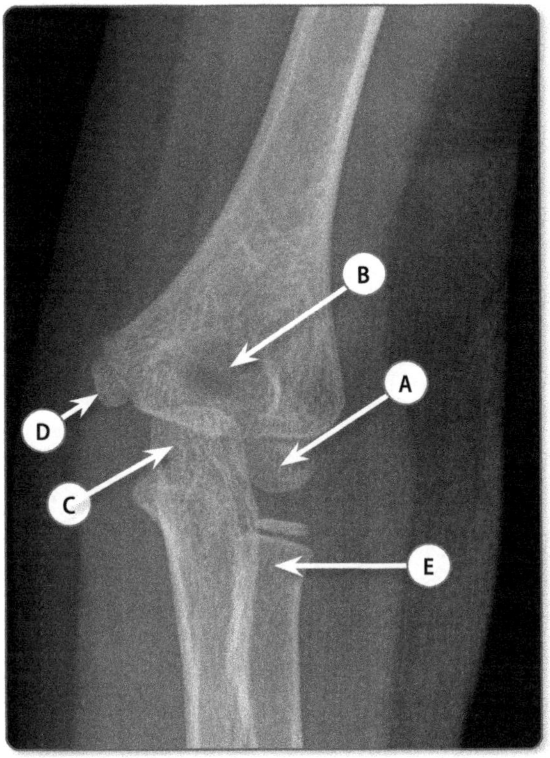

Case 5.10

QUESTION		WRITE YOUR ANSWER HERE
A	Name the structure labelled A.	
B	Name the structure labelled B.	
C	Name the structure labelled C.	
D	Name the structure labelled D.	
E	Name the structure labelled E.	

Case 5.11

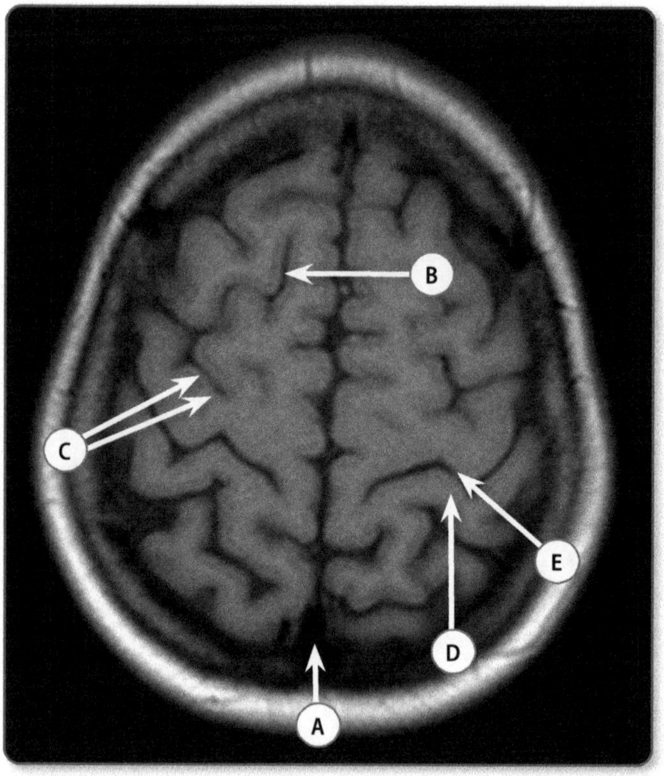

Case 5.11

QUESTION		WRITE YOUR ANSWER HERE
A	Name the structure labelled A.	
B	Name the structure labelled B.	
C	Name the structure labelled C.	
D	Name the structure labelled D.	
E	Name the structure labelled E.	

Case 5.12

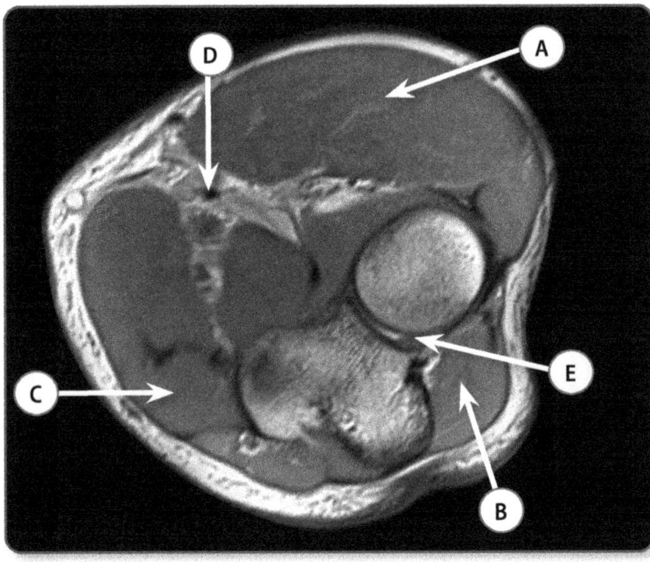

Case 5.12

QUESTION		WRITE YOUR ANSWER HERE
A	Name the structure labelled A.	
B	Name the structure labelled B.	
C	Name the structure labelled C.	
D	Name the structure labelled D.	
E	Name the structure labelled E.	

Case 5.13

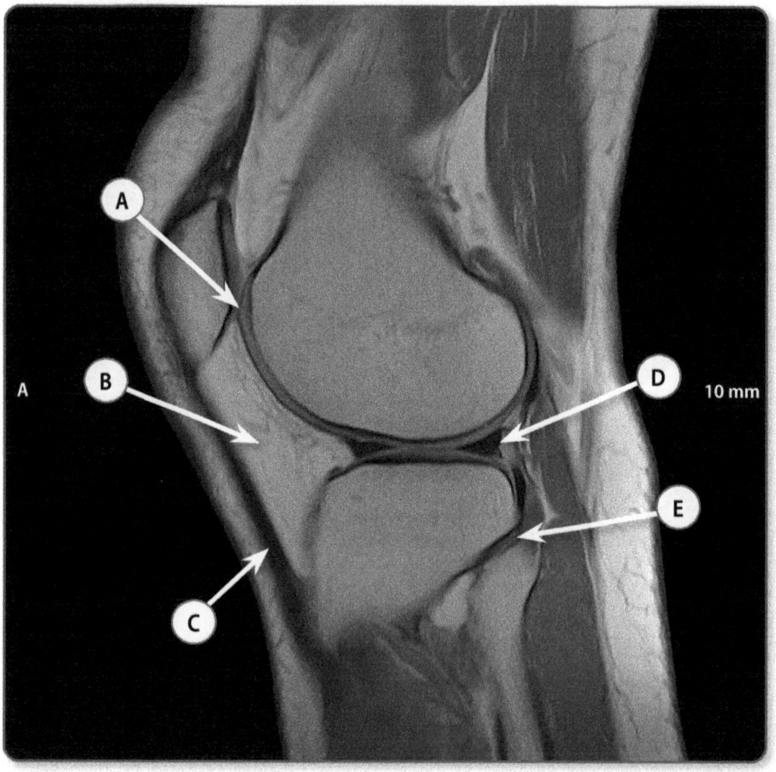

Case 5.13

QUESTION		WRITE YOUR ANSWER HERE
A	Name the structure labelled A.	
B	Name the structure labelled B.	
C	Name the structure labelled C.	
D	Name the structure labelled D.	
E	Name the structure labelled E.	

Case 5.14

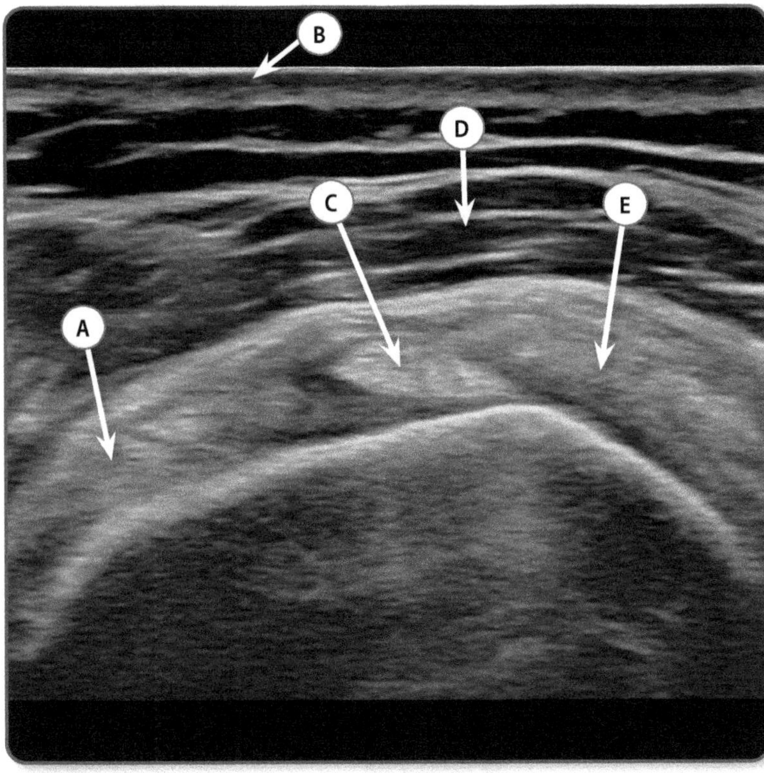

Case 5.14

QUESTION		WRITE YOUR ANSWER HERE
A	Name the structure labelled A.	
B	Name the structure labelled B.	
C	Name the structure labelled C.	
D	Name the structure labelled D.	
E	Name the structure labelled E.	

Case 5.15

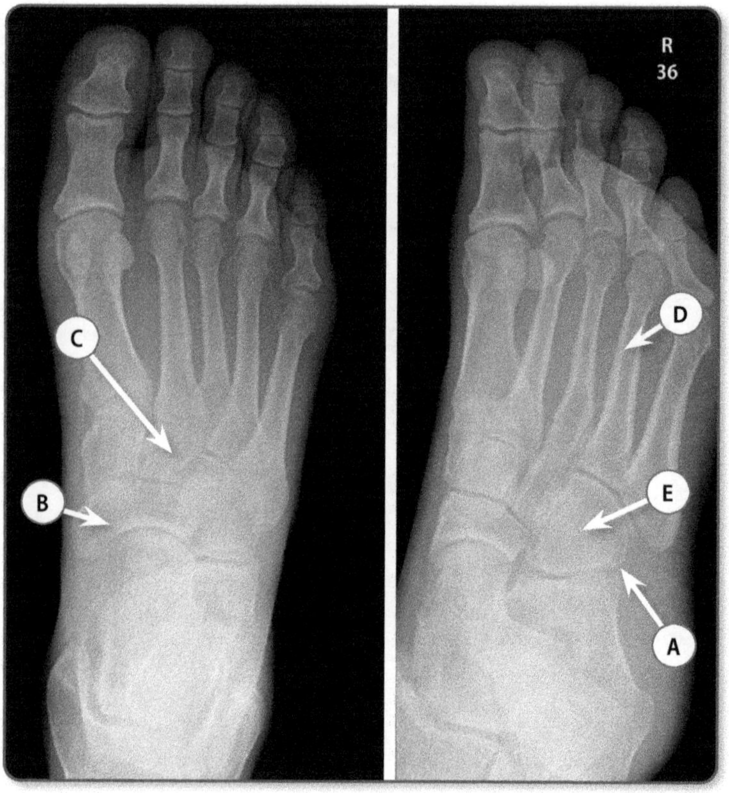

Case 5.15

QUESTION		WRITE YOUR ANSWER HERE
A	Name the structure labelled A.	
B	Name the structure labelled B.	
C	Name the structure labelled C.	
D	Name the structure labelled D.	
E	Name the structure labelled E.	

Case 5.16

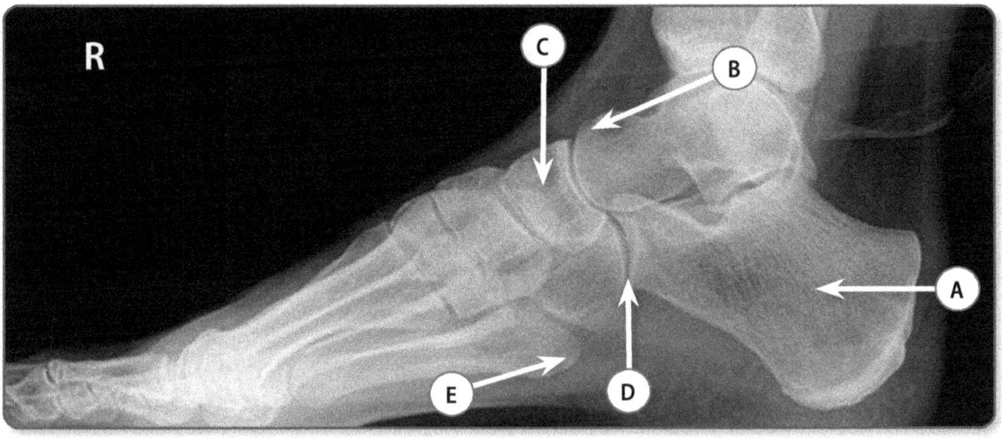

Case 5.16

QUESTION		WRITE YOUR ANSWER HERE
A	Name the structure labelled A.	
B	Name the structure labelled B.	
C	Name the structure labelled C.	
D	Name the structure labelled D.	
E	Name the structure labelled E.	

Case 5.17

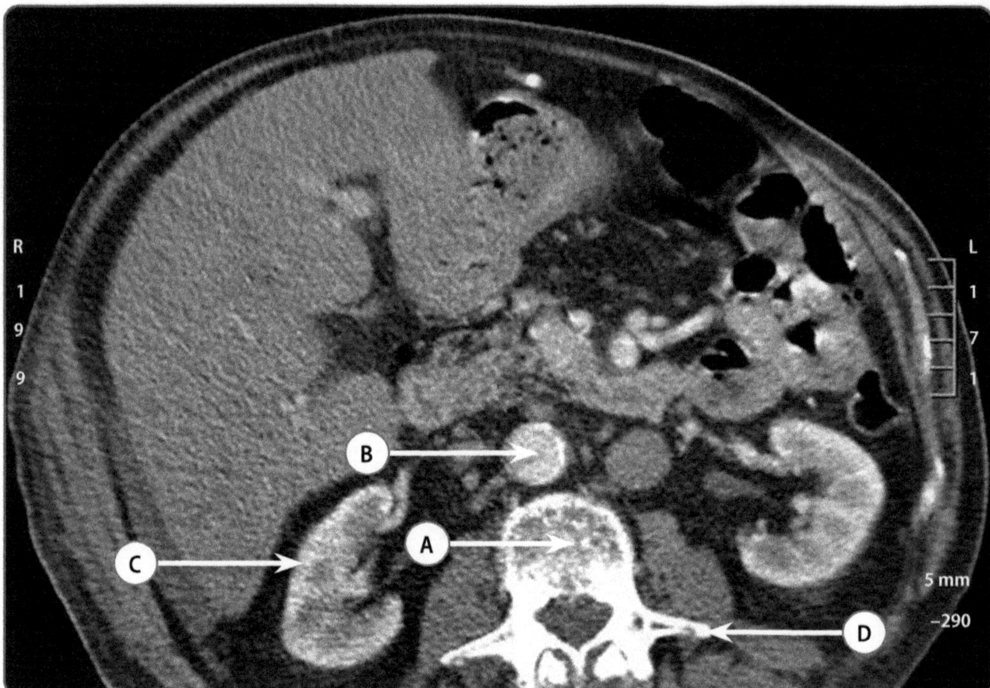

Case 5.17

QUESTION		WRITE YOUR ANSWER HERE
A	Name the structure labelled A.	
B	Name the structure labelled B.	
C	Name the structure labelled C.	
D	Name the structure labelled D.	
E	Which normal variant is demonstrated?	

Case 5.18

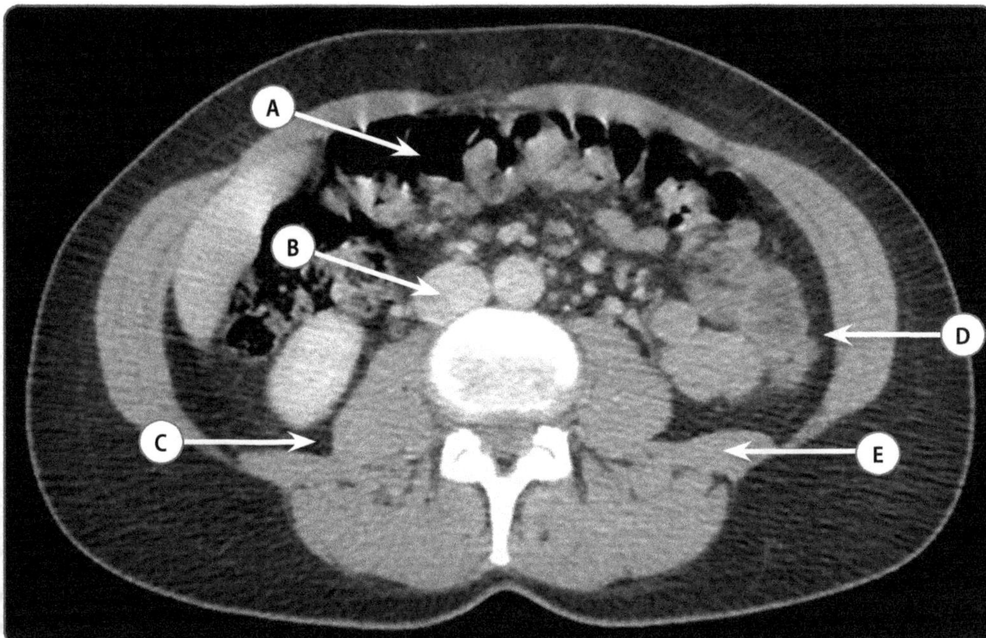

Case 5.18

QUESTION		WRITE YOUR ANSWER HERE
A	Name the structure labelled A.	
B	Name the structure labelled B.	
C	Name the structure labelled C.	
D	Name the structure labelled D.	
E	Name the structure labelled E.	

Case 5.19

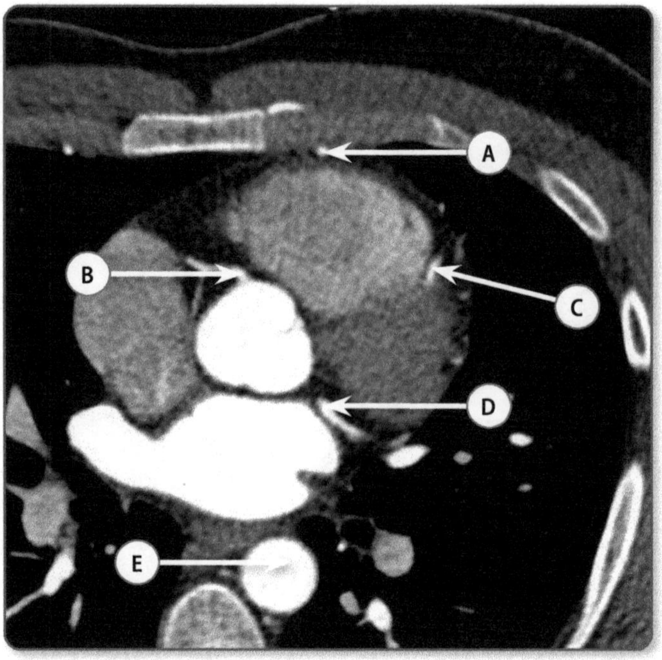

Case 5.19

QUESTION		WRITE YOUR ANSWER HERE
A	Name the structure labelled A.	
B	Name the structure labelled B.	
C	Name the structure labelled C.	
D	Name the structure labelled D.	
E	Name the structure labelled E.	

Case 5.20

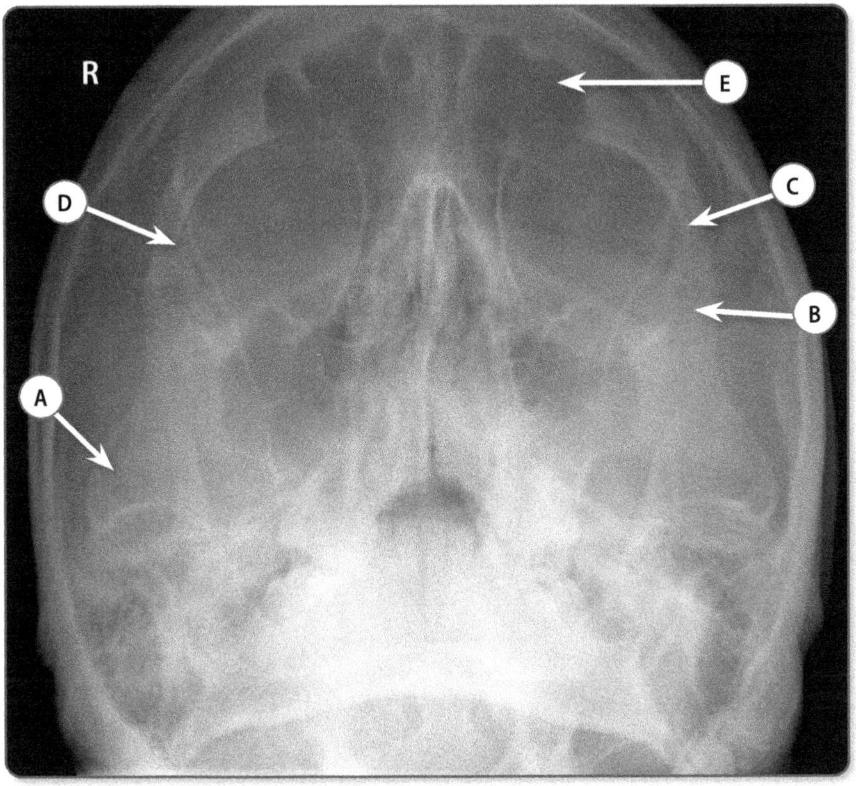

Case 5.20

QUESTION		WRITE YOUR ANSWER HERE
A	Name the structure labelled A.	
B	Name the structure labelled B.	
C	Name the structure labelled C.	
D	Name the structure labelled D.	
E	Name the structure labelled E.	

Answers

Case 5.1

A Right 10th rib

B Left scapula

C Left costophrenic angle

D Right clavicle

E Name the normal variant: Right aortic arch

Frontal radiograph of the chest.

For further discussion see Chapter 2, Cases 2.26–2.32.

Case 5.2

A Left vertebral artery

B Left posterior inferior cerebellar artery

C Basilar artery

D Left superior cerebellar artery

E Left posterior cerebral artery

Angiogram of the left vertebral artery.

For further discussion see Chapter 1, Cases 1.14–1.17.

Case 5.3

A Pyloric canal

B Areae gastricae

C First part of duodenum/duodenal cap

D Second part of duodenum

E Valvulae conniventes

Spot film from a barium meal, taken at an oblique angle.

For further discussion see Chapter 3, Case 3.6.

Case 5.4

A Right diaphragmatic crus

B Right adrenal gland

C Coeliac axis

D Vessels at splenic hilum (splenic artery)

E Left adrenal gland

Axial contrast-enhanced CT.

For further discussion see Chapter 3, Cases 3.14, 3.48 and 3.49.

Case 5.5

A Duodenum, junction of D2 and D3

B Hepatic flexure of large bowel

C Gastric fundus

D Left renal vein

E Abdominal aorta

Coronal contrast-enhanced CT of the abdomen and pelvis.

For further discussion see Chapter 3, Cases 3.6 and 3.12.

Case 5.6

A Right anterior cerebral artery

B Right posterior cerebral artery

C Basilar artery

D Left internal carotid artery

E Left middle cerebral artery (MCA)

MR angiogram of the brain.

For further discussion see Chapter 1, Cases 1.14–1.17.

Case 5.7

A Basion

B Epiglottis

C Opisthion

D Ligamentum nuchae

E Ligamentum flavum

MR cervical spine.

Weir J, Abrahams P, Spratt JD, et al. Imaging Atlas of Human Anatomy, 6th edition. UK: Elsevier, 2021:59.

Butler P, Mitchell AWM, Healy JC. Applied Radiological Anatomy, 2nd edition. Cambridge: Cambridge University Press, 2012:83.

Case 5.8

A Pedicle

B Spinous process

C Inferior vertebral notch

D Facet joint

E Intervertebral disc

Lateral radiograph of the thoracic spine.

For further discussion see Chapter 4, Cases 4.19–4.31.

Case 5.9

A Frontopolar artery

B Pericallosal artery

C Pituitary gland

D Cerebellar vermis

E Clivus

Midline sagittal T1-weighted MRI of the brain.

For further discussion see Chapter 1, Cases 1.1–1.5.

Case 5.10

A Secondary ossification centre of the capitulum

B Olecranon fossa

C Olecranon process

D Secondary ossification centre of the medial epicondyle

E Proximal radial metaphysis

Anteroposterior radiograph of the left elbow (child).

For further discussion see Chapter 4, Case 4.34.

Case 5.11

A Superior sagittal sinus

B Right superior frontal sulcus

C Right precentral sulcus

D Left postcentral gyrus

E Left central sulcus

Axial MRI of the central sulcus.

For further discussion see Chapter 1, Case 1.6.

Case 5.12

A Brachioradialis

B Anconeus

C Flexor carpi ulnaris

D Median nerve

E Proximal radioulnar joint

Axial MRI of the proximal radioulnar joint.

For further discussion see Chapter 4, Case 4.35.

Case 5.13

A Patellofemoral joint

B Hoffa's (infrapatellar) fat pad

C Patellar tendon

D Posterior horn of the lateral meniscus

E Proximal tibiofibular joint

MR knee left

Weir J, Abrahams P, Spratt JD, et al. Imaging Atlas of Human Anatomy, 6th edition. UK: Elsevier, 2021:232.

Butler P, Mitchell AWM, Healy JC. Applied Radiological Anatomy, 2nd edition. Cambridge: Cambridge University Press, 2012:344.

Case 5.14

A Subscapularis

B Skin

C Biceps tendon

D Deltoid muscle

E Supraspinatus

US shoulder right – rotator interval.

Weir J, Abrahams P, Spratt JD, et al. Imaging Atlas of Human Anatomy, 6th edition. UK: Elsevier, 2021: 76–78.

Butler P, Mitchell AWM, Healy JC. Applied Radiological Anatomy, 2nd edition. Cambridge: Cambridge University Press, 2012:290.

Case 5.15

A Right calcaneocuboid joint

B Right navicular

C Right middle cuneiform

D Right 4th metatarsal

E Right cuboid

Dorsoplantar and dorsoplantar oblique radiographs of the right foot.

For further discussion see Chapter 4, Cases 4.1 and 4.2.

Case 5.16

A Right calcaneus

B Head of the right talus

C Right navicular

D Right calcaneocuboid joint

E Base of the right 5th metatarsal

Lateral weight bearing radiograph of the right foot.

For further discussion see Chapter 4, Cases 4.1 and 4.2.

Case 5.17

A Vertebral body

B Aorta

C Cortex of right kidney

D Left transverse process

E Name the normal variant: Left inferior vena cava

Axial CT at the level of the kidneys.

For further discussion see Chapter 4, Cases 4.1 and 4.2.

Case 5.18

A Transverse colon

B Inferior vena cava

C Right posterior pararenal space

D Left paracolic gutter

E Left quadratus lumborum

Axial contrast-enhanced CT of the abdomen.

The paracolic gutters (also known as the paracolic recesses) are found lateral to the ascending and descending colon. They are formed by two peritoneal recesses which run adjacent to the ascending and descending colon. Both paracolic gutters are continuous with the rectouterine and rectovesical spaces in the pelvis. The right paracolic gutter tends to be larger than the left, and is in communication with the right subphrenic and subhepatic spaces. The phrenicocolic ligament forms a partial barrier between the left paracolic gutter and the subphrenic spaces on the left.

Quadratus lumborum is one of the muscles of the posterior abdominal wall. It has attachments to the 12th ribs, the transverse processes of the lumbar vertebrae, the iliolumbar ligament, and the iliac crest. The arcuate ligament is formed from a focal thickening of the fascial covering of quadratus lumborum superiorly. The iliolumbar ligament is formed from a thickening of this fascial layer inferiorly, and runs between the transverse processes of L5 to the iliac crests.

Butler P, Mitchell AM, Ellis H. Applied Radiological Anatomy. Cambridge: Cambridge University Press, 1999: 193, 277.

Case 5.19

A Left internal mammary artery

B Right coronary artery

C Left anterior descending artery

D Circumflex artery

E Descending thoracic aorta

Axial CT of the chest.

For further discussion see Chapter 2, Cases 2.1–2.18.

Case 5.20

A Right zygomatic arch

B Frontal process of left zygoma

C Zygomatic process of left frontal bone

D Right zygomaticofrontal suture

E Left frontal sinus

Occipitomental radiograph.

For further discussion see Chapter 1, Case 1.27.

Chapter 6

Practice paper 2

Case 6.1

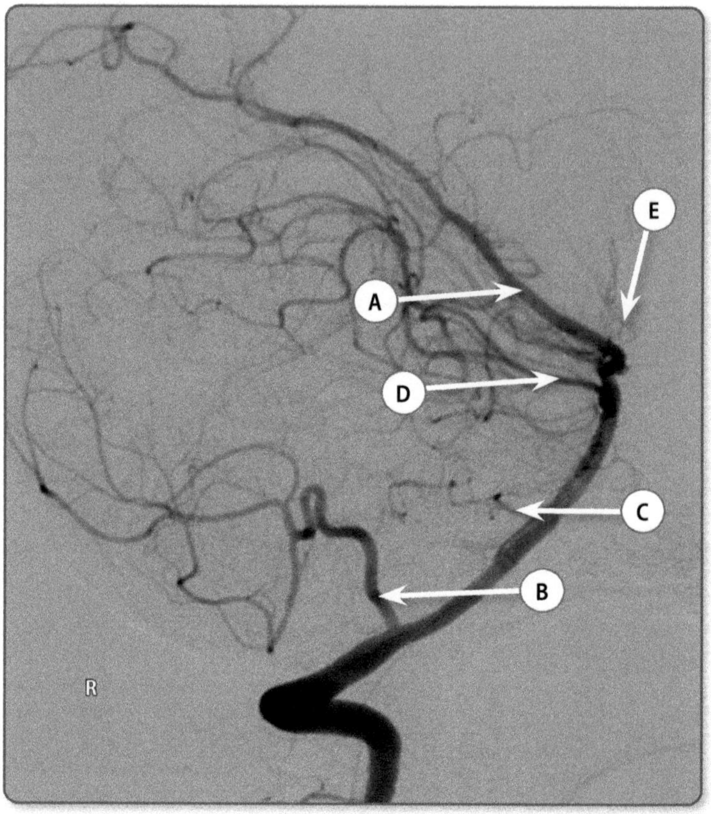

Case 6.1

QUESTION		WRITE YOUR ANSWER HERE
A	Name the structure labelled A.	
B	Name the structure labelled B.	
C	Name the structure labelled C.	
D	Name the structure labelled D.	
E	Name the structure labelled E.	

Case 6.2

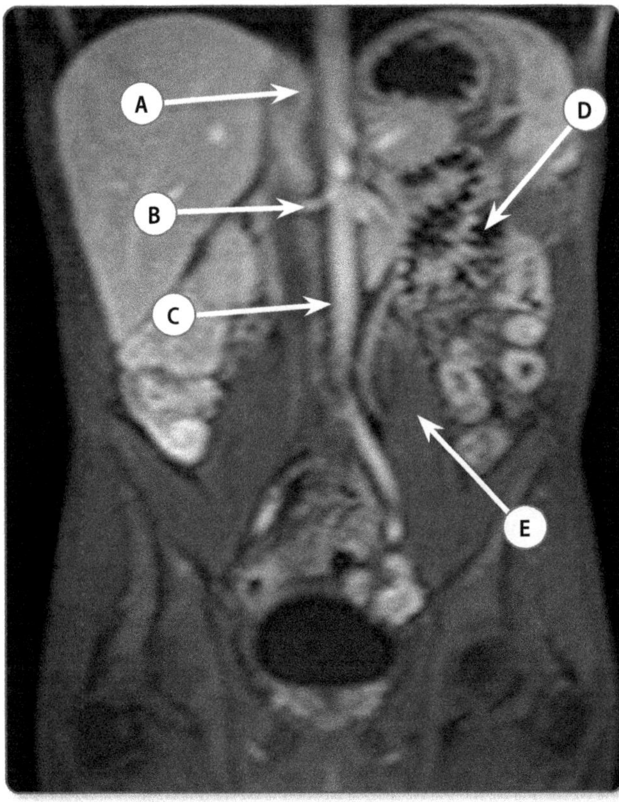

Case 6.2

QUESTION		WRITE YOUR ANSWER HERE
A	Name the structure labelled A.	
B	Name the structure labelled B.	
C	Name the structure labelled C.	
D	Name the structure labelled D.	
E	Name the structure labelled E.	

Case 6.3

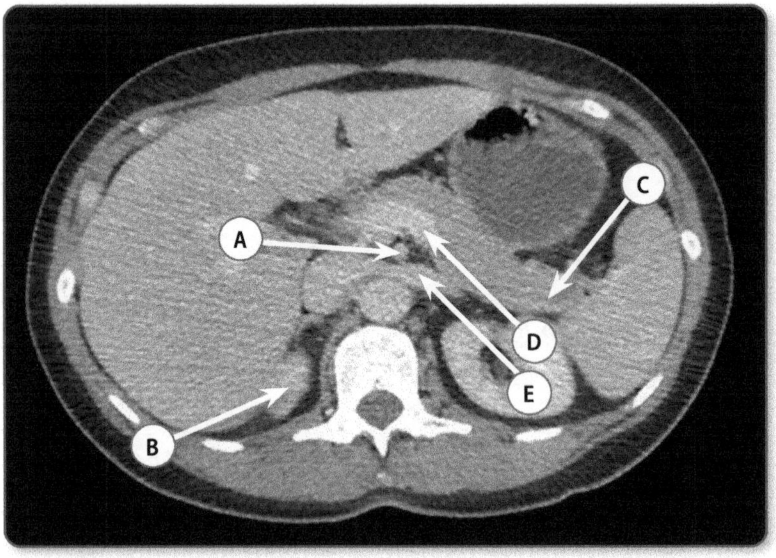

Case 6.3

QUESTION		WRITE YOUR ANSWER HERE
A	Name the structure labelled A.	
B	Name the structure labelled B.	
C	Name the structure labelled C.	
D	Name the structure labelled D.	
E	Name the structure labelled E.	

Case 6.4

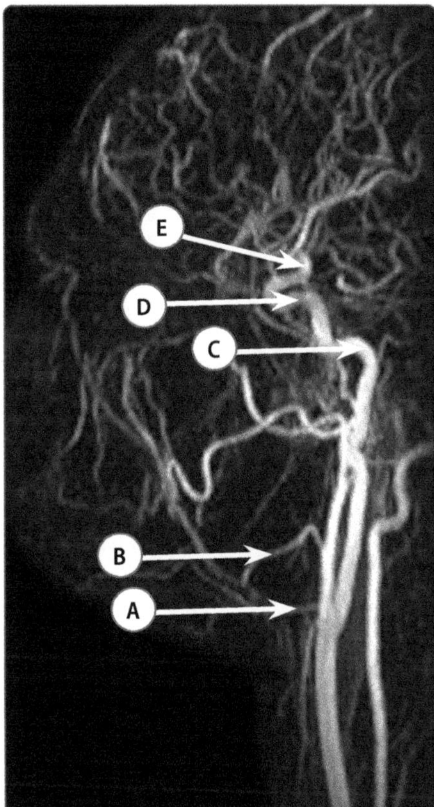

Case 6.4

QUESTION		WRITE YOUR ANSWER HERE
A	Name the structure labelled A.	
B	Name the structure labelled B.	
C	Name the structure labelled C.	
D	Name the structure labelled D.	
E	Name the structure labelled E.	

Case 6.5

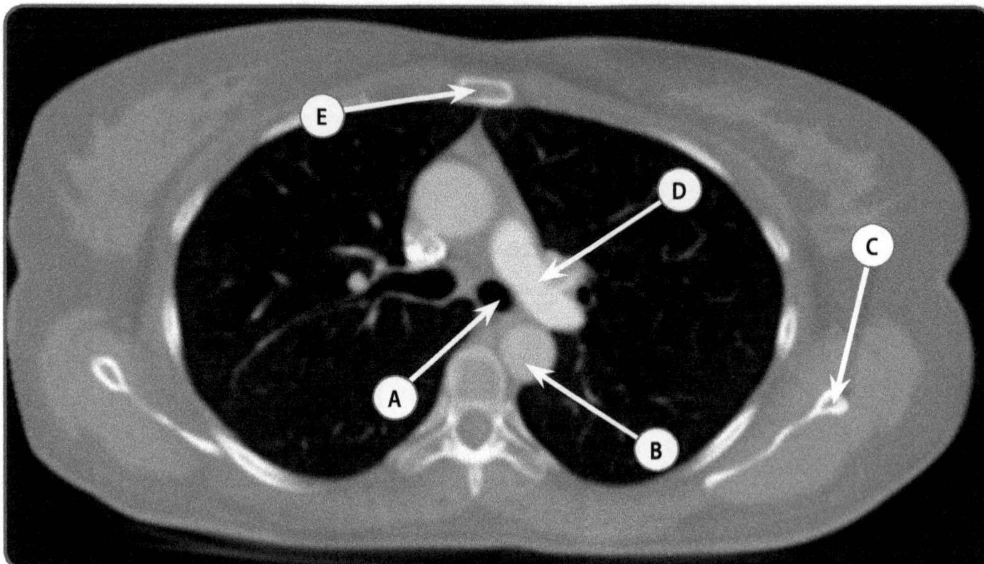

Case 6.5

QUESTION		WRITE YOUR ANSWER HERE
A	Name the structure labelled A.	
B	Name the structure labelled B.	
C	Name the structure labelled C.	
D	Name the structure labelled D.	
E	Name the structure labelled E.	

Case 6.6

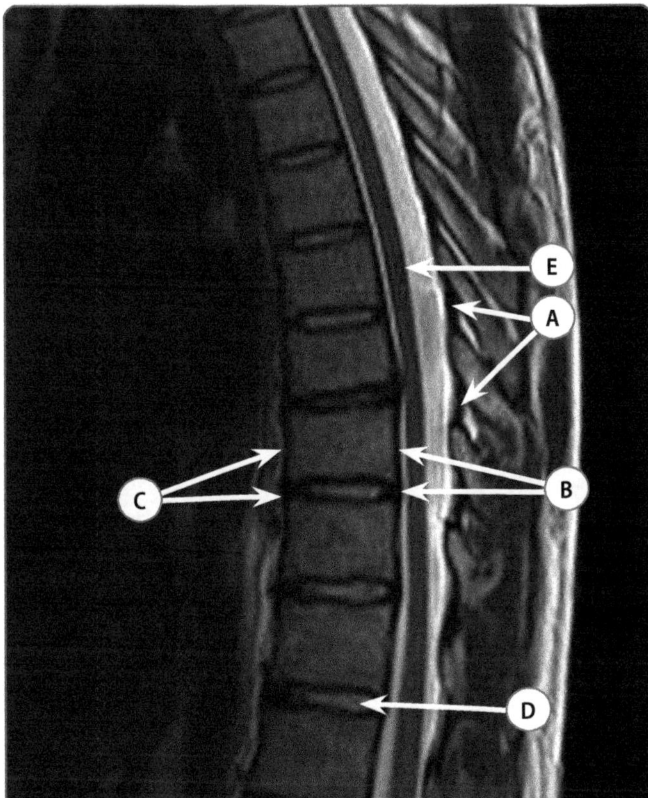

Case 6.6

QUESTION		WRITE YOUR ANSWER HERE
A	Name the structure labelled A.	
B	Name the structure labelled B.	
C	Name the structure labelled C.	
D	Name the structure labelled D.	
E	Name the structure labelled E.	

Case 6.7

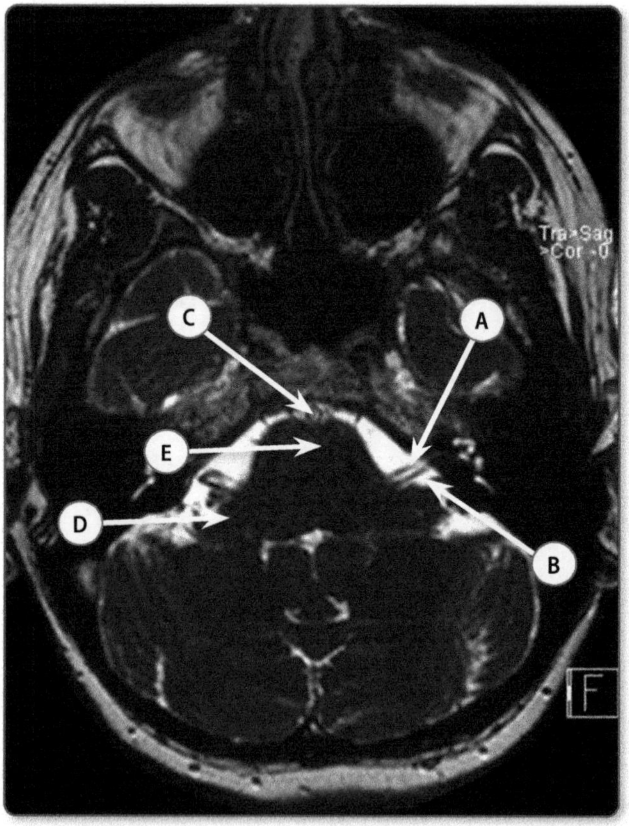

Case 6.7

QUESTION		WRITE YOUR ANSWER HERE
A	Name the structure labelled A.	
B	Name the structure labelled B.	
C	Name the structure labelled C.	
D	Name the structure labelled D.	
E	Name the structure labelled E.	

Case 6.8

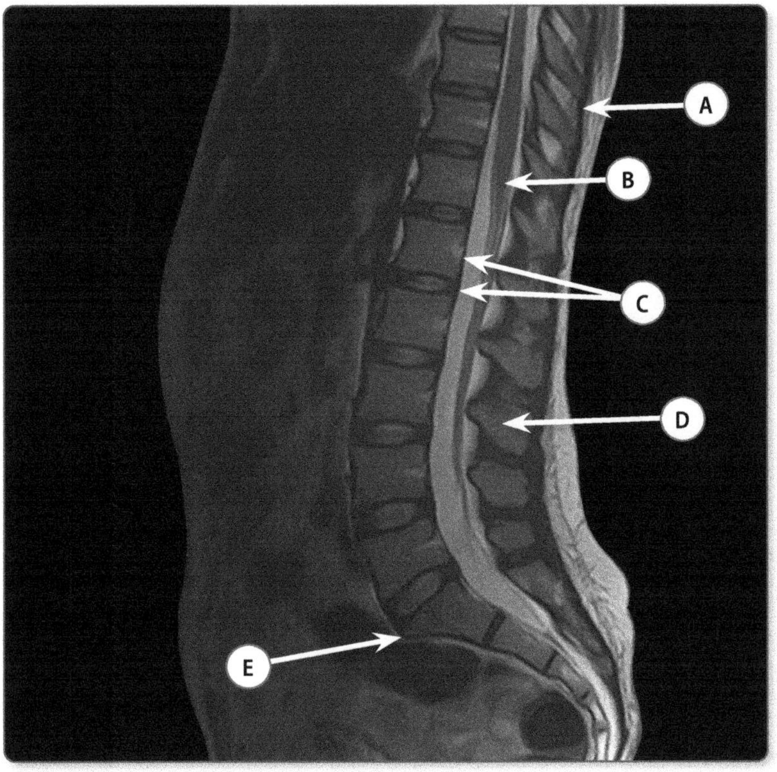

Case 6.8

QUESTION		WRITE YOUR ANSWER HERE
A	Name the structure labelled A.	
B	Name the structure labelled B.	
C	Name the structure labelled C.	
D	Name the structure labelled D.	
E	Name the structure labelled E.	

Case 6.9

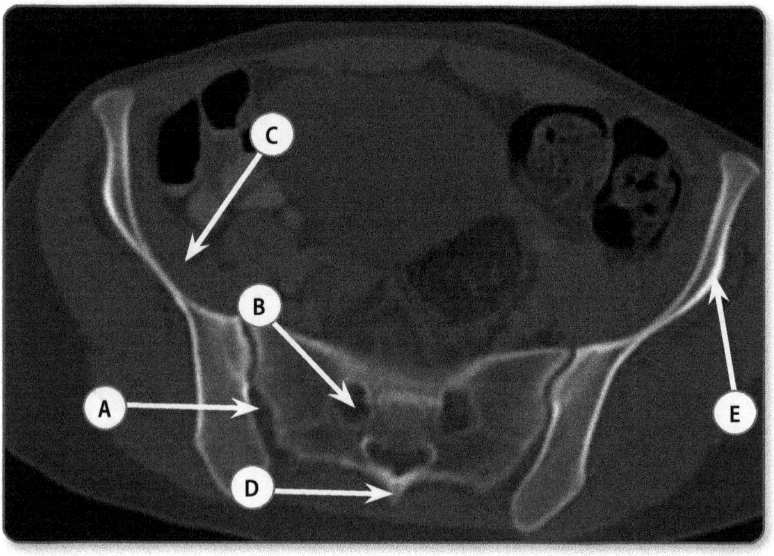

Case 6.9

QUESTION		WRITE YOUR ANSWER HERE
A	Name the structure labelled A.	
B	Name the structure labelled B.	
C	Name the structure labelled C.	
D	Name the structure labelled D.	
E	Name the structure labelled E.	

Case 6.10

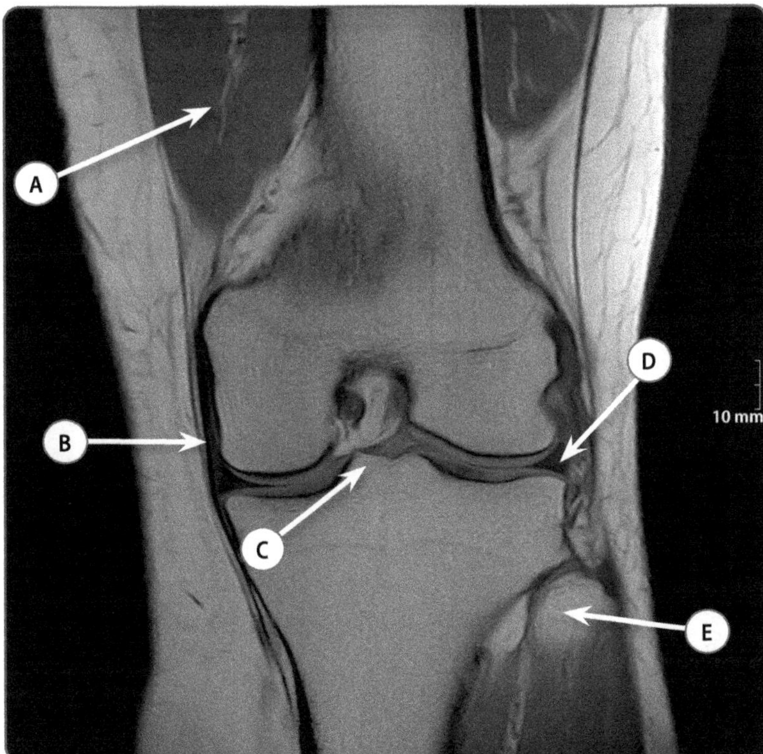

Case 6.10

QUESTION		WRITE YOUR ANSWER HERE
A	Name the structure labelled A.	
B	Name the structure labelled B.	
C	Name the structure labelled C.	
D	Name the structure labelled D.	
E	Name the structure labelled E.	

Case 6.11

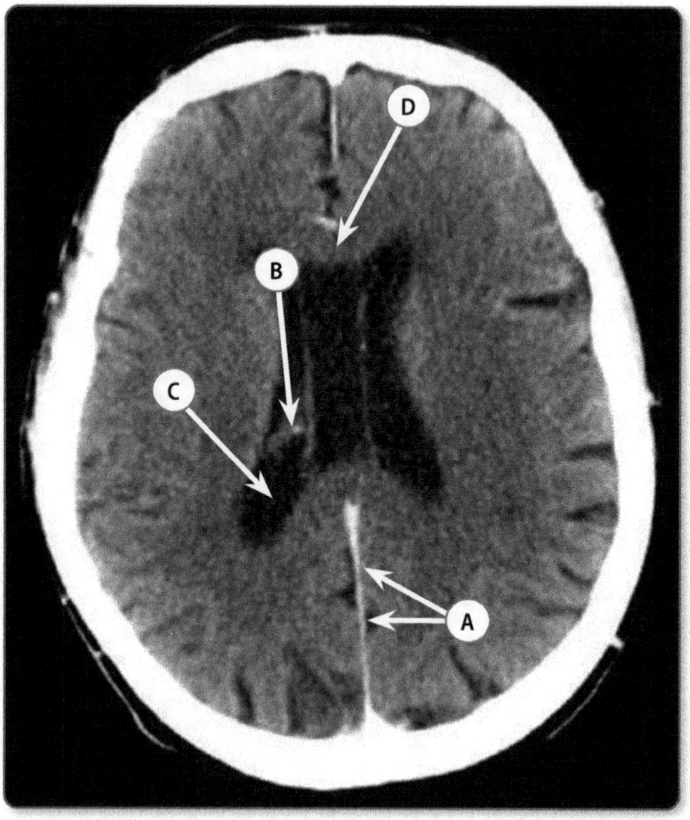

Case 6.11

QUESTION		WRITE YOUR ANSWER HERE
A	Name the structure labelled A.	
B	Name the structure labelled B.	
C	Name the structure labelled C.	
D	Name the structure labelled D.	
E	Which normal variant is demonstrated?	

Case 6.12

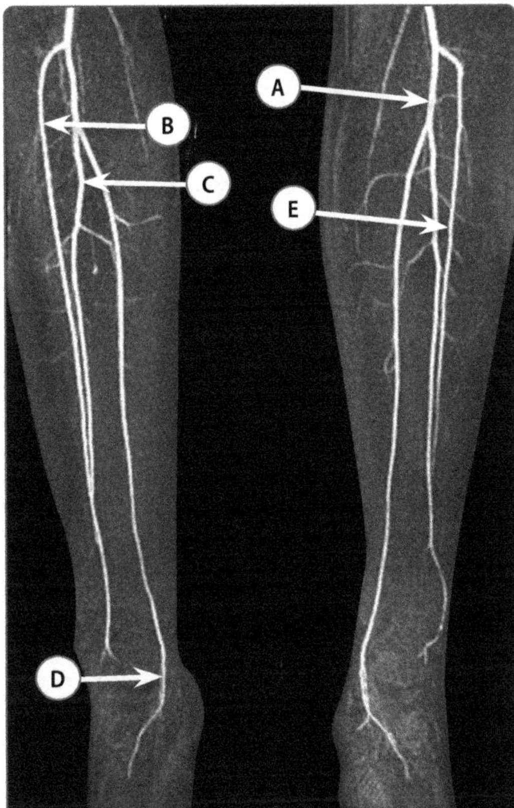

Case 6.12

QUESTION		WRITE YOUR ANSWER HERE
A	Name the structure labelled A.	
B	Name the structure labelled B.	
C	Name the structure labelled C.	
D	Name the structure labelled D.	
E	Name the structure labelled E.	

Case 6.13

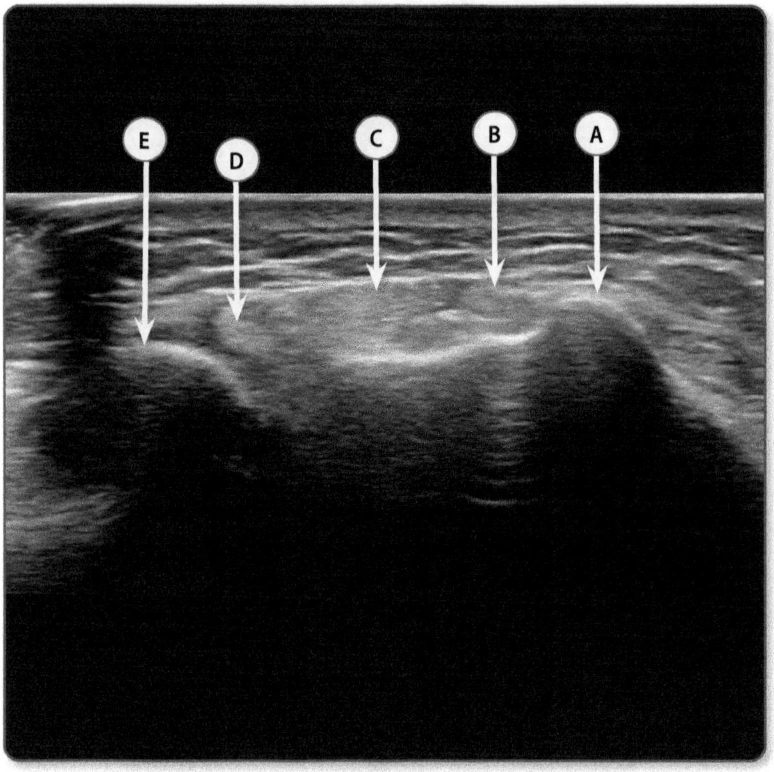

Case 6.13

QUESTION		WRITE YOUR ANSWER HERE
A	Name the structure labelled A.	
B	Name the structure labelled B.	
C	Name the structure labelled C.	
D	Name the structure labelled D.	
E	Name the structure labelled E.	

Case 6.14

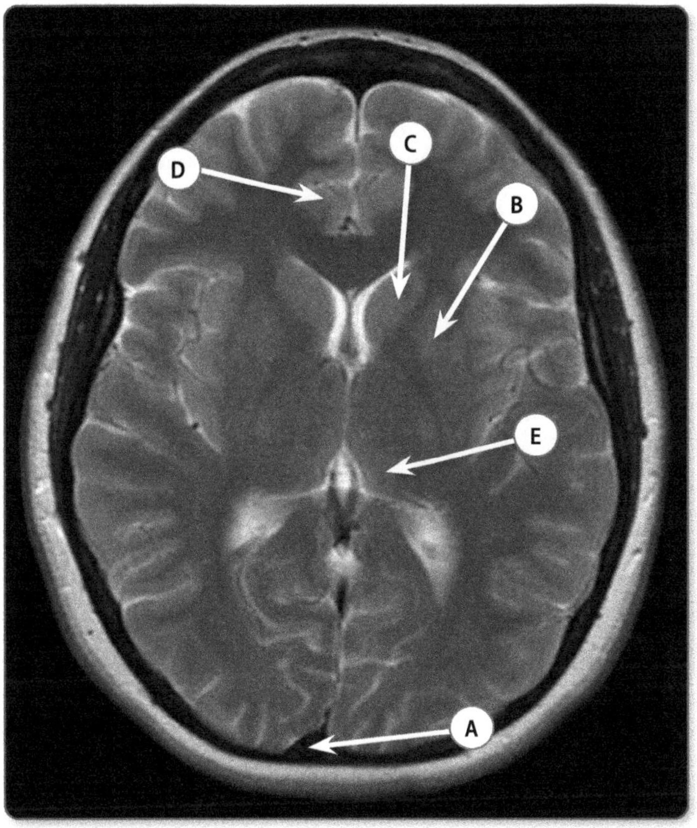

Case 6.14

QUESTION		WRITE YOUR ANSWER HERE
A	Name the structure labelled A.	
B	Name the structure labelled B.	
C	Name the structure labelled C.	
D	Name the structure labelled D.	
E	Name the structure labelled E.	

Case 6.15

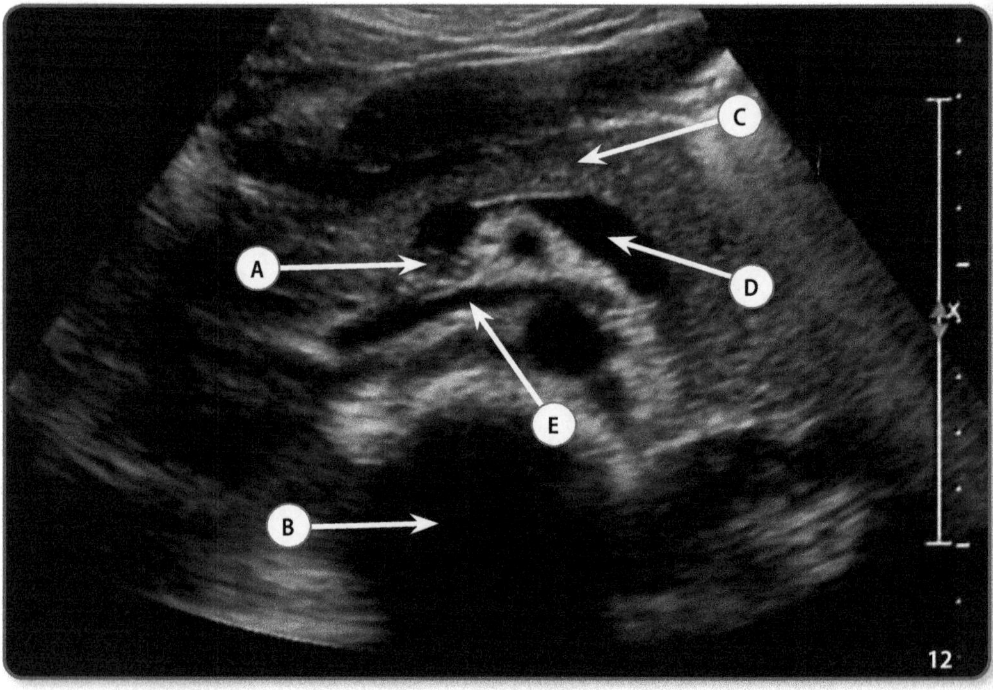

Case 6.15

QUESTION		WRITE YOUR ANSWER HERE
A	Name the structure labelled A.	
B	Name the structure labelled B.	
C	Name the structure labelled C.	
D	Name the structure labelled D.	
E	Name the structure labelled E.	

Case 6.16

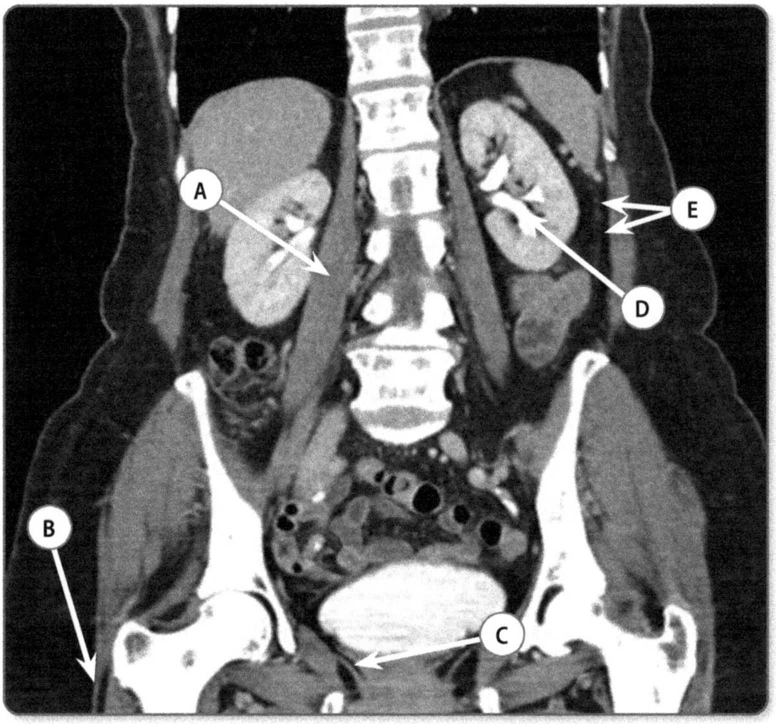

Case 6.16		
QUESTION		WRITE YOUR ANSWER HERE
A	Name the structure labelled A.	
B	Name the structure labelled B.	
C	Name the structure labelled C.	
D	Name the structure labelled D.	
E	Name the structure labelled E.	

Case 6.17

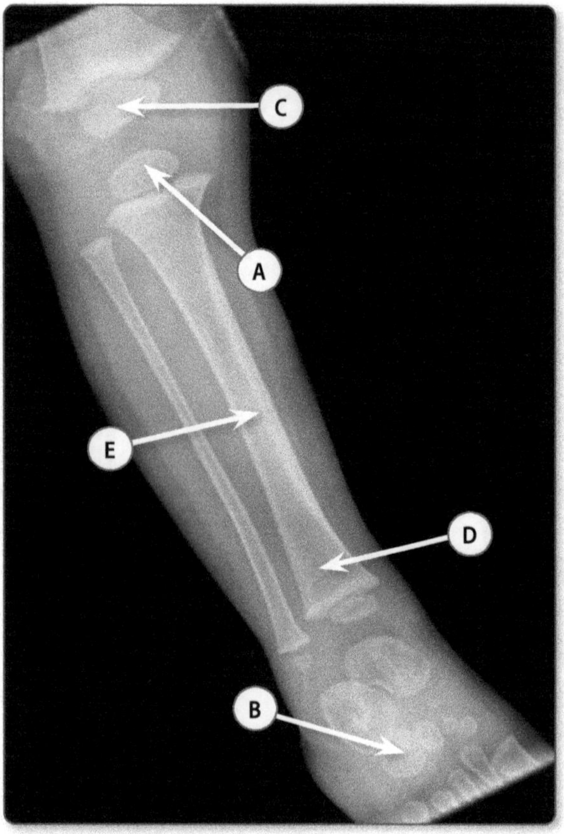

Case 6.17

QUESTION		WRITE YOUR ANSWER HERE
A	Name the structure labelled A.	
B	Name the structure labelled B.	
C	Name the structure labelled C.	
D	Name the structure labelled D.	
E	Name the structure labelled E.	

Case 6.18

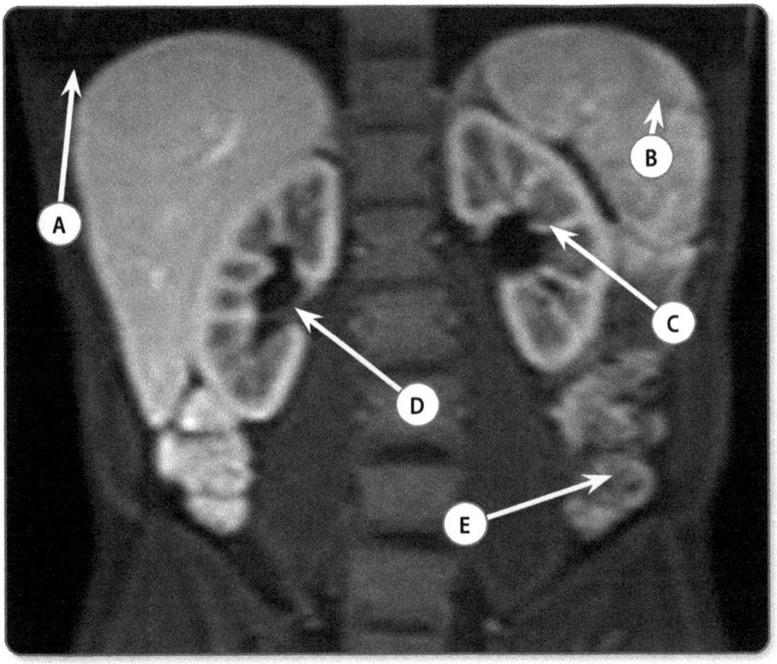

Case 6.18		
QUESTION		WRITE YOUR ANSWER HERE
A	Name the structure labelled A.	
B	Name the structure labelled B.	
C	Name the structure labelled C.	
D	Name the structure labelled D.	
E	Name the structure labelled E.	

Case 6.19

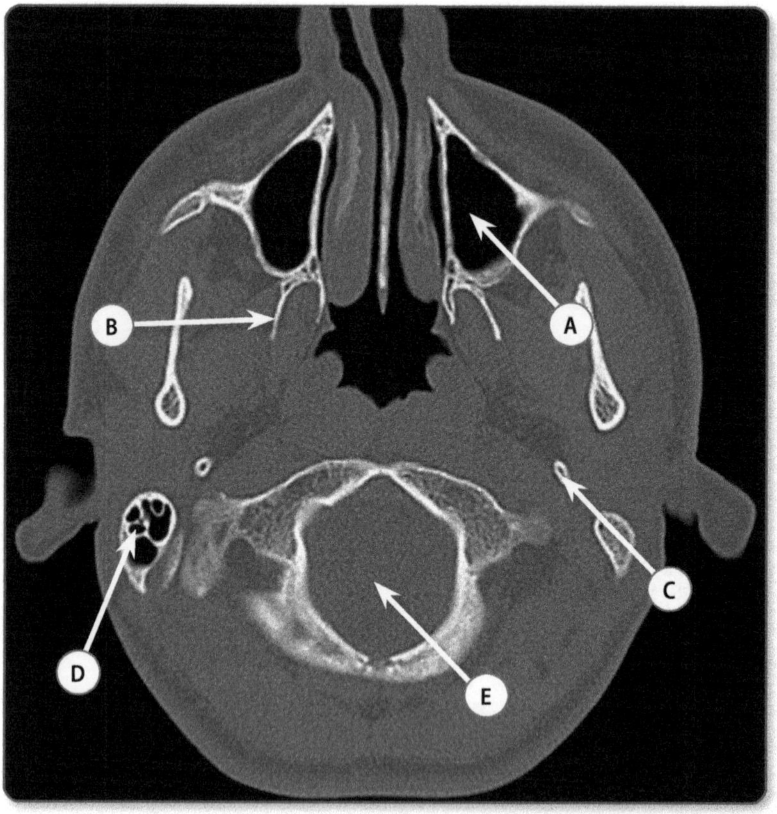

Case 6.19

QUESTION		WRITE YOUR ANSWER HERE
A	Name the structure labelled A.	
B	Name the structure labelled B.	
C	Name the structure labelled C.	
D	Name the structure labelled D.	
E	Name the structure labelled E.	

Case 6.20

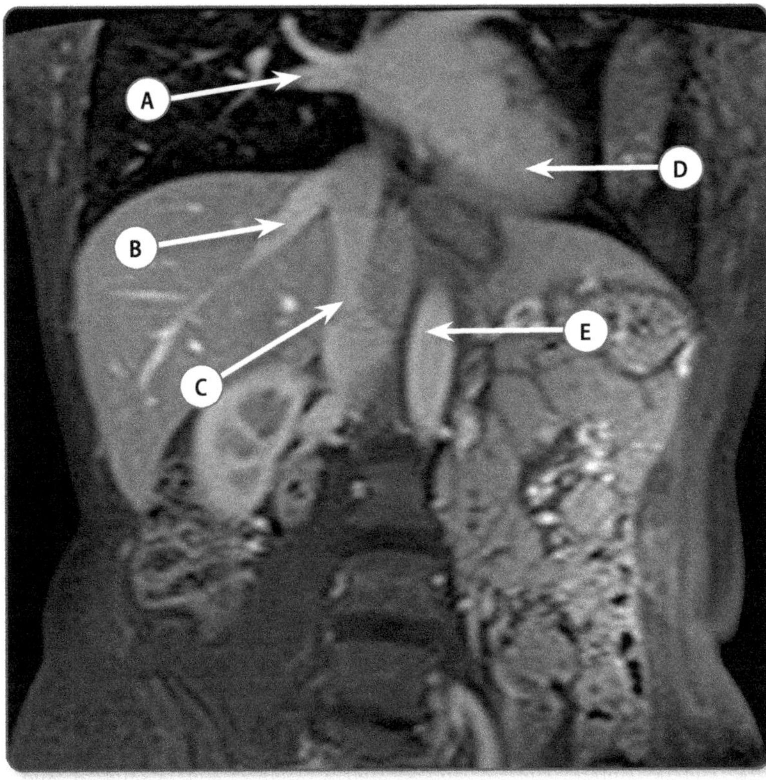

Case 6.20

QUESTION		WRITE YOUR ANSWER HERE
A	Name the structure labelled A.	
B	Name the structure labelled B.	
C	Name the structure labelled C.	
D	Name the structure labelled D.	
E	Name the structure labelled E.	

Answers

Case 6.1

A Right posterior cerebral artery

B Right posterior inferior cerebellar artery (PICA)

C Right anterior inferior cerebellar artery (AICA)

D Left superior cerebellar artery

E Thalamostriate/thalamoperforating arteries

Angiogram of the right vertebral artery.

For further discussion, see Chapter 1, Cases 1.14–1.17.

Case 6.2

A Intrahepatic inferior vena cava

B Right renal artery

C Abdominal aorta

D Jejunal loop

E Left psoas major

Coronal abdominal MRI.

For further discussion, see Chapter 3, Cases 3.10 and 3.12.

Case 6.3

A Superior mesenteric artery

B Upper pole of right kidney

C Pancreatic tail

D Splenic vein

E Left renal vein

Axial contrast-enhanced CT.

For further discussion, see Chapter 3, Case 3.3.

Case 6.4

A Left lingual artery

B Left facial artery

C Petrous portion of left internal carotid artery

D Cavernous portion of left internal carotid artery

E Supraclinoid/intracranial portion of left internal carotid artery

MR angiogram of the neck.

For further discussion, see Chapter 1, Cases 1.14–1.17.

Case 6.5

A Left main bronchus

B Descending aorta

C Left scapula

D Left main pulmonary artery

E Body of sternum

Axial CT of the chest.

For further discussion, see Chapter 2, Cases 2.19–2.25.

Case 6.6

A Ligamentum flavum

B Posterior longitudinal ligament

C Anterior longitudinal ligament

D Intervertebral disc

E Thoracic spinal cord

Sagittal MRI of the spine.

For further discussion see Chapter 4, Cases 4.19–4.31.

Case 6.7

A Left facial nerve

B Left vestibulocochlear nerve

C Basilar artery

D Right middle cerebellar peduncle

E Pons

Axial T2-weighted MRI of the cerebropontine angle.

For further discussion see Chapter 1, Cases 1.1–1.19.

Case 6.8

A Supraspinous ligament

B Conus medullaris

C Posterior longitudinal ligament

D L3 spinous process

E Sacral promontory

MR lumbar spine.

Weir J, Abrahams P, Spratt J, et al. Imaging Atlas of Human Anatomy, 6th edition. UK: Elsevier, 2021:60.

Butler P, Mitchell AWM, Healy JC. Applied Radiological Anatomy, 2nd edition. Cambridge: Cambridge University Press, 2012:82–86.

Case 6.9

A Right sacroiliac joint

B Right sacral foramen

C Right iliacus

D Spinous process of S1

E Left iliac blade

Axial CT of the sacroiliac joint.

The sacroiliac joint is a synovial joint formed by the articular surface of the sacrum and the articular surface of the iliac bone. Unlike most synovial joints, the surfaces that make up the sacroiliac joint are irregular.

The sacrum is composed of five vertebrae which are fused together in the mature skeleton. The sacral foramina represent the intervertebral foramina. The bone is expanded laterally to these foramina to form the lateral masses of the sacrum.

Iliacus arises from the inner surfaces of the ileum and fuses with the psoas to form the iliopsoas which inserts into the lesser trochanter of the femur.

Ryan S, McNicholas M, Eustace SJ. Anatomy for Diagnostic Imaging, 3rd edition. Edinburgh: Saunders, 2010:290–291.

Case 6.10

A Vastus medialis

B Medial collateral ligament

C Medial intercondylar tubercle (eminence)

D Lateral meniscus

E Fibular head

MR knee right.

Weir J, Abrahams P, Spratt J, et al. Imaging Atlas of Human Anatomy, 6th edition. UK: Elsevier, 2021:231.

Butler P, Mitchell AWM, Healy JC. Applied Radiological Anatomy, 2nd edition. Cambridge: Cambridge University Press, 2012:345.

Case 6.11

A Falx cerebri

B Choroid plexus in the right lateral ventricle

C Occipital horn of the right lateral ventricle

D Genu of the corpus callosum

E Cavum septum pellucidum

Axial CT of the brain.

Cavum septum pellucidum is a variant of the septum pellucidum where there is a separation between the septal laminae.

For further discussion see Chapter 1, Cases 1.7–1.9.

Case 6.12

A Left tibioperoneal trunk

B Right anterior tibial artery

C Right peroneal artery

D Right posterior tibial artery

E Left anterior tibial artery

Lower limb MR angiogram.

For further discussion see Chapter 4, Cases 4.16–4.18.

Case 6.13

A Lister's tubercle

B Extensor pollicis longus

C Extensor digitorum

D Extensor digiti minimi

E Ulna

US wrist right extensor compartments 3, 4 and 5.

Weir J, Abrahams P, Spratt J, et al. Imaging Atlas of Human Anatomy, 6th edition. UK: Elsevier, 2021:85.

Butler P, Mitchell AWM, Healy JC. Applied Radiological Anatomy, 2nd edition. Cambridge: Cambridge University Press, 2012:313.

Case 6.14

A Superior sagittal sinus

B Left lentiform nucleus

C Head of left caudate

D Right cingulate gyrus

E Left thalamus

Axial CT of the brain at the level of the basal ganglia.

For further discussion see Chapter 1, Cases 1.7–1.9.

Case 6.15

A Uncinate process of pancreas

B Vertebral body

C Body of pancreas

D Splenic vein

E Left renal vein

Transverse image from an abdominal ultrasound.

For further discussion see Chapter 3, Case 3.3.

Case 6.16

A Right psoas

B Right iliotibial tract

C Right levator ani

D Infundibulum of left lower pole calyx

E Left lateral conal fascia

Coronal CT urogram.

For further discussion see Chapter 3, Cases 3.13 and 3.53.

Case 6.17

A Right proximal tibial epiphysis

B Right cuboid

C Right distal femoral epiphysis

D Right distal tibial metaphysis

E Right tibial diaphysis

Anteroposterior radiograph of the right tibia/fibula (child).

For further discussion see Chapter 4, Cases 4.2–4.8.

Case 6.18

A Right costophrenic angle

B Spleen

C Column of Bertin, interpolar region left kidney

D Right renal pelvis

E Descending colon

Fat-sat coronal MRI of the abdomen.

For further discussion see Chapter 3, Case 3.9.

Case 6.19

A Left maxillary antrum

B Right lateral pterygoid plate

C Left styloid process

D Right mastoid air cells

E Foramen magnum

Axial CT of the head.

For further discussion see Chapter 1, Cases 1.32–1.38.

Case 6.20

A Right inferior pulmonary vein

B Right hepatic vein

C Intrahepatic inferior vena cava

D Left ventricle

E Abdominal aorta

Coronal MRI of the abdomen.

For further discussion see Chapter 3, Case 3.39.

Chapter 7

Practice paper 3

Case 7.1

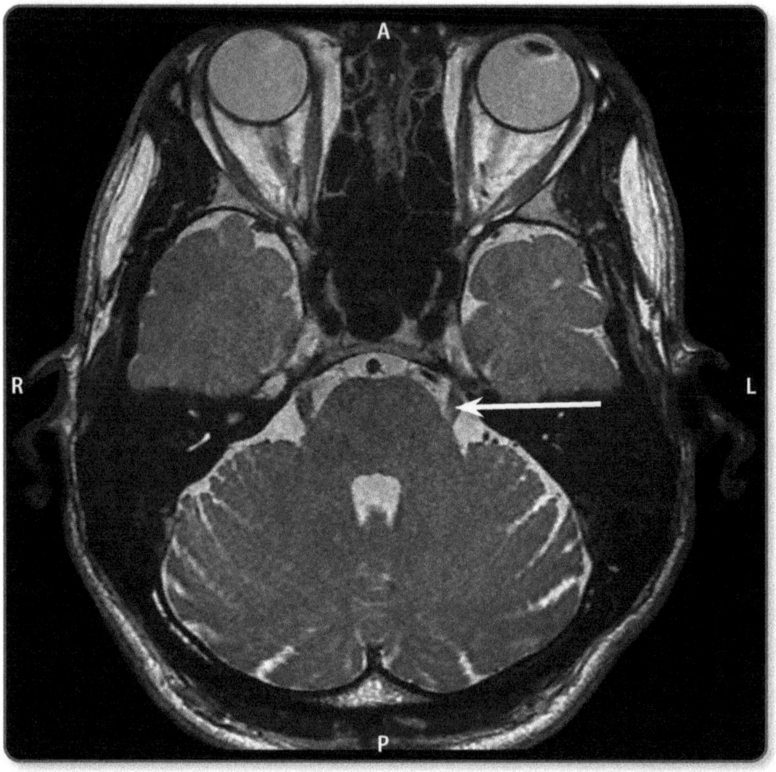

Case 7.1	
QUESTION	WRITE YOUR ANSWER HERE
Name the arrowed structure.	

Case 7.2

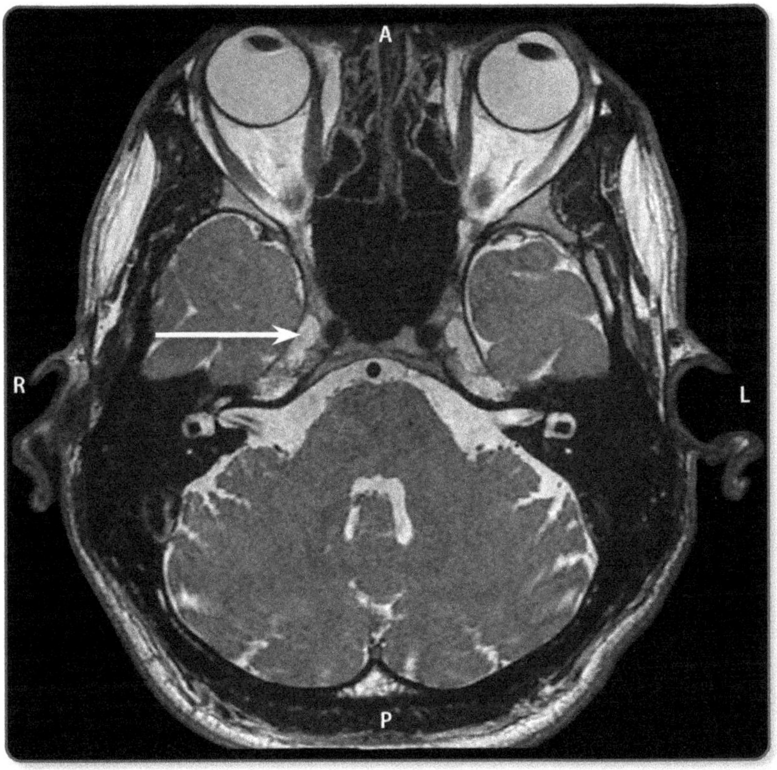

Case 7.2

QUESTION	WRITE YOUR ANSWER HERE
Name the arrowed structure.	

Case 7.3

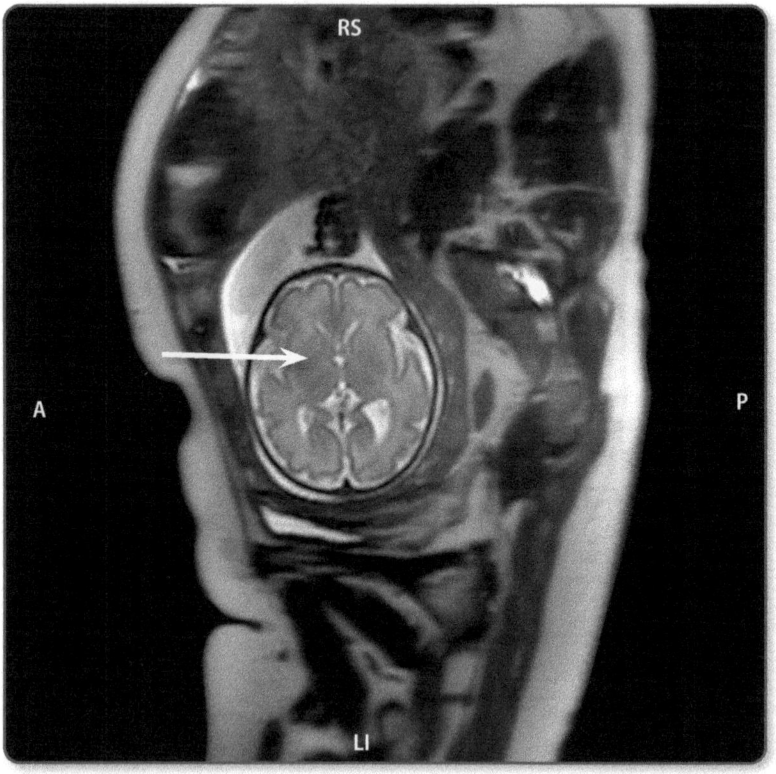

Case 7.3

QUESTION	WRITE YOUR ANSWER HERE
Name the arrowed structure.	

Case 7.4

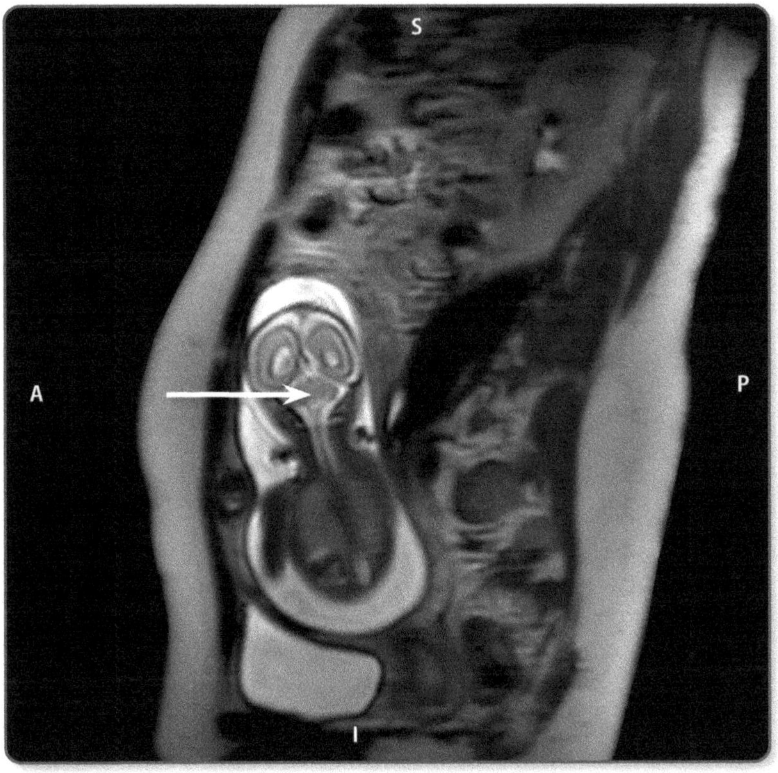

Case 7.4	
QUESTION	WRITE YOUR ANSWER HERE
Name the arrowed structure.	

Case 7.5

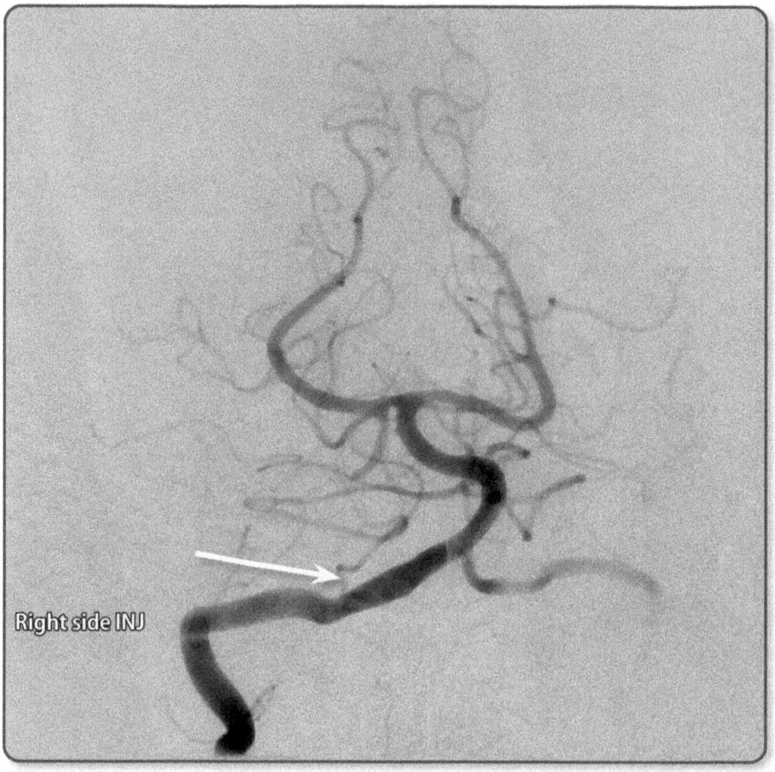

Case 7.5

QUESTION	WRITE YOUR ANSWER HERE
Name the arrowed structure.	

Case 7.6

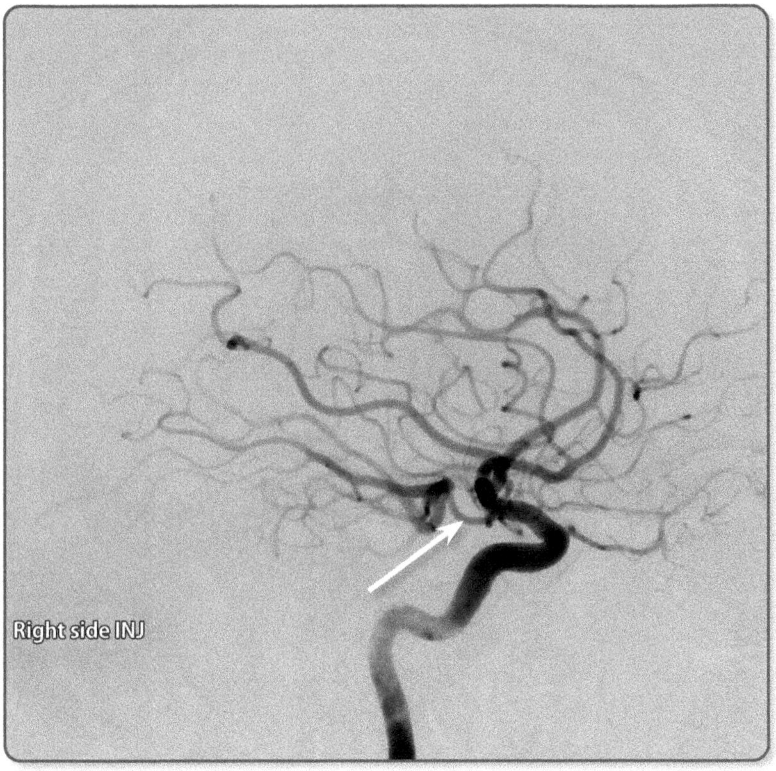

Case 7.6

QUESTION	WRITE YOUR ANSWER HERE
Name the arrowed structure.	

Case 7.7

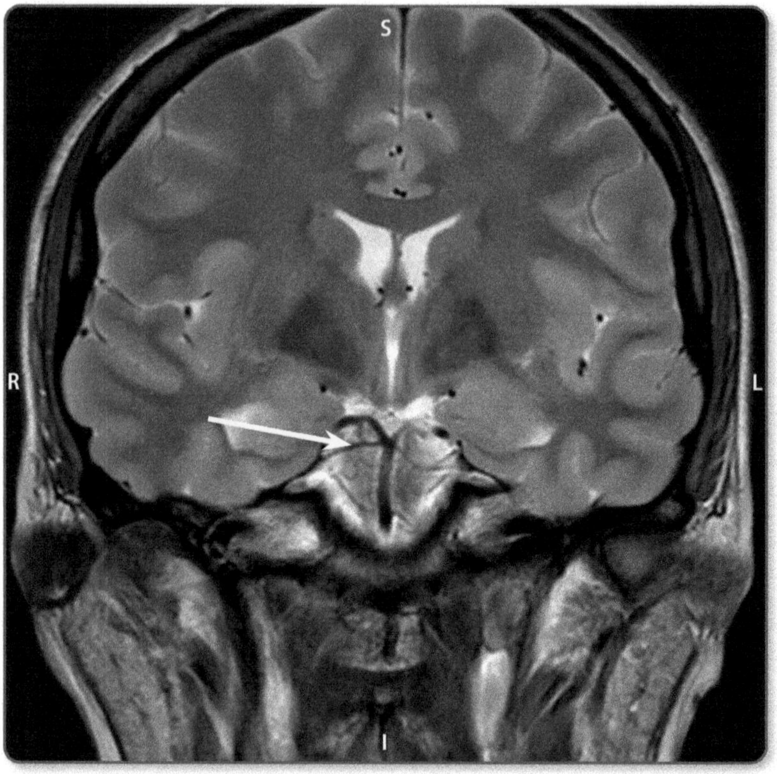

Case 7.7

QUESTION	WRITE YOUR ANSWER HERE
Name the arrowed structure.	

Case 7.8

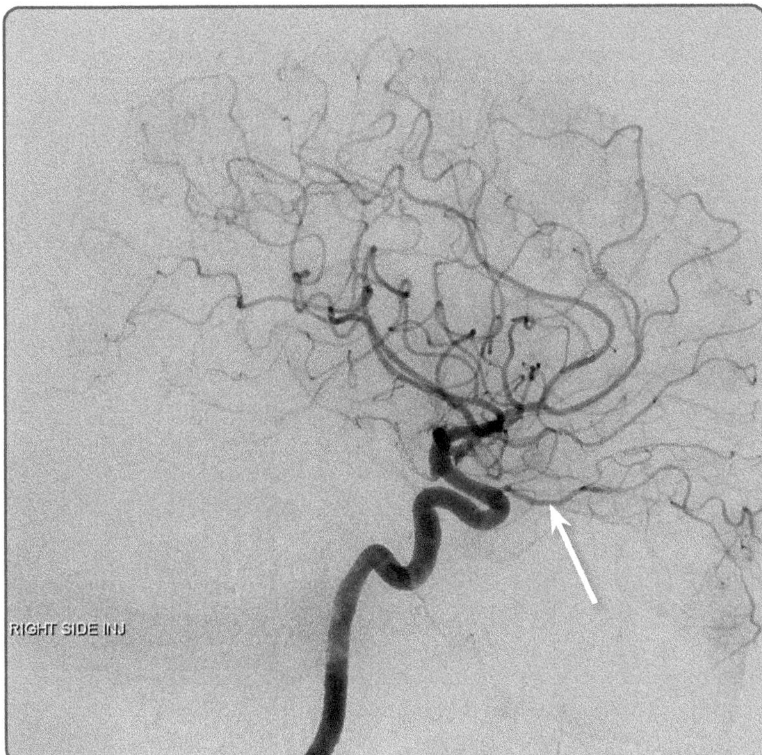

Case 7.8

QUESTION	WRITE YOUR ANSWER HERE
Name the arrowed structure.	

Case 7.9

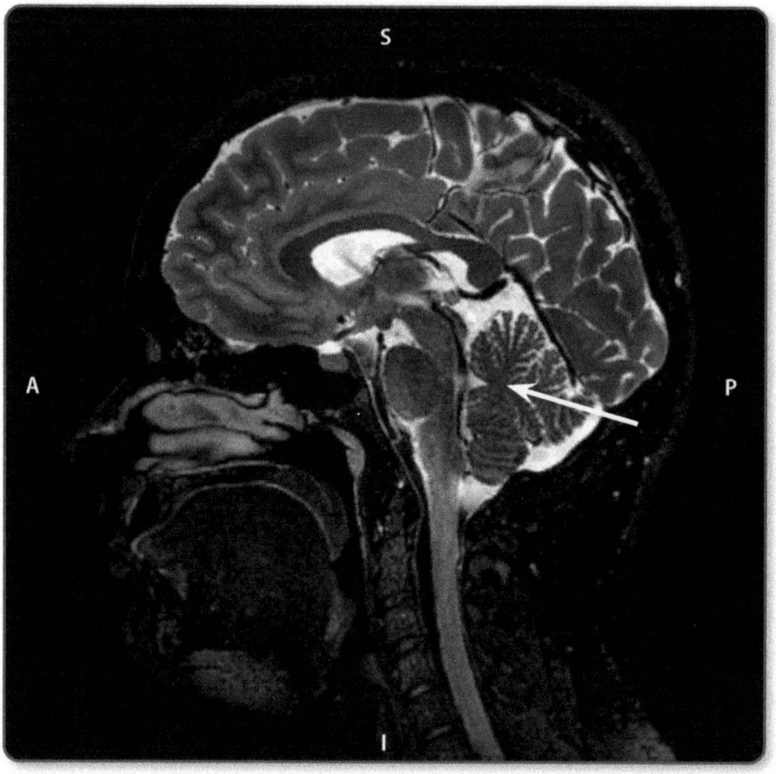

Case 7.9

QUESTION	WRITE YOUR ANSWER HERE
Name the arrowed structure.	

Case 7.10

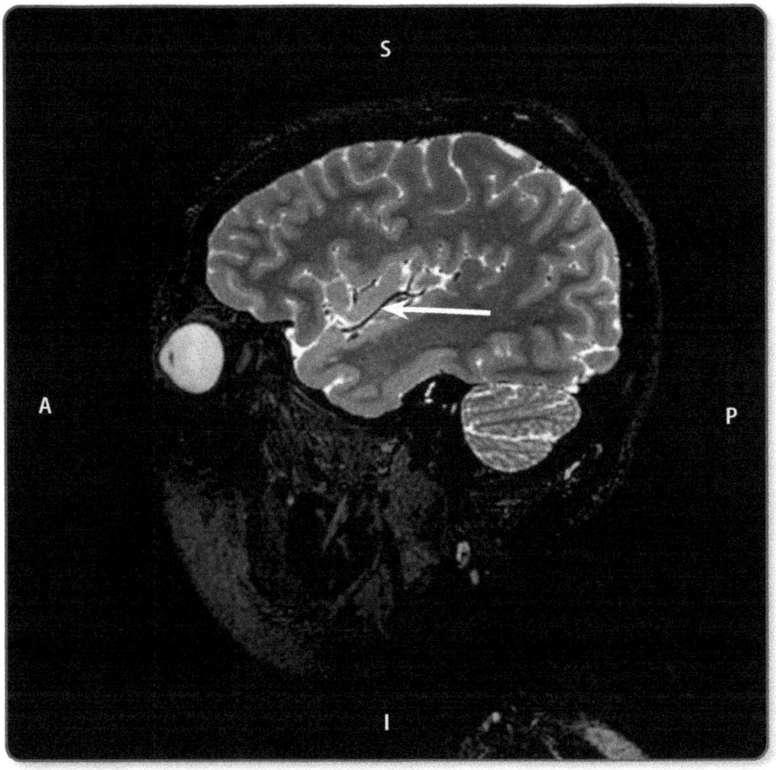

Case 7.10	
QUESTION	WRITE YOUR ANSWER HERE
Name the arrowed structure.	

Case 7.11

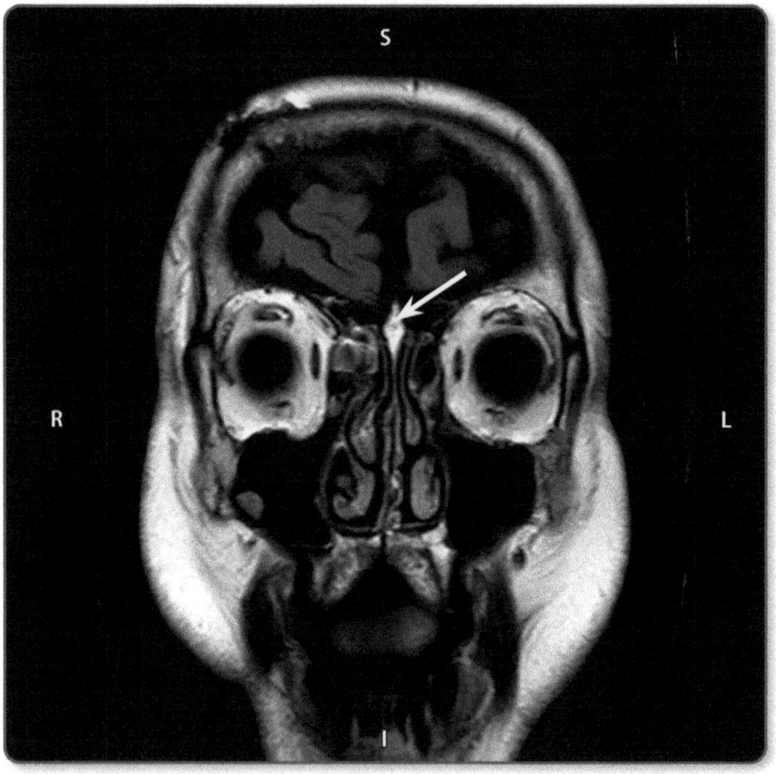

Case 7.11

QUESTION	WRITE YOUR ANSWER HERE
Name the arrowed structure.	

Case 7.12

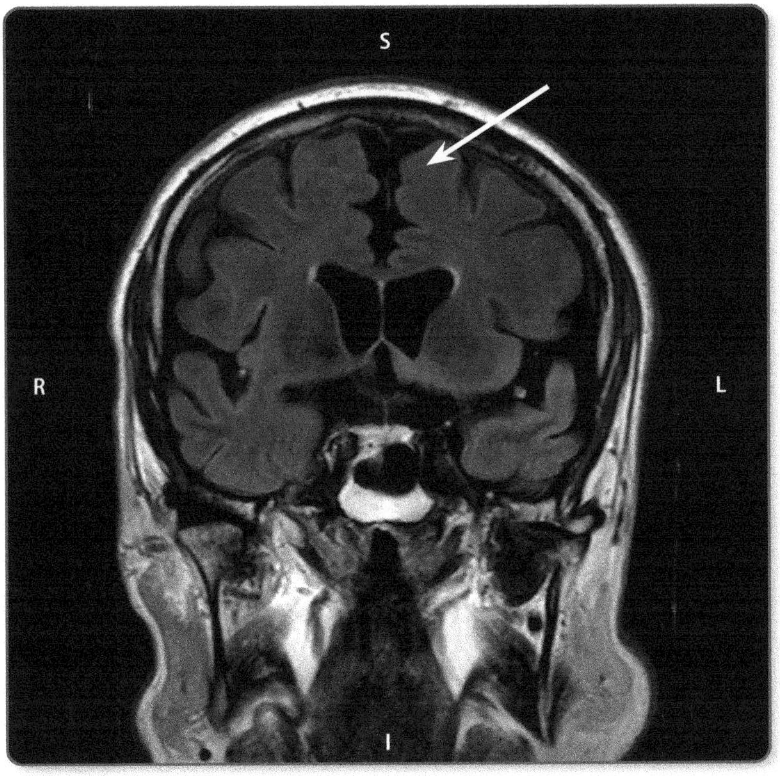

Case 7.12

QUESTION	WRITE YOUR ANSWER HERE
Name the arrowed structure.	

Case 7.13

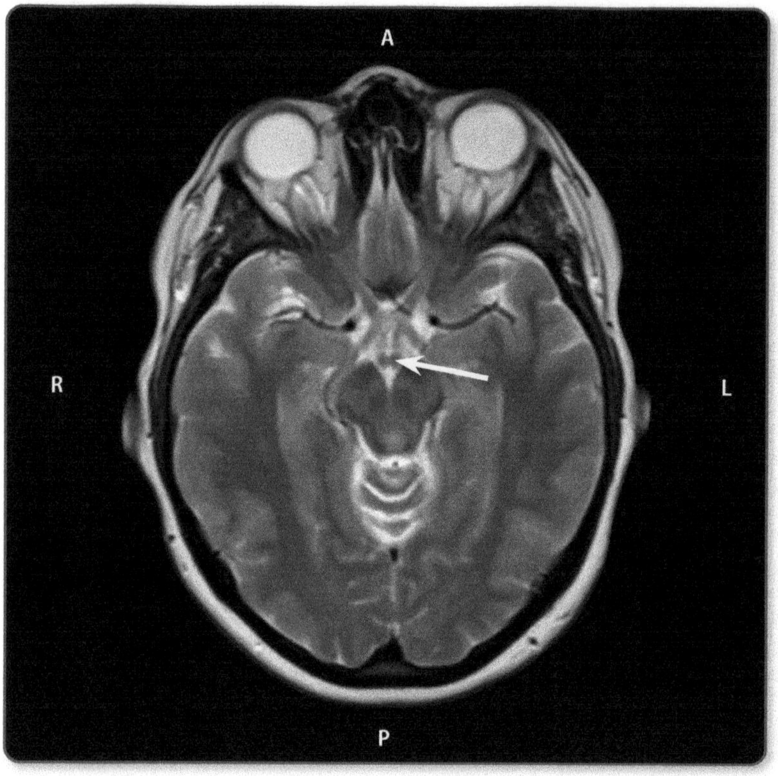

Case 7.13

QUESTION	WRITE YOUR ANSWER HERE
Name the arrowed structure.	

Case 7.14

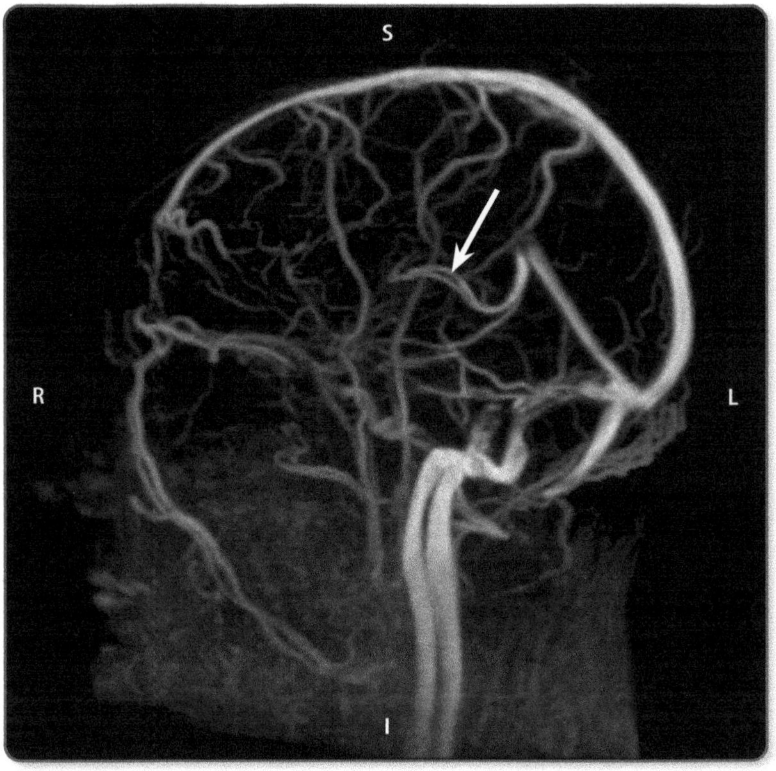

Case 7.14	
QUESTION	WRITE YOUR ANSWER HERE
Name the arrowed structure.	

Case 7.15

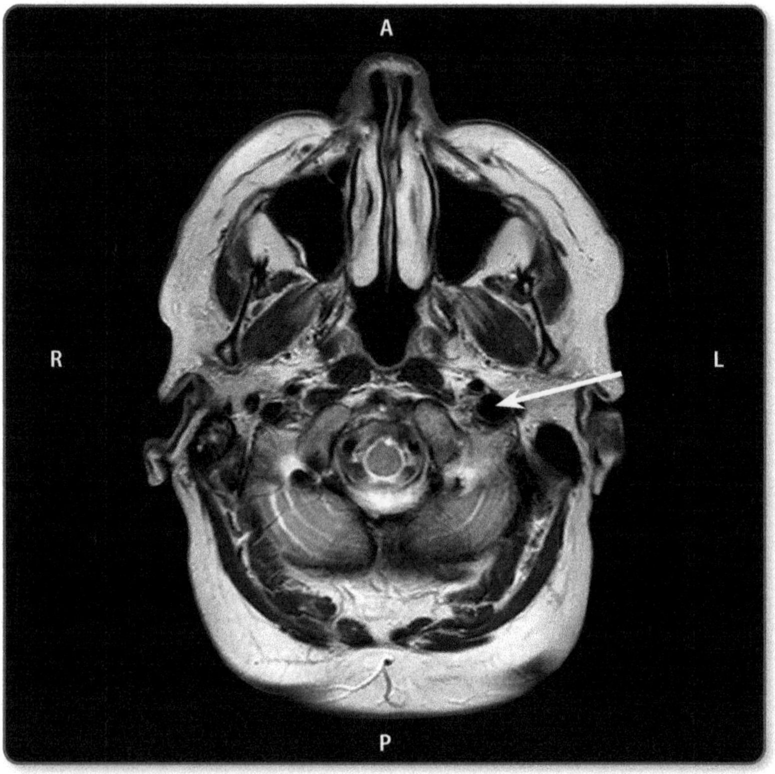

Case 7.15

QUESTION	WRITE YOUR ANSWER HERE
Name the arrowed structure.	

Case 7.16

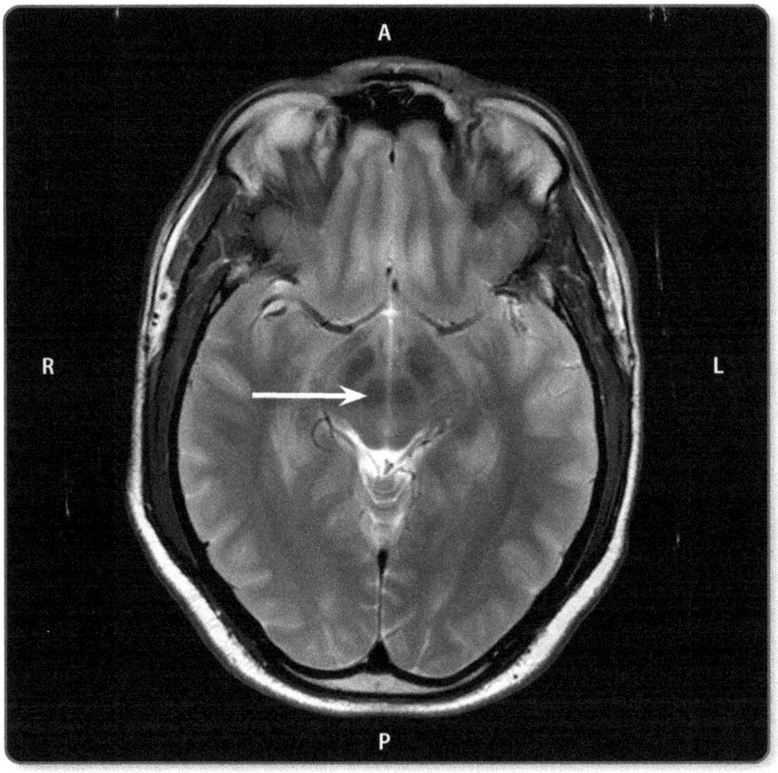

Case 7.16	
QUESTION	WRITE YOUR ANSWER HERE
Name the arrowed structure.	

Case 7.17

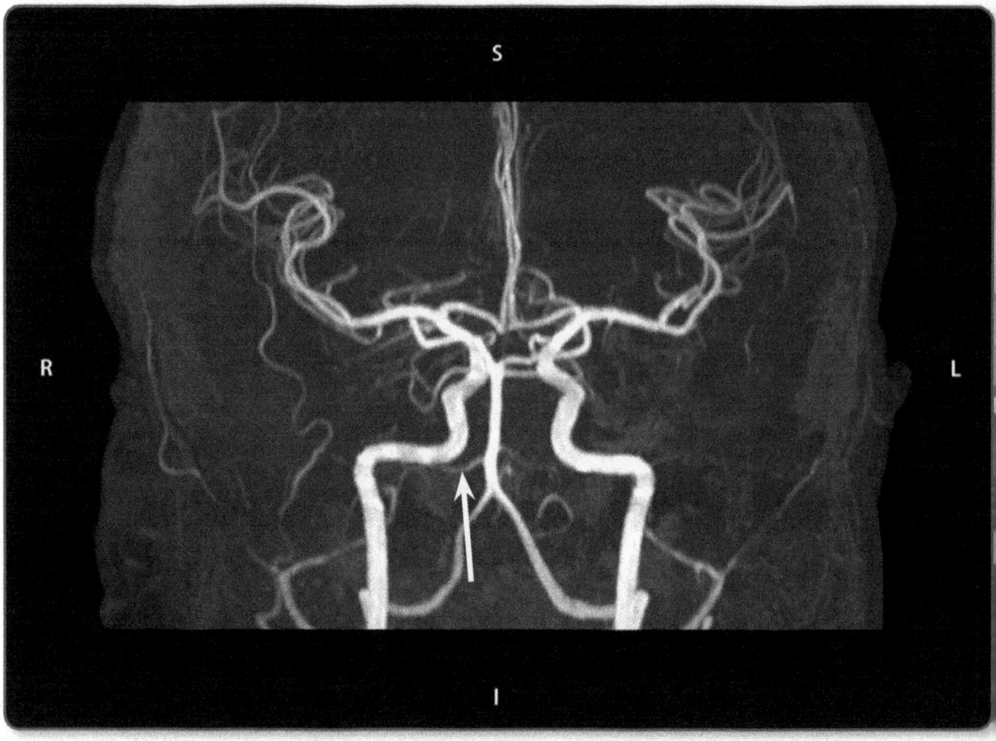

Case 7.17

QUESTION	WRITE YOUR ANSWER HERE
Name the arrowed structure.	

Case 7.18

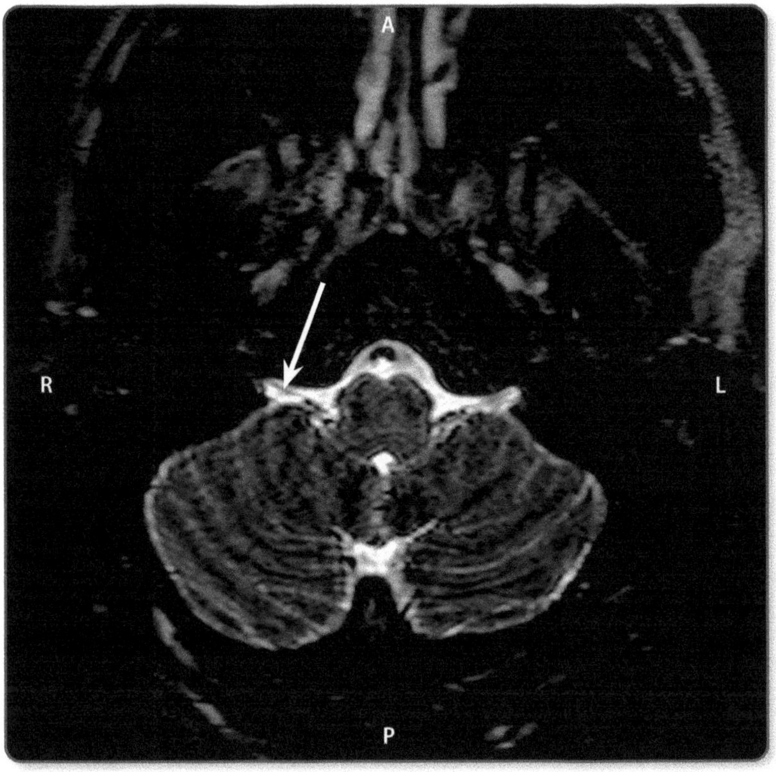

Case 7.18

QUESTION	WRITE YOUR ANSWER HERE
Name the arrowed structure.	

Case 7.19

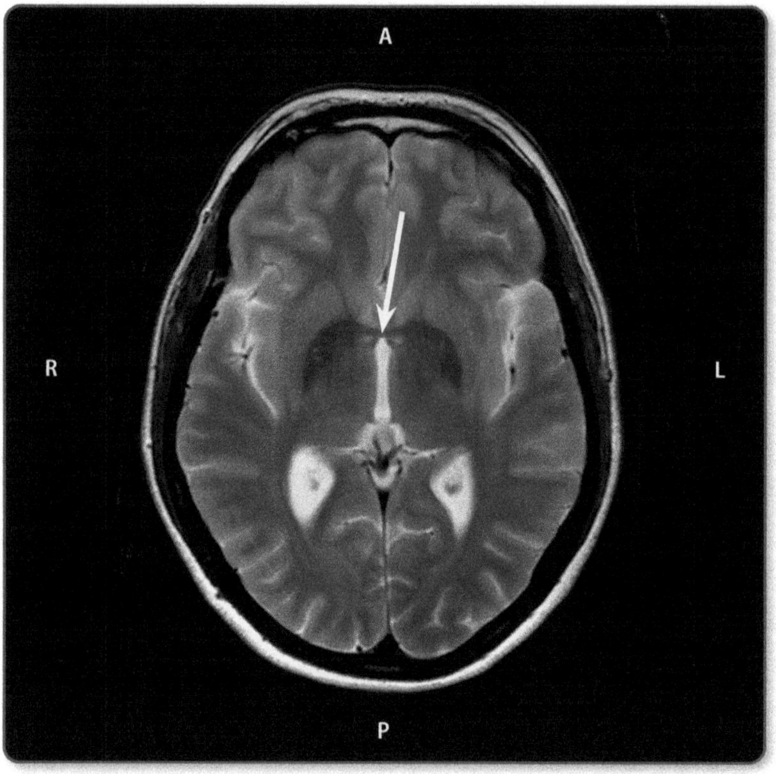

Case 7.19	
QUESTION	WRITE YOUR ANSWER HERE
Name the arrowed structure.	

Case 7.20

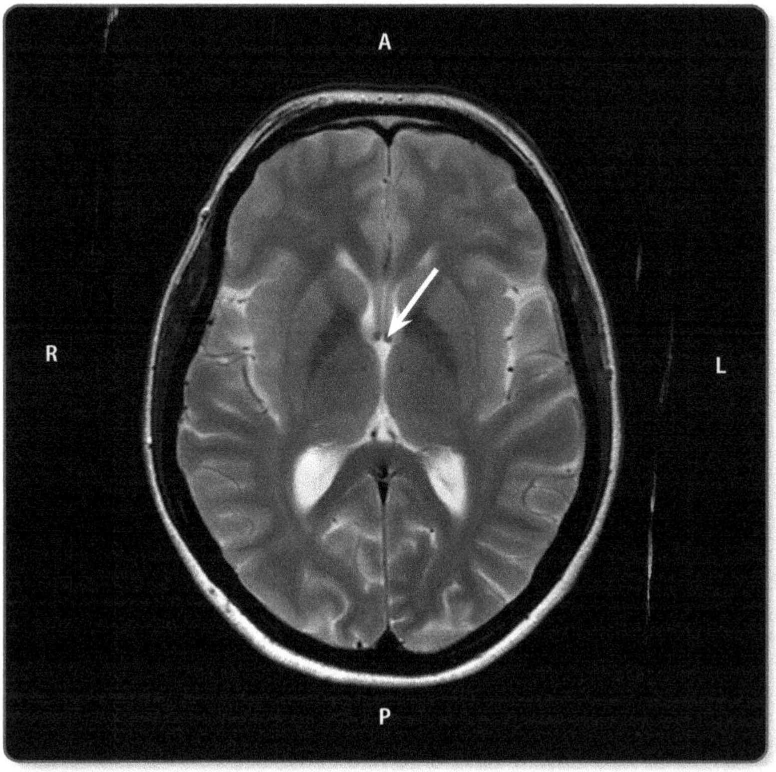

Case 7.20

QUESTION	WRITE YOUR ANSWER HERE
Name the arrowed structure.	

Case 7.21

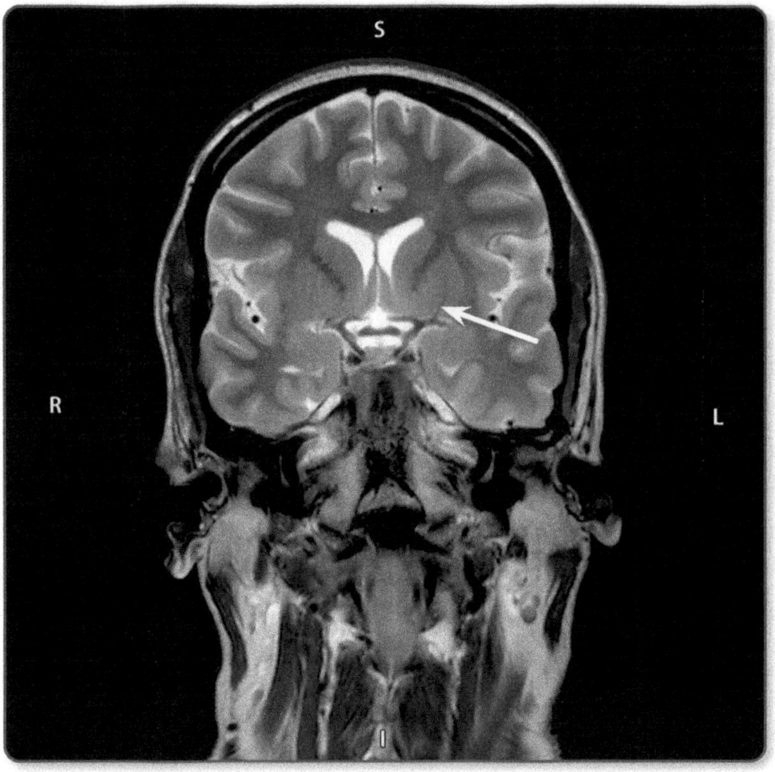

Case 7.21	
QUESTION	WRITE YOUR ANSWER HERE
Name the arrowed structure.	

Case 7.22

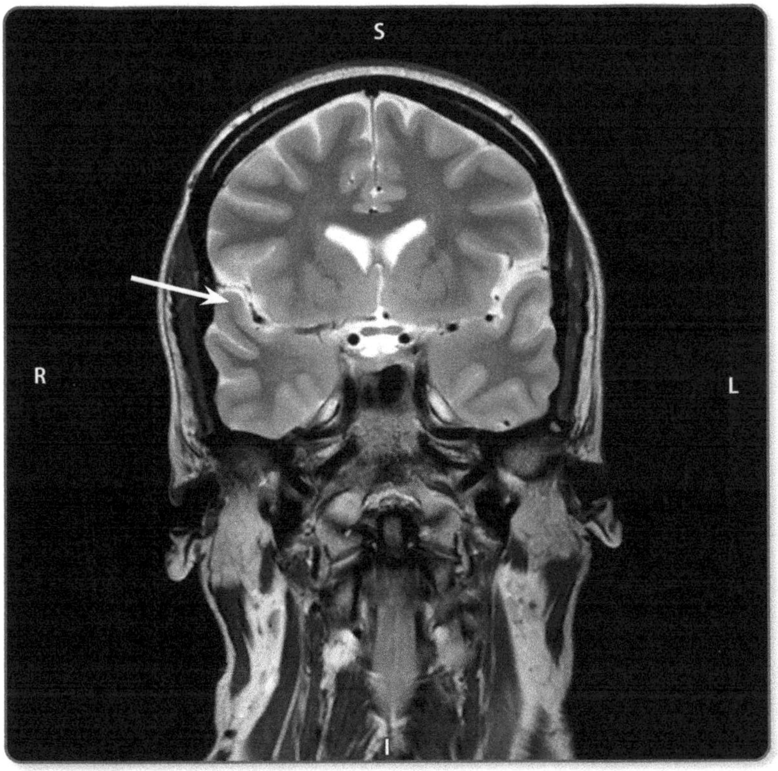

Case 7.22

QUESTION	WRITE YOUR ANSWER HERE
Name the arrowed structure.	

Case 7.23

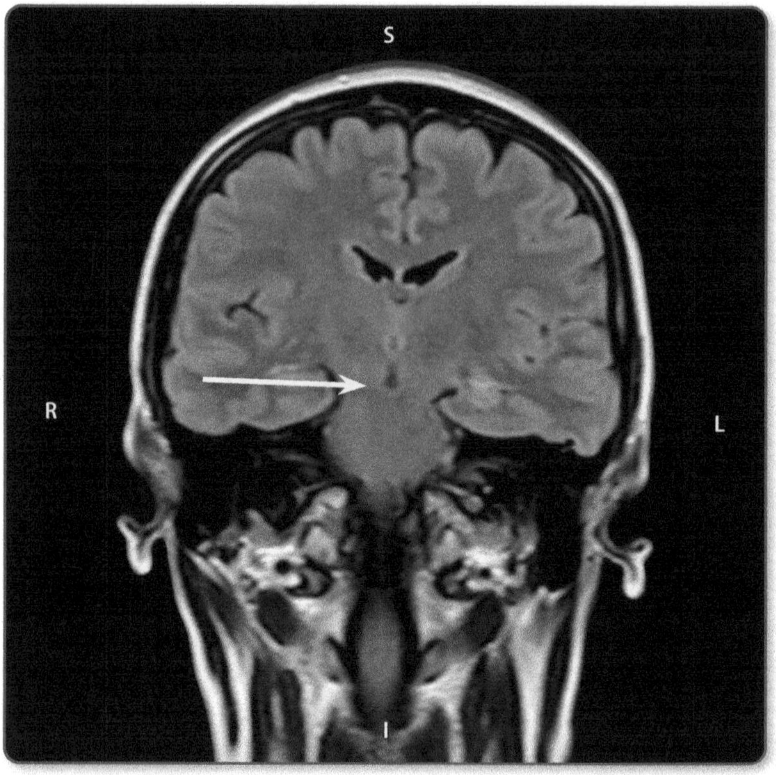

Case 7.23	
QUESTION	WRITE YOUR ANSWER HERE
Name the arrowed structure.	

Case 7.24

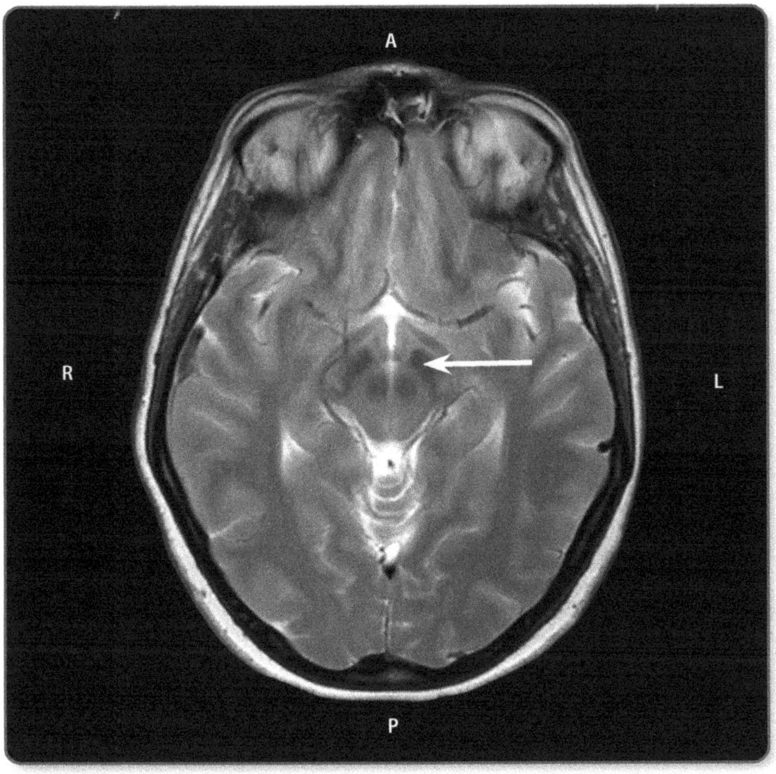

Case 7.24

QUESTION	WRITE YOUR ANSWER HERE
Name the arrowed structure.	

Case 7.25

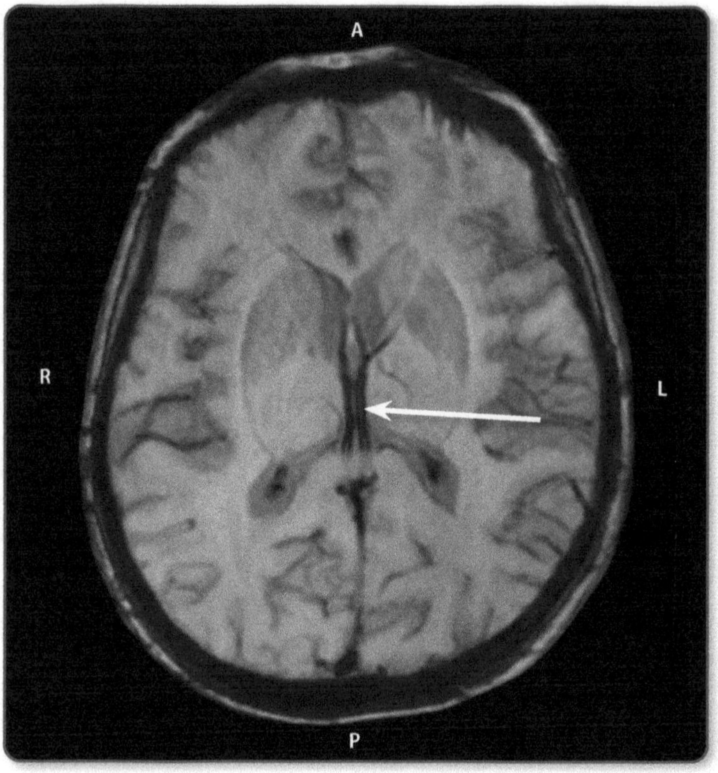

Case 7.25

QUESTION	WRITE YOUR ANSWER HERE
Name the arrowed structure.	

Answers

Case 7.1

Left trigeminal nerve

Case 7.2

Right Meckel's Cave

Case 7.3

Putamen (lentiform nucleus)

Case 7.4

Cerebellum

Case 7.5

Right posterior inferior cerebellar artery (PICA)

Case 7.6

Right posterior communicating artery

Case 7.7

Right superior cerebellar artery (SCA)

Case 7.8

Right ophthalmic artery

Case 7.9

Cerebellar vermis

Case 7.10

Middle cerebral artery (MCA)

Case 7.11

Crista galli

Case 7.12

Left superior frontal gyrus

Case 7.13

Left mammillary body

Case 7.14

Internal cerebral vein

Case 7.15

Left internal jugular vein

Case 7.16

Right red nucleus

Case 7.17

Right anterior inferior cerebellar artery (AICA)

Case 7.18

Right hypoglossal nerve (cranial nerve XII) in right hypoglossal canal

Case 7.19

Anterior commissure

Case 7.20

Left fornix

Case 7.21

Left lenticulostriate artery (arising from left middle cerebral artery).

Case 7.22

Right superior temporal gyrus

Case 7.23

Right cerebral peduncle

Case 7.24

Left subthalamic nucleus

Case 7.25

Left internal cerebral vein

Index

Note: Page numbers in **bold** or *italic* refer to tables or figures respectively.

D

E

F

G

J

K

L

Q

R

S

W

X

Z

EU GSPR Authorised Reprsentative
Logos Europe, 9 rue Nicolas Poussin
1700, La Rochelle, France
Phone: +33 (0) 6 67 93 73 78
E-mail: contact@logoseurope.eu

www.ingramcontent.com/pod-product-compliance
Ingram Content Group UK Ltd.
Pitfield, Milton Keynes, MK11 3LW, UK
UKHW051044120926
8556IPUK00041B/1222

* 9 7 8 1 7 8 7 7 9 1 7 9 4 *